"Almost a Man of Genius"

LIVES OF WOMEN IN SCIENCE

Founding Editor: Pnina Abir-Am
Series Editor: Ann Hibner Koblitz

VOLUMES IN THE SERIES

A Convergence of Lives
Sofia Kovalevskaia—Scientist, Writer, Revolutionary,
by Ann Hibner Koblitz

A Matter of Choices
Memoirs of a Female Physicist,
by Fay Ajzenberg-Selove

Creative Couples in the Sciences,
edited by Helena M. Pycior, Nancy G. Slack,
and Pnina G. Abir-Am

"Almost a Man of Genius"
Clémence Royer, Feminism, and Nineteenth-Century Science,
by Joy Harvey

"Almost a Man of Genius"

Clémence Royer, Feminism, and Nineteenth-Century Science

Joy Harvey

R

Rutgers University Press
New Brunswick, New Jersey, and London

Library of Congress Cataloging-in-Publication Data

Harvey, Joy Dorothy.
"Almost a man of genius" : Clémence Royer, feminism, and nineteenth-century science / Joy Harvey.
p. cm. — (Lives of women in science)
Includes bibliographical references (p.) and index.
ISBN 0-8135-2397-4 (alk. paper)
1. Royer, Clémence, 1830–1902. 2. Naturalists—France—Biography.
I. Title. II. Series.
QH31.R787H38 1997
509' .2—dc21 96-39286
[B] CIP

British Cataloging-in-Publication information available

Translations from the French are by the author.

Manufactured in the United States of America

To the memory of
my mother,
Dorothy Hanfling Colby,
a woman of intellect and courage

Contents

Foreword

Readers at the interface of history of science and women's studies are by now familiar with Joy Harvey's superb essay on Clémence Royer, published almost a decade ago in *Uneasy Careers and Intimate Lives: Women in Science, 1789–1979,* a collection of essays that played a key role in Rutgers University Press's establishing a series dedicated specifically to the lives of women in science.[1] Now Harvey expands the scope of that essay to encompass the first book-length study in English of Royer, a nineteenth-century French woman thinker, who wrote extensively on science, philosophy, feminism, and their interaction, for both specialist and popular audiences.[2] Harvey explores the "anomaly" of Royer's life and work as a pioneering woman of science whose scientific ideas and professional career had to come to terms with the problem of gender and science, most notably in connection with the widely debated implications of Darwin's theory of evolution for man and woman's place in both nature and society.[3]

As Harvey demonstrates in impressive archival and analytical detail, Royer's life is uniquely situated to illuminate the complex and shifting relationship between gender and science, especially throughout the second half of the nineteenth century, a period that witnessed major changes in the social and political organization of both science and society. Royer's life reflects the rise of female emancipation, of professional science, and of their interaction in the context of the major political changes in Europe in the second half of the nineteenth century. Indeed, it is one of Harvey's many strengths to account for Royer's emergence as a renowned woman of science pronouncing on matters of both science and society, in terms of her long-term association with the Société d'Anthropologie of Paris. Through her membership in this major scientific institution, which served as a sociopolitical forum for the transfer and application of scientific, positivist, and evolutionist ideals, Royer ensured that the standpoint of women and of their gender difference had a voice in the scientific and hence authoritative issues of the day.

Royer's life is shown by Harvey to be a landmark in female scientific creativity and its relationship to female social and political emancipation, not only in her native France but also in other European countries in which she lived and worked, especially in Britain, Italy, Switzerland, and Belgium. Like other pioneering women of science in the nineteenth century, most notably the American astronomer Maria Mitchell, the Russian mathematician Sophia Kovalevskaia, and the British physicist Hertha Ayrton,[4] Royer had to struggle to reconcile her fascination with and talent for science with her membership in the "second sex." That sex was considered by the patriarchy of her time to be unequal, inferior, and altogether unsuited for the scientific pursuits that held the key to the understanding and control of both nature and the social order. As a commentator and translator of Darwin, Royer was well placed to notice and comment on the social implications of evolutionist ideas, especially as they related to gender.

The specific manifestations of Royer's life in history, so meticulously researched and insightfully discussed by Harvey in the context of nineteenth-century science, can be seen both as the culmination of a succession of creative female role models and an apogee of female discrimination in science. Royer's "career" seems to combine themata from the lives and works of culturally creative women preceding her that range from Mme d'Hondt (a seventeenth-century linguist active in the Académie des Sciences, who was denied formal membership despite her high qualifications); Mme du Châtelet, the eighteenth-century author of physics texts, translator of Newton, and collaborator of Voltaire, whose influence Royer acknowledged directly; Sophie Germain, the nineteenth-century author of mathematical texts and interlocutor of Gauss; to Marie and Irène Curie, mother and daughter, the twentieth-century Nobelists in physics and chemistry.[5]

Royer found a measure of power, but also suffered the fragility of the sociocultural space for female celebrity like other independent women, especially writers and feminists. Germaine de Staël, George Sand, the actress Rachel, and those she knew personally, Marie d'Agoult, Maria Deraismes, Marguerite Durand among others in France and George Eliot, Barbara Bodichon, Harriet Martineau, Margaret Fuller in Britain all impinged directly and indirectly on Royer's challenging goals in scientific and social analysis. Harvey sketches the rich trajectory of profound personal change undergone by Royer, largely by her own agency: the daughter of staunch royalists turned fierce republican, the convent-educated girl turned atheist, the French patriot turned cosmopolitan European turned frequent exile by the political upheavals of the mid-nineteenth century, the bourgeois moralist turned practitioner of amour libre and motherhood out of wedlock, the autodidact commentator and translator (an accepted avenue for female entree into science) turned heroic challenger of the greatest nineteenth-century proponents of scientific systems, most notably Newton, Rousseau, Comte, Darwin, and Spencer.

Harvey's book is particularly valuable for her acute insights into the history of Darwinian evolution, its reception, and its social implications (Harvey was one of the editors of the *Correspondence of Charles Darwin*), as well as for her absorbing and compassionate telling of Royer's difficult personal life, with its distinct stages of intellectual and emotional growth and turmoil. Harvey's discussion of Royer's multidisciplinary contributions to a wide range of topics—philosophy, economics, anthropology, biology, and politics—is a revelation. So is Harvey's attentiveness to the social, cultural, and political grounding of Royer's gender as it creatively enabled and constrained the expression of her genius and passion for science. Royer's originality, so vividly captured by Harvey, is a unique testimony to the emancipatory role of science for women and, conversely, to the enrichment and "debiasing" of science by thought grounded in the historical specificities of the female existence.

As is often the case in history of science, the relevance of Royer's ideas to the different preoccupations of her twentieth-century followers, both women and men, ranges from anticipating modern trends to espousing ideologies considered nowadays to be politically incorrect. Hence, Harvey's decision to conclude her book with a guided tour of how Royer's main ideas have been received by her various biographers is a particularly remarkable feature of her book. It lets us see how much of the "body of work" of a given thinker is inextricably linked to the shifting scientific and sociopolitical agendas of her readers. Though not all of Royer's views are currently upheld in the many fields to which she contributed, her never-ceasing creativity greatly advanced the cause of female emancipation. As Harvey conveys in her restrained tone, Royer's life and work were heroic in overcoming, however imperfectly, the double standard that continues to plague creative women even today, in and out of science. It is a much-needed reminder of just how long and how much of Royer's vision remained utopian for reason of persistent gender inequality.

Pnina G. Abir-Am
Series Editor

Acknowledgments

Many debts have accumulated over the years since this project began to emerge parallel to the research for my Ph.D. thesis at Harvard on the Société d'Anthropologie de Paris under the direction of Everett Mendelsohn, who first introduced me to many scholars in France. I would like to begin by acknowledging the importance of the small community of scholars who have studied and published works on Clémence Royer. Firstly, I owe much to the friendship and assistance of Claude Blanckaert in Paris, with whom I discussed Royer since we first worked through the archives of the Société d'Anthropologie together and came across her suppressed memoir in 1979. A year later, we examined Royer's archives at the Marguerite Durand Library, then in the *mairie* of the fifth *arrondissement.* We have continued to talk and argue about Royer since that time, and I have always gained a great deal from those conversations, and still more from Blanckaert's careful scholarship in the history of French anthropology and from his beautifully wrought publications. I am also grateful for the assistance of Linda Clark, who first directed me to Royer's archives in the Marguerite Durand Library and pointed me in the direction of other source material. She discussed her own research on Royer with me and shared her studies of French education and feminism. I met Yvette Conry at the beginning of my research, and she was extraordinarily helpful; I regret that in subsequent years I spoke to her only over the telephone. When in 1985 I briefly met Geneviève Fraisse, my conversation with her led me to her book on Royer that had just been published, a continuing inspiration and delight to me over the years. I had some excellent discussions many years ago with Robert Richards about Royer and Spencer. He then put his student Sara Joan Miles in communication with me and over the years, we have continued to exchange both papers and ideas. Her careful analysis of Royer's publications, particularly the Darwin prefaces and translations, have proved very useful, although we have often agreed to disagree. She kindly gave me a copy of her dissertation on Royer.

I recognize the vital importance of the year I spent at the Department of History of Science at the University of Oklahoma on a Rockefeller Fellowship (1989–1990), during which I was able to dedicate myself to finishing the first version of this book. My discussions there with Robert and Mary Jo Nye about the scientific interests of nineteenth-century French men and women were unfailingly useful. Marilyn Ogilvie shared with me her insights about the delights and problems of writing the biographies of women in science. I would also like to acknowledge the help of James Allen, who led me to the archives of Céline Renooz.

Over the past fifteen years, I gained more than I can ever repay from the hospitality and intellectual support of my friends in Paris: Anne-Marie Moulin, Claude and Armelle Debru, Marc and Sophie Lallemand, Jean and Elisabeth Gayon, Claire Ambroselli, Serge and Gabrielle Netchine, and Claude and Martine Blanckaert, all of whom gave me insights into life and attitudes in France and corrected many mistaken views about French society and my errors in the French language. They have all coupled their friendship with generous introductions to other historians and philosophers of science, as well as scientists in Paris. I would like to make a special mention of the loss I feel in the absence of Rosalind Rey, recently deceased, whose friendship and conversation I sorely miss.

I would also like to acknowledge the importance of the friendship and encouragement of my friends and former colleagues Ann LaBerge, Doris Zallen, Muriel Lederman, Mordecai Finegold, and Richard Burian at Virginia Polytechnic Institute and State University and their assistance in allowing me time and space to complete this project in the Center for the Study of Science in Society. I thank as well my former colleagues on the Darwin Correspondence Project, especially Frederick and Anne Burkhardt, Duncan Porter, and Jonathan Topham. Most especially, I would like to thank Thomas Junker, who shared with me his understanding of nineteenth-century German Darwinism.

A number of people have played an editorial role in the final production of this book. I owe a debt to Pnina Abir-Am, who encouraged me to begin this project many years ago and has continued to believe in it, to Dorinda Outram, who first read and edited the article on Royer that appeared in her and Pnina Abir-Am's volume *Uneasy Careers and Intimate Lives* and remains a strong supporter. I cannot express my gratitude sufficiently to Nick Gill, whose work in redirecting the emphasis and editing the first chapters of this book gave me the courage to continue. I also thank Karen Reeds, science editor of Rutgers University Press, who has urged me to write and rewrite this book and provided me with many helpful suggestions. Thanks as well to Doris Zallen and Terry Murray, who read the final version of the first four chapters. In addition, I thank Geneviève Fraisse, whose careful reading of and commentary on the complete manuscript aided me beyond measure. Of course, any errors that remain are my own.

To the many librarians and archivists in France, Britain, Switzerland, and Italy who have aided me over the years I would like to express my gratitude and recognition. I also recognize a debt to Denise Ferembach, former secretary-general of the Société d'Anthropologie de Paris, who many years ago made it possible for me to use the invaluable archives of that society. Thanks are also due to the following libraries and institutions for permission to cite from archival resources or to reproduce illustrations: The Syndics of Cambridge University, Cambridge, England, for materials held in the Darwin Archive, including reproduction of the memorandum from Clémence Royer; Houghton Library, Harvard University, Cambridge, Massachusetts, for reproduction of the Clémence Royer caricature; Archives Nationales de France, Paris, for materials in the Ministry of Education files, the Victor Considérant archive, and the Jules Simon papers; Bibliothèque Marguerite Durand, Paris, for materials from the Dossier and Correspondence of Clémence Royer; Bibliothèque Nationale de France, Paris, for materials in the François Lenoir, Ernest Havet, and Félix Nadar archives and permission to reproduce the photograph of Clémence Royer; Préfecture de Police de Paris for permission to cite materials from the Pascal Duprat and Clémence Royer dossiers; Bibliothèque Publique et Universitaire, Geneva, Switzerland, for materials held in the Ernest Naville, Carl Vogt, and René-Édouard Chaparède archives. I would also like to thank the Société d'Anthropologie de Paris, and its secretary general, Alain Fromont, in particular, for permission not only to cite materials held in its archives, but to translate the suppressed memoir of Clémence Royer and to reproduce her photograph published in the *Bulletin et Mémoirs de la Société d'Anthropologie.*

Finally, I would like to thank Janet Browne, whose deep knowledge of nineteenth-century Darwinism, skill as writer and Darwin biographer, and attentive ear as a friend has proven a spur and an encouragement to me and to this project over many years. To my children, who have endured Clémence Royer in her many forms since their adolescent years and well into their maturity, I offer here my gratitude for their interest and patience. I cannot overlook the assistance and encouragement of all the editors at Rutgers University Press, especially my former editor Karen Reeds, and my copyeditor Ingrid Muller. To the many other friends and associates who have helped me over the years I apologize for not recognizing them by name here and offer my thanks.

"Almost a Man of Genius"

Introduction

"She was almost a man of genius," the French linguist and critic Ernest Renan said of Clémence Royer. The double description of her as "almost a man" and "almost a genius" was not lost on her feminist friends two years before her death, who asked, "Why almost? Why a man?"[1] It has proven impossible to locate Renan's quotation in anything but secondary sources. Royer reported to a friend that this often used quotation came from a conversation she had with Renan about his work *The Future of Science* (*L'Avenir de science*). The question comes up for the biographer: why use such a title? Yet this designation encapsulates issues that pursued this woman throughout her life. How could one be an active, innovative woman thinker in a period when women assumed passive and noncreative roles or ran the risk of being seen as masculinized or desexed? How could one be a brilliant woman when women had been and still were characterized by male friends and colleagues as dangerous, even monstrous, when they were too clever? How could one have a child and retain one's creative life? Most importantly, how could one study science, adopt it as a philosophy, and be taken seriously by scientists as well as philosophers at a period when women were routinely excluded from the field of science by their education? Royer's life is the story of a woman struggling with these questions, at times consciously reformulating them and coming up with her own answers.

Although she continues to be best known for her Darwin translation and the startling preface with which she introduced it, Clémence Royer believed her most important contribution to future generations to have been a reinterpretation of matter and life. She undervalued the importance of her continual commentary on women's issues and the questions surrounding women in science, although these are the most "modern" elements of her thought. No voice in the nineteenth century is comparable to hers on this issue. As a rebel, constantly challenging what she read, she was considered not quite a participant in science, although she belonged to some important anthropological societies and was read seriously by some physicists and mathematicians. She was, however, a continual promoter, critic, and philosopher of science.

Into every one of her intellectual productions during most of her life she inserted the question of woman's varied roles in society. Whether she was discussing taxation in an economics book, revolutionary movements in a novel, the application of Darwin's ideas to human society in prefaces to her Darwin translations, or the falling birth rate before the Anthropological Society of Paris, she insisted that the concerns of women be addressed. At the end of her life, even while she considered elementary particles underlying all matter, the possibility that one could be creative and a woman lay embedded in her scientific writings. Even in her cosmological writings she raised the problem of genderized descriptions of matter. And she retained her right to challenge the great male scientists including both Newton and Darwin. These themes were explicit in her regular column for the feminist paper *La Fronde* during the last five years of her life, but they can be found in her earliest published writings.

In her younger years Royer seems to have shared the belief of her century that she "thought like a man." One of her colleagues in the Société d'Anthropologie has reported that she thought this meant she had a "masculine brain." Yet her view of women's intellectual capacities went beyond this. Women had a kind of genius peculiar to themselves, she believed, and in her own writings we see again and again her insistence that men have radically underestimated woman's capacity for action, for creativity, for science. In her novel she split her male protagonist into twins, one passive, private, mystical, scholarly, almost asexual, and the other active, scientific, sexual, political, and social. It is clear from her autobiographical statements that she saw these two sets of characteristics as representing her own double nature, and she deeply resented that women were being assigned a passive role. She saw herself as a rebel against much of her society but she did not see herself as a freak or an anomaly. What she had done intellectually, she believed, all women could do if they were willing to use logic and mathematics as rigorously as she had done.

When one writes about a well-known man or woman, one can take many things for granted. A biographer of Charles Darwin or Coleridge, Oscar Wilde or Mary Wollstonecraft can put the subject's last name alone in the title and expect immediate recognition. A lesser-known figure requires an apologia, an explanation of who this is, why one has bothered to write a biography about her. Carolyn Heilbrun has signaled the special issues surrounding women's biographies that compound the issue of "importance."[2] For a woman working in the field of science, the question is not only: "what did she write?" and "was she important?" but "what was her major discovery?" In Royer's case, because she was a philosopher and critic of science rather than a working scientist, there are no "discoveries" to which one can point. Instead we have a woman encountering science and attempting to rethink the fundamental basis of this mode of thought at a time when few women had the opportunity to become scientists. She is unique for her century in the manner in which she insisted on her right to challenge male authority, whether that authority was social, scientific, or political.

A biographer runs into many difficulties, not the least of which is a close identification with the subject, which leads one either to excuse or explain away the contradictions in a complex life. Richard Holmes observes in his study of Coleridge that some of the best biographers have been hostile to their subject.[3] We have all seen the dangers of hagiography. Hostility preserves some distance, as Holmes insists. Often the biographer would like to ask the subject questions about some contradiction in the subject's writings or life that remain unexamined or are inexplicable. One longs for the freedom of the oral historian to inquire, "Why did you do or say that?" On the other hand, too close as well as too great a distance leads one to ignore the subtle explanations of a life that the biographical subject herself provides, dropping a hint here and there, as she describes herself in her letters and in her work.

In Royer's biography, an underlying issue is the problem of female scientific literacy, an issue that Clémence Royer herself consistently raised. In the nineteenth century male nonscientists, amateur scientists, and philosophers had a special, often close, relationship with science, which they felt their basic education had prepared them to understand. Royer, who also felt a close tie to science, continually expressed her regret that as a woman she had been prevented first from being educated in science, then from obtaining a serious audience, then from getting a chair in philosophy or science, so that her entire life, active and productive as it was, hovered on the edge of poverty.

Royer never saw herself in the role of science popularizer, although she wanted to make science more accessible to the ordinary person, nor did she try simply to report on the science of her day. Her mission, as she saw it, was to construct a philosophy that would make the world comprehensible, using science as a tool to do so. As she declared in her autobiography, "What she was looking for was a doctrine for herself, not professional methods."[4] She insisted in her Darwin preface at the age of thirty that, far more than Darwin, she had "dared hypotheses," and she continued to dare them until her death.[5] At the age of forty, Royer began to rethink Newtonian physics. Never had she felt such happiness, she said, as when she saw a way to reinterpret Newton's physics. This delight in the life of the mind makes her always interesting to read, as she draws the reader into sharing her pleasure.

Royer's constant cry for priority over male scientists and her insistence on her originality derived in part from a desire to reverse the common nineteenth-century judgment that women, regardless of education or intelligence, lacked creative capacities except for childbearing. Tennyson stated this in its bluntest form in his well-known poem "The Princess." "They hunt old trails, said Cyril, very well. But when did woman ever yet invent?"[6] This negative judgement was repeated by well-known women scientists of the day. Mary

Somerville, for example, although affirming her work in science and her love for both astronomy and mathematics, denied that she had produced really original work. "I have perseverance and intelligence but no genius: that spark from heaven is not granted to the sex."[7] In reaction to this widespread view, Royer was driven to insist that women had a special feminine genius that could be applied to science as well as to the arts.[8] At the end of her life she reversed her old complaint about the difficulties she had experienced as a woman, conceding that her originality derived from her experience as a woman struggling with "unwomanly" aspects of thought, with profound questions about the nature of the universe, of life, of human origins.[9] Had she been a man, she noted, specialization would have prevented her from trying to look beyond a small corner of knowledge. If her answers were not as directly useful to biology and physics as she expected them to be, they were and are nonetheless profoundly intriguing. Even sophisticated scientific critics of her own day had to grant her that much.

Although her name is not familiar to the general reader, every decade or so the writings of Clémence Royer have been rediscovered and reinterpreted. An attempt will be made in the afterword to show the various interpretations of Royer as a writer and thinker by her first biographer, Albert Milice, in the period between the two world wars, then by her old colleagues and associates at *La Fronde* in 1930 and again in 1954. A revival of interest in Royer began among historians of science with the study of French Darwinism by Yvette Conry in 1974 and five scholars in France and the United States in the 1980s: Geneviève Fraisse, Linda Clark, Claude Blanckaert, and myself, followed by Sara Joan Miles's dissertation. (See afterword for a detailed discussion of these.) The publication in France of a previously unknown and unpublished manuscript by Royer about women, sexuality, and the diminished birthrate, first located in the archives of the Société d'Anthropologie by Claude Blanckaert and myself (a translation of which I have appended here), has helped to reopen the discussion of her as a fascinating and controversial figure.

CHAPTER 1

A Fire of the Mind: Family, Childhood, and Youth of Clémence Royer

"One rarely takes enough account of the evolution of the mind of a child, of the variety and nature of the images which the child stores up in the still sleeping conscious memory," wrote Clémence Royer in her autobiography.[1] There are no independent sources to tell us about Clémence Royer as a child. We have to depend on Clémence Royer's own recollections, first in this unpublished autobiography, then in the comments she made on a published biographical article.[2] The only other source is her novel written just before she turned thirty, which gives us insight into her view of how the life of an independently minded young woman should proceed.

Clémence Royer was born on 21 April 1830 in Nantes, Brittany, rue Montesquieu, but her father and mother married only seven years later. She was, therefore, born Augustine-Clémence Audouard and only became Royer when she was legitimized by this marriage in 1837. Her mother, like herself, may have been legitimized only after her birth. Did Royer know of her initial illegitimacy? The answer is probably yes.[3] All her life, she considered the loyalty of men and women to each other far more important than formal marriage. One of the rights she felt children should have was the right to search for their father, which was forbidden under the Napoleonic Code.[4]

She had no need to search for her own father, Augustin-René Royer. He had been a captain in the light infantry in his early forties, stationed at Belle-Île-en-Mer in Brittany, where he met her mother, Joséphine-Gabrielle Audouard, a bright young woman of twenty-four. As a very young officer under Napoleon, Royer had become a captain three years before the restoration of the Bourbon monarchy in 1815 and had sworn an oath to uphold the royal family. Following the July revolution of 1830, the Orleanist "citizen king"

Louis-Philippe came to the throne. In January 1831, Augustin Royer took a leave from the army and joined the rebels who surrounded the "legitimist" group of royalists. The duchesse du Berry, a young and attractive widow and mother of the young comte d'Artois, later the comte de Chambord, led this rebellion. In 1832, in the company of a group of artistocratic supporters, she had the young pretender crowned as Henry V of France in a cathedral in Prague. Brittany was a center for the revolt, and hundreds died in the royalist uprising in that region.

Captain Royer may have hoped to make his name and fortune by associating himself with this rebellion. The duchesse du Berry had signed a brevet making him one of her royal guards, something Clémence was proud of, even in later life, in spite of her republicanism.[5] Later he became embittered when the Bourbon restoration failed to materialize. Born on 1 March 1788, he grew up in a bourgeois village (Saint-Pierre-la-Coeur) in the canton of Rais, in the La Mayenne area of Maine, where some member of his family had been mayor for a number of generations. His father, René Royer, was a wood merchant, quite well-to-do, who after the death of his first wife, Augustin-René's mother, married a servant girl.[6] This remarriage dismayed the young man; he joined the army at the age of nineteen in 1809 and was rapidly advanced to officer. When the Bourbon restoration took place, he was only in his early twenties. By the time he was thirty he was a captain in a regiment of light infantry and had not advanced further ten years later, although he was treasurer of his regiment. He may have felt that opportunities for further advancement were even more limited under the new July monarchy. On the other hand, he may have been led to rebel, as his daughter believed, from an almost anachronistic sense of "honor."

Clémence Royer's mother, Joséphine-Gabrielle Audouard, was working as a seamstress in Nantes when she and Captain Royer first met, according to one source, but she was no grisette.[7] She had been the favorite daughter of a Breton naval officer, captain of the port of Brest. As a young man, Royer's grandfather, Joseph Louis Audouard, had fought in many sea battles from 1778 to 1798 and was wounded in two of them. He was one of the first members of the Legion of Honor, to which he was admitted in June 1804.[8] Royer later described her mother as having inherited her grandfather's courage and spirit and being accustomed from her early childhood not to flinch when the canons were fired to signal the arrival of ships in port. She even learned to light the fuses herself, but the subsequent report broke one of her eardrums, resulting in partial deafness.

Clémence Royer considered herself a true Breton because of her mother and her grandfather. She seriously believed that "race characteristics" were carried by the maternal line, yet Joséphine-Gabrielle's own mother was a beautiful Flemish girl, Wilhelmina Griffith, whom the Breton sailor had met on a voyage to Flessing. Joséphine-Gabrielle's father described her conception and birth in nautical terms, telling her that she had been "built in the dockyards at Flessing and launched in the sea at Brest." Perhaps because she was her father's favorite, Joséphine Audouard's mother resented the mutual affection of father and daughter. After the naval captain's death, when Joséphine was only fifteen, she found herself playing the part of Cinderella in the household. Since she was the oldest child and a girl, her beautiful Flemish mother left all the work to her, including the care of her "lazy" younger brothers. Perhaps to escape from this domination, she developed her skills as an embroiderer and lace maker, which could give her economic independence. She passed this craft on to her daughter, Clémence, who practiced it throughout her life. The daughter identified with her mother's paternal heritage, believing that a child belonged to the mother far more than to the father. It is a curiosity of her identification of herself as a Breton that she saw no contradiction in her ideas and—as far as one can tell—simply dismissed her own Flemish ancestry on her mother's side.[9]

Brittany had a history of rebellion against the central government since the time of the French Revolution, when the Breton "Whites" sided with the king. As a true daughter of independent Brittany, Clémence's mother may have encouraged Captain Royer to join the Bourbon rebellion. She certainly supported him in the revolt. Joséphine-Gabrielle, treasuring her childhood as the daughter of a naval captain, may have wanted her lover to play a courageous part. Soon after Clémence was born, the July revolution occurred, toppling the Bourbon dynasty and replacing it with the more liberal Orléans citizen-king Louis-Philippe. Recovering from childbirth, the young woman did not follow Captain Royer to Prague where he had joined the eager rebels at the coronation of the young aspirant to the throne. The father's experience of that dramatic moment never left him.

Mother and daughter soon came to join the captain in Savoy, where he spent his days plotting the rebellion with his fellow conspirators. They returned to France, where Clémence took her first steps on a terrace of the Park of Versailles, and learned to navigate stairs on the "three pink marble steps of which Musset has sung."[10] The rebellion failed in 1832; France as a whole did not rise to restore the Bourbons a second time. Captain Royer was condemned to death along with his fellow conspirators and fled to Switzerland.

Clémence's first memories were of the beautiful area around Lake Léman at Panda near Lausanne, where her parents stayed at the house of a friend, Dr. Marcel. Traveling from Paris, which they left during the cholera epidemic, they passed through Lyon, Chambray, Annecy, to Geneva and through most of Switzerland. As a little girl she had crossed the famous glacier, the "Mer de Glace," on her mother's lap. This experience left her with bewildered memories and a "confused and dramatic sense of the power of nature."[11] Her early vision of mountains and ice had affected her with an intensity that no later impression could equal. No artistic representations of nature could ever quite equal those recalled images. Throughout her life, she felt "a sense of her powerlessness to produce beauty," aggravated by severe myopia which, from her early childhood, insulated her from the outside world.[12] She later believed that her nearsightedness was the main reason that she had chosen a contemplative life.

From an early age she had been forced to analyze "with remarkable precision" the central core of things. Her attempt to penetrate to the heart of things, she later claimed, led to an internal exploration and made her a philosopher interested in science rather than an artist or a poet. Her myopia may also explain why her longest artistic attempt, a novel, was singularly devoid of detailed physical descriptions of human beings, their surroundings, or nature, except for the most dramatic spectacles: mountains, volcanos, dramatic caves, vast stretches of water, or ice.

When Clémence was five, her father returned to Orléans and gave himself up to the judicial courts, hoping to pay a penalty and end his exile. He was jailed for a few months while awaiting trial. Clémence's mother, visiting him in jail on Saint Henri's Day, along with the wife of another member of the conspiracy, displayed her own bravado by distributing hot wine to any prisoner who would shout "Long Live Henri V." At the trial, Clémence, a child of five, sat on the knees of one of her father's friends. She remembered her father standing before the judges, proudly insisting that he had acted as "a man of honor." In spite of Captain Royer's outspoken admission of his participation in the rebellion, he was acquitted by the judges' unanimous vote. His lawyer expressed great surprise at this outcome after the captain's unwise insistence on his right to act as he had done. There may have been a prior decision of the government not to prosecute the rebels or punish them too severely, since the judges were lenient with most of the minor figures involved in the rebellion.

Captain Royer was not punished financially for his act of rebellion. He was awarded a pension of Fr 1,400 a year by the army in recognition of his years of army service. This was of course not the major financial source for him, since he had inherited some properties in La Mayenne. For the next seven years Clémence lived like a little Parisian, playing happily in the gardens of the Tuileries, allowed in the salon if she behaved, listening intently to adult conversation. Her parents and friends called her "the little mouse" both because of her small size and her high-pitched, nervous cry as she ran about at play. She alternated between being a shy, even timid, child devoted to reading and a born chatterer seeking adult companionship. She described herself as both "very restless and very reflective," and the double aspect of her personality remained throughout her life. During this same period, her mother and father, who appear to have been quite dedicated to each other in their early years, finally married.

Royer later described the strong personalities of her parents in vivid terms. She depicted her mother as "very intelligent, very active, with a very strong will," although without much formal education. Her father, on the other hand, had a character "of tempered steel." He was well educated, devoting himself to mechanical inventions in his civilian life rather than politics. He hoped to make a name for himself through a successful patent on one of his inventions once his political and military career was over. More than once his daughter described him as a "hero behind his time," "quixotic in his loyalty," "a liberal legitimist of the Chateaubriand school." He had described himself in Chateaubriand's terms as "a monarchist by reason, Bourbon by honor, republican by nature."[13]

Clémence Royer's early education was sporadic. She learned to read from her mother and to calculate and play mathematical games from her father, who was pleased that she had inherited his mathematical abilities. Until she was ten, she remained at home, occasionally attending small local schools. "Well-chosen readings" and the conversation of the adults around her had made her sensitive to language and to learning.

During her childhood, her parents substituted a love for theater for their lost political life. They loved musical theater especially, often singing together at home. They even tried their hands at song writing and instructed their little girl in the rules of verse making, which gave her an early facility in turning out occasional verse. She shared their love for the theater, sometimes attending plays with them, sometimes taken by her nurse.

Although Royer describes her early life as "sparkling" and "very Parisian" in its emphasis on pleasure and society, the attempt to live at the level of their aristocratic friends soon proved disastrous. Her father found himself short of money because of his unsuccessful metallurgical inventions and his political misfortunes. His patent to utilize the heat given off in the process of glass making to cast iron failed to bring him the fortune he expected, disappointing his ambition once again. He blamed his wife for not having brought a dowry into the marriage and for not having been economical enough. In turn, she blamed her husband for having spent his inheritance on political adventures. They decided to leave Paris and live in his native village to save money, a decision that put a further strain on an embittered marriage.

When they left for the provinces, the captain placed his daughter, now ten years old, in a convent school at Mans (Sacré-Coeur du Mans). This school catered to the daughters of aristocrats like the more famous Sacré-Coeur of Paris, which Marie d'Agoult (Daniel Stern) has described so vividly in her memoirs.[14] Some of Captain Royer's political friends had sent their daughters to this convent, and he may have seen this as a way of providing an entree for his daughter into the aristocratic society he so admired. It must have become evident, all too soon, that her family was neither wealthy nor aristocratic, and she had no friends except for a little Spanish girl, the daughter of another failed rebel.

Clémence had had little prior religious training, in spite of her father's association with the "legitimists," who were staunch supporters of the Catholic Church. She had attended mass with her parents where she "behaved herself quietly like a good little girl allowed in the salon." She didn't ask why it was necessary to go to church on Sunday, although she believed, as she had been told, that there was a grand old man with a long white beard living above the clouds, watching what was going on on earth. She addressed prayers to him before going to bed. An "old pious servant," who later retired to a convent, gave her holy medals, pictures of the saints, and statues of the Virgin. Her mother, a woman of the world, quite frankly enjoyed balls more than religious services and observed fasts only because it was customary. The young Clémence Royer confused religious miracles with fairy tales and *The Arabian Nights:* she thought they were all the same. When she was ten, she promised a novena to the Virgin if she would give her Aladdin's lamp. She saw herself as a second Joan of Arc, conjuring up the genie of the lamp to make the comte de Chambord the new king of France, and so validating her father's rebellion.[15]

Fifteen years later, the image of the heroic Maid of Orléans spurred her in her own rebellion, this time directed against the authority of the church. The little tale of praying for a magic lamp told by Clémence demonstrates not only her confusion about religion but the degree to which she identified her father's political ambitions with her own wishes. She may have sensed the desperation of his failed ambitions, the degree to which they had put a wedge between her parents. The strongest memory of her father was of him standing at attention during the mass given by a Polish priest at Saint-Roch in Paris. Although she admitted he preferred this twenty-minute service because of its brevity, she described his appearance with reverence: "With his straight body, his arms crossed, his beautiful appearance, his arresting features, his thin, tight lips, carrying in his hand a prayer book that he never consulted," she saw him as a soldier on guard before his Lord.[16] To less loving eyes he may have seemed to be more like Hans Christian Andersen's "steadfast tin soldier." She was to love the same characterics many years later in her lover, Pascal Duprat, who had the same tall, thin, quixotic appearance coupled with a more sparkling personality but the same inability to succeed in business.

In her convent school, Clémence at ten years was "a dreamy child," with only one friend. She must have been a very lonely child as well, ignored by the older girls. She started out triumphantly, winning prizes and advancing rapidly through the classes. But she soon developed a dramatic reaction to the heavy Catholic religious training that was part of her preparation for First Communion. Attending Communion classes a year earlier than most children in the school because she seemed intellectually precocious, she was shocked at the possibility of sinning without knowing it and imagined herself to be guilty of unmentionable sins. At first, visualizing Paradise and Hell to herself, she sought mystical experiences, imagining herself as destined for sainthood. The other girls were oblivious to her dreams of grandeur, "never suspecting what was going through my head, seeing in me neither someone elected by the Lord or the devil."[17] When she failed to experience religious ecstasy, she fell into a depression. Later she described her feelings: "The invocations and the transports of mystical love containing ardent formulas for the incarnate God that she fed upon overexcited her tense nerves and made her aspire to unknown sensations that did not come and that she couldn't produce. When her nature resisted and rejected ecstasy, she concluded that she was an unworthy being and tortured herself about this."[18]

The result of her self-torture was a sense of depression and an inability to learn. She felt her mind full of darkness and thought nothing earthly was of any importance. "Her reason and her precocious imagination were awakened by all those things seen or heard during a nomadic and agitated childhood." If she could only die "in the odor of sanctity" before she was eighteen, maybe she could escape the terrors of a life that had been pictured to her as somber and serious. "One mortal sin could compromise all eternity, and legions of invisible demons were unceasingly encouraging one to commit one. How horribly sad."[19]

Her love of theatrical images may have helped fire her imagination. One priest, trying to impress the dangers of secular life, described a girl at a ball dancing with a man who dies in her arms. She finds she is dancing with a corpse. The priest repeated this final scene three times with increasing dramatic intensity. Clémence was horrified at the consequences of secular enjoyment. She began to have incessant headaches, possibly migraines, which may have been associated with early puberty. She had entered the convent school as a clever pupil, winning all the prizes; eighteen months later she seemed to have forgotten everything she had ever learned. Her parents were very concerned about the change in mental and physical health and decided to pull her out of the convent before she completly "lost her mind" (*tourner à l'idiotisme*).[20]

The head of the convent realized that she had a little rebel on her hands. After all, one form of rebellion is to carry out unwelcome orders to their ridiculous extremes, as more than one satirical novel has portrayed. Royer commented many years later that "the director of the boarding school, a woman of rare energy, judged me intelligent, but said of me, 'Pride will be her downfall.' From her point of view she was right. Under the submissive believer she detected the rebellious reasoner."[21] Throughout her life, pride in her knowledge, her reasoning abilities, and her logical interpretations would continue to cause her trouble. Even Darwin sighed at Royer's stubborn pride. One should add that she always considered rebellion as a positive good and described herself as a rebel in the preface to her one novel.

Even after she left the convent, she continued her extreme mystical religious practices, wearing a hair shirt under her dress. She became reserved and defiant with her parents, believing that they weren't pious enough, and scorned their rather casual Catholicism; in the young child's eyes they were already damned. If the catechism was literal truth, it had to be followed to its logical conclusion. After all, Royer observed, "If you believe in Paradise and the way to get there, then of course you want to have first place. Everything else is a contradiction."[22] Her comment as an adult illustrates her intense ambition as well as her religious beliefs. The logic of her interpretation of religion had made her "a stupid rebel who lived waiting for death," perhaps again in unconscious imitation of her father's heroics.[23] Her father tried to bring her out of her depression by inviting her to the theater. When she defiantly refused, he slapped her face, the only time he struck her. She took this blow like a martyr, but secretly resented it.[24] This period of preadolescent depression seems to have lingered for another six months. She recovered only when her family, missing the excitement of the capital, returned to Paris in 1843. Now thirteen, she saw the Tuileries and the other places where she had played as a child. She burst into tears when she realized she was no longer a little girl in short skirts. This realization seems to have purged her of her depression. Suddenly she felt freed from the sense of sin. "It seemed to her that she was leaving a prison in which she had lived confined for three years."[25]

The world was pleasurable and beautiful to her, full of balls in the winter and country parties and picnics on the grass with "amiable and gay people" in the summer. Later she spoke of the dances she attended as helping to dissipate "the black butterflies of devotion."[26] She threw herself into dancing polkas and quadrilles with the energy she had previously had for religion, tapping out the rhythm of the music even when she wasn't dancing. Her world had changed. She was caught up in feverish activity, with a taste for the wordly life she had dreaded. The priests, who had alarmed her with the image of a young woman dancing with a corpse, diminished in importance. Her adolescence had arrived, and she became active in the social world with which her parents surrounded her.

She did not give up the contemplative side of her life. She read everything she could find, but she was not yet a scholar. She did not try to attend the public lectures at the Sorbonne or the Collège de France, nor did she know about them. She did not have the ambition to study medicine that some of the bright young women of the following generation would develop. "The word 'doctor' applied to a woman seemed to me a monstrosity, as it did to all those around me."[27]

At fifteen, novels and plays had the greatest influence on her. She read Mme de Staël's great novel *Corinne,* which describes the tragic life of a woman, half-English and half-Italian, who amazes her society with inspired, dramatic declamations and then abandons this life because of her unlucky love for an Englishman. The young girl burst into tears as she read it.[28] The literary critic Moers has shown the importance of this novel as a "children's book for a special kind of nineteenth-century child—girls of more than ordinary intelligence or talent and rising ambition to fame beyond the domestic circle. Reading *Corinne* made an event of their youth—for some a catalyst to their own literary development—which in later years they could not wholly reject unless willing also to deny their own enthralling, painful awakening as women of genius—their own 'days of Corinne' in Matthew Arnold's phrase."[29]

"Days of Corinne" might almost serve as an epigram for the adolescence of Clémence Royer. Her own novel written fifteen years later reveals her devotion to that book and to the image of female genius. Italy, where the novel is set, became for Royer, as well as many other nineteenth-century women, a symbol of a country where both creativity and freedom could flourish.[30] Years later she was to evoke Corinne again as she received the homage of her friends.

She loved poetry, as well as prose and drama. She divided her time between reading and more feminine accomplishments of the day including music—for which she said she had an indifferent gift, although she later received a certificate in music—and needlework, in which she excelled. Propped up on her embroidery frame were plays of Racine or Corneille, from which she learned great female roles, dressing herself up in the tablecloth to recite before the mirror. "That is because I had seen Rachel," she explained.[31] This great mid-nineteenth-century actress appeared to Clémence like a living representation of Corinne, one of Rachel's most famous roles.

The actress Rachel was unequaled in her tragic representations of great heroines, with a deep and vibrating voice, excelled in the century only by Sarah Bernhardt. The portrait of Clémence Royer at eighteen, reprinted in *La Fronde* on the hundredth anniversary of her birth, shows a sweet young girl with her hair loosely pulled back and with a shy smile on her face. In hairstyle, costume, and expression the portrait resembles contemporary portraits of Rachel: like her she was small and dark-haired with bright eyes and a good complexion. Her identification with heroic ideals was to retain a theatrical dimension.

For all her love of theater, Clémence could never have gone on the stage. The life of an actress was no possibility for a girl raised as Clémence was in a middle-class environment. Rachel was famous not just as a great actress but, like most actresses of the period, as a courtesan, patronized by the great names of the July Monarchy and the Second Empire. Among Rachel's best remembered roles besides Corinne was her performance of Jeanne d'Arc and her dramatic representation of Liberty when, upon declaration of the Second Republic, she wrapped herself in the tricolor and sang the Marseillaise. She died rather tragically from tuberculosis while still young, living in comparative poverty with two children born outside of marriage.[32] Rachel may also have been the model for the actress-courtesan Léona in Royer's only novel.

Two events were to change Clémence's life: her father's absence from her life and the 1848 revolution. Her parents' quarrels came to a head. Her father, now in his late fifties, began to display a "paranoid and monomaniacal" jealousy of his much younger wife.[33] Without divorce as an option, the only solution was separation of husband and wife. The aging former captain returned to La Mayenne to live in his native village, where he still had some small property. In many ways, his departure freed Clémence from the direct exposure to her father's unhappiness. His intense, unfulfilled ambitions and his tragic sense of being a failed hero must have been a burden to his family. Her mother was livelier and more practical and, as Royer later put it, "had a clearer sense of reality," a sense that the young girl imbibed as she watched her mother face the changes in her life.

The absence of her father may have reinforced the sense of rebellion she retained all her life. Fifteen years later she described a mother endorsing rebellion in her daughter as a positive step in society, helping to eliminate future social despotism. "I acted today towards my daughter as our mother should have acted formerly towards me. . . . I counseled her in rebellion against her father's wishes. . . . There is certainly a vice in the constitution of the modern family. . . . The impractical sharing of moral power, which by its nature is indivisible, results only in sapping the root of the child's confidence and obliges her to choose between two guides. . . . Like you, I have the conviction . . . that children belong to their mothers."[34]

The 1848 revolution, soon after her eighteenth birthday, came as an illumination to Clémence. She experienced an intellectual awakening, later described as both a "renaissance or an evolution." Her faith in her father's political beliefs was shattered, and she adopted republican convictions, which she defended coherently against her relatives. Those around her were either legitimists or Orleanists, who "had nothing in common but the fear of the republic."[35] Although she initially knew about this revolution only through journals, news events, posters, and town criers, she was inspired by reading the poet and historian Lamartine who supported the Second Republic. In his speeches on behalf of the revolution he enlarged upon his views of social change as he had described them in his great history of the first French revolution.[36] When her father heard from a relative that she was "turning into a red," she passionately defended her ideas to him in a twelve-page letter. Instead of being annoyed at her, as she must have expected, he congratulated her for her eloquence. Her father's response was of great significance to her: "This was the first serious thing that I wrote," she says of her letter.[37]

Her adoption of republican ideas was accompanied by a re-examination of all her other beliefs. Clémence began to substitute the "vague but large and gentle Deism" of Lamartine for her previously "narrow and austere congregational devotions."[38] This process of "substitution" must have been much more difficult than those words imply. She later described her anger and rage when she began to lose her Catholic belief. In her mid-twenties she looked back on her childhood and saw herself "betrayed," accusing the church of deliberately lying to her and "darkening her childhood."[39]

She was more directly influenced by an old family friend, who was a deputy and a republican strongly attached to clerical beliefs. She never identified the man, only saying that he was a councilor of state for the Empire until his death. This friend took the young girl under his wing, taking her to debates at the National Assembly and escorting her to public ceremonies of the republic (fig. 1). When she described her newly acquired adherence to the republic to the deputy, he expressed his surprise "to hear the little daughter of committed royalists speak out so boldly."[40] He brought her additional books that expanded her mind, increasing her devotion to republicanism until it surpassed that of her mentor, through, as she put it, "a logical deduction."[41] She wrote enthusiastic patriotic verses. Two years later, at the age of twenty, she even recited one of her verses to her idol, Lamartine.

Must I, at twenty, to earn a little gold,
Stop my advance towards beautiful ideals?
Because the world scoffs or I fear sarcasm
Should I stifle holy enthusiasm in my heart?
Against prejudice I stiffen my reason.
Even if it brings me death, I will drink the poison.
I aspire to goodness, to truth, to dreams of glory.
No, I no longer wish to believe in vain terrors.
To battle, my mind calls out, blessing you.
Like a horseshoe striking granite, it throws
A thousand sparks into the night,
Struggle produces nothing but renewed ardor.
Attentive to their voices, I hear the Gods' commands.
March! they cry to me, find your crown in heaven.[42]

She never lost her devotion to the image of the Second Republic, and her later enthusiasm about the group of exiled republicans she met in Switzerland must have derived from this early commitment. The election of Louis Napoléon as president was to prove the downfall of the republic. Clémence commented that this was no surprise to her, since her father had voted for Louis Napoléon, convinced that this would result in an empire.[43] He died before he could see his prediction come true and Louis Napoléon proclaim himself Napoléon III.

Augustin-René Royer died in August 1849, at the age of sixty-one, returning from a walk to check on his properties at Deounière. He seems to have had a stroke or heart attack. Only the barking of his dog brought passers-by to his side. Clémence must have felt both sorrow and a sense of freedom. She could now live her life in her own way, with the small inheritance of a piece of property for her dowry.

We shall find reasons in the next chapter to raise questions about the apparent straightforwardness of Clémence Royer's transition from her late teens to her early twenties, and to investigate the dangerous situations to which the loss of her father may have exposed her. The novel she wrote ten years later describes in vivid detail the rape of a young girl by her cousin at the age of eighteen. Like Clémence, this young woman has just lost her father. Like her, she decides to become a teacher. No hint of this is given in her autobiography. In that account, she moves swiftly on, making a rational choice not to marry. She later explained her refusal to consider possible suitors as a result of her view of her parents' unhappy marriage. Marriage was at best a " kind of dangerous lottery" in which big winnings were rare.[44] In a culture where almost all marriages were arranged, she realized that, with her limited dowry, the exceptional young men she dreamed about were unlikely to come forward. Nor did she have the kind of beauty or social position that would make a promising young man forgo a dowry. The few potential husbands that were suggested she unhesitatingly rejected, not wanting to make a "marriage of convenience," a possibility that raised in her an "instinctive distrust."[45] She realized that the only result would be to limit the independence that her mother had already extended to her.

At twenty she felt she had begun to "recreate" herself, as she later put it. She was certain that she was going to accomplish something significant, although she was not certain what that would be. Although she had been able to place some short pieces of poetry in small reviews, when she tried to write in prose, she discovered that she had no real knowledge of the rules of her own language and knew nothing about fundamental mathematical laws, what Royer termed the "metaphysics of language and numbers."[46] In the process she also discovered her own "natural logic," which "in one bound led her to extreme consequences of any principle and which undoubtedly rendered her invincible in every discussion." The "invincibility" of her logic, she believed, had made enemies for her, although she dismissed this as being due to a world "in which inconsequence and contradiction reign in perpetuity."[47]

For the next three years she decided to study arithmetic and French in order to obtain one of the only professional diplomas then available to women, the prestigious certificates just instituted by the Hôtel de Ville, the municipal government of Paris, which would qualify her as a secondary-school teacher. In two years she passed three examinations, including the music examination—although she considered herself an indifferent musician—and was awarded her certificates with honors.[48] During this period of self-taught study, she had been impressed by two pieces of scholarship more than any others: one of them was the great French historian Jules Michelet's book on Roman history.[49] The other was the publication of Antoine Becquerel's public lectures on physics given at the Conservatoire des Arts et Métiers, which first made her aware of the atomic structure of matter.[50] As she later put it, "The latter was the negation of all miracles and the former the negation of all Christian history if one applied the same rules to it."[51] Michelet had caused her to rethink the biblical story and would soon have a major impact upon her understanding of religion. Becquerel's lectures had an even longer lasting influence, but it was not until forty years later that she made a full analysis of his atomic theories and made her own attempts to synthesize the physical understanding of the universe.[52]

Now twenty-three, with her professional certificates, she put her name up for a position in France or England. As we will see, changes in the laws regulating secondary instruction of young women precluded her careful preparation for a career from being a sure guarantee of a safe economic future: the new laws had weakened if not destroyed the importance of her qualifications. Her response to these obstacles to her teaching career would change her life and precipitate her forward as a writer and intellectual. Within seven years she would become a major spokeswoman for the two fields of economics and Darwinian evolutionism.

The first effect of the new laws on Royer was her decision to teach in Britain. While many women thought the changes in French education were temporary, Royer may have been eager in any case to seize an opportunity to see another country. Young Frenchwomen were always in demand to teach French in Britain. An enterprising woman, Sarah Lewis, offered Clémence Royer a position in the school she was starting in English-speaking Wales. She planned to offer girls mathematical and map-making skills, in addition to the usual trio of subjects generally offered to British girls: French, music, and English. Royer saw an opportunity to travel as well as learn English, and welcomed this chance. Knowing that the Celtic Welsh had some historical relationship with the Bretons, she may have been curious about these people related to her mother's paternal ancestry. Whatever the combination of reasons, in January 1854 Royer took the train that would take her to the English Channel, to London, and finally to an English-speaking Welsh city in western Wales.

As recently as late December 1853, the first train ever to travel from London to west Wales had arrived at its terminus in the city of Haverfordwest. It was possible even then to leave London at 9:40 in the morning and arrive by 6:00 in the evening. The significance of the city as a trading center was consequently enhanced, while its importance as a port diminished. Immediately after the establishment of the first regular train service from London, an advertisement appeared in the *Pembrokeshire Herald* that a Mrs. Lewis announced the opening of a school.[53] She would share the teaching with a foreign lady. The two women proposed to teach a wide variety of subjects.

By February 1854, a new liberal paper, the *Haverfordwest and Milford Haven Telegraph,* had been started in opposition to the *Pembrokeshire Herald,* which represented entrenched Toryism. In the first issue of this paper, a more detailed advertisement was published, and a prospectus was offered. This seminary "for young ladies" was to be "conducted by Mrs Lewis." It read, "The course of English studies embraces English Grammar and Composition;

Writing; Arithmetic including Mental Calculation; Geography, Natural and Physical; the Globes; the Construction of Maps; Chronology, History Ancient and Modern; Plain and Ornamental Needlework." For extra fees it was possible to take "French, German, Italian, Music, Drawing, Painting in various styles." The concluding words, "a Foreign lady resides in the house," were set off from the rest of the advertisement as a great inducement (fig. 2).[54]

The school was situated on a fashionable street, Castle Terrace, and was located in one of a series of handsome attached three-story houses with recessed doorways and rooms with high ceilings. Members of the gentry and clergy, including a respectable widow and a surgeon, resided in the street, which lay just below the old Norman castle near the highest point of the town. The ruined castle, built in the reign of King Stephen by Gilbert de Clare, first earl of Pembroke, dominated the small city, which had more of the appearance of a Continental town than an English one. Part of its ancient keep recently had been turned into the county jail, and a "parade" extending from the castle for some distance had become a public walk with a dramatic view overlooking the river.[55]

The class lines of the city of Haverfordwest were well established, from Lord Milford nearby in Picton, who dined and hunted with the local county families, to the poor Irish and Welsh families who worked as navvies at the docks both in town and in Milford Haven. Although many winding streets remained, climbing up the hill on which the city was built, other streets had been enlarged by destroying deteriorating buildings. A fashionable broad street was constructed, named Victoria in the young Queen's honor.

The oldest church, St. Martin's, with its Elizabethan structure and small churchyard, was within a block of Castle Terrace. On a parallel street, on another high point, was the other major Church of England edifice, St. Mary's, built on the site of an old Norman church and echoing its Gothic structure. The church was just up the road from the fashionable Mariners and Castle Hotels. Dissenting chapels were also prominent in the area, especially those belonging to the Baptists and the Methodists, which they were in the process of rebuilding. A Society of Friends had existed at the end of the eighteenth century, but the old Quakers had married women in the Church of England and become absorbed into establishment religion. Some of these Quaker families were still prominent in the city, although others, the Starbucks for example, lived outside the city. Many of the dissenters were liberal professionals, members of the clergy, physicians, lawyers, or middle-class journalists. Their views were prominently represented in the new newspaper, which incorporated the changing interests of the new middle class. The conflict between various sects and the struggle between the dissenting sects and the established church in Britain provided the context for Clémence Royer to rethink her own beliefs.

A number of progressive societies had been started, both to encourage scientific and literary learning among the professionals and to educate members of the respectable working class. A Mechanics Institute had been inaugurated in the town in 1850 to provide lectures to respectable laborers on the topics of science, literature, and philosophy, but this was absorbed into the far more successful Milford Haven Mechanics Institute. Many of the leading professionals came to lecture on such topics as "The Microscope" or "The State of Medical Knowledge." A Scientific and Literary Society had been formed and offered a reading room as well as regular lectures on interesting topics during the winter session to its members. Another society, an Archaeological Association, regularly met to look at nearby ruins in Ruthin and St. David's.[56]

Every Sunday, using her Catholicism as an excuse for not attending Protestant church services, Royer would go for long, solitary walks, examining the beautiful historic ruins nearby or walking along the seaside, impressed by the dramatic rock outcroppings near the town.[57] Five miles from the town lay Milford Haven and the sea, where Royer would explore dramatic caves, as she would later describe in her novel. Only fifteen miles from Haverfordwest were the ruins of a great cathedral at St. David's, which had been such a famous place of pilgrimage in the Middle Ages that William the Conqueror himself had come as a penitent. In the mid-nineteenth century a new cathedral was built over the old Gothic ruins. Here the bishop of the Church of England celebrated Communion and confirmed the youth of the area in Welsh as well as in English.

Royer's year in Wales may well have stimulated her interest in biblical criticism. This was, after all, the period of debate about Strauss's *Life of Jesus,* followed some years later by Renan's *Vie de Jésus,* which both attempted to reinterpret Jesus as a historical figure.[58] The established Church of England also had its critic in Bishop Colenso, who had begun to look critically at the Bible.[59] Samuel Wilberforce, bishop of Oxford, was one of the fiercest opponents of Colenso and his public opposition contributed to Colenso's removal to a missionary outpost in South Africa among the Zulus, where he served as bishop of Natal. Young women, like Bessie Raynes Parkes, wrote searching letters to their friends about the religious doubts that Strauss and Colenso had raised in their minds.[60] Royer would more than once refer to the bishop of Oxford's later attack on T. H. Huxley.

Biblical criticism, soon to be of great interest to Royer, was mingled with lectures on Shakespeare as a moral philosopher in the liberal newspaper. Shakespeare, said the lecturer Naylor, inculcated charity in an intolerant age and advocated peace principles in a warlike age.[61] The playwright was characterized as more in accord with the New Testament than those who spoke from the pulpit. It is not surprising to find that, when Royer came to write her novel, she also saw herself as presenting moral as well as intellectual ideas.[62] The newspaper reported also on the debates within the Dissenting Churches. Excerpts from the analysis of ecclesiastical history by the Christian Socialist Frederick D. Maurice also formed a regular feature.[63] One series of articles on burial superstitions, which had appeared under the pseudonym "Nat Noncon," berated the division of a burial ground into two parts, one consecrated and one not—and reads almost like an anticipation of Royer's later discussion of burial practices.[64]

Royer arrived at a period when agitation over girls' education had just begun in England. This concern would culminate in the reports of the late 1860s.[65] There were at the time two notable girls' schools in all of England: Cheltenham, run by Dorothea Beale and patronized by both the great art critic John Ruskin and the founder of the Working Men's College, Frederick D. Maurice; and Frances Buss's North London Collegiate in London. Even these two great girls' schools were weak in mathematics, as the local examinations would soon reveal. The lesser girls' schools taught little except English, music, and French with some training in dancing and art. It is surprising to find Royer teaching in one of the few girls' schools in which both mental and practical arithmetic would be offered. She loved mathematical games all her life, but it is not evident how easily she could have taught such topics, given her very limited knowledge of the English language on her arrival. There may, in fact, have been little call for her skills, since the curriculum in girls' schools was often tailored to those who attended them and the desires of their mothers. Few women considered mathematics a necessary part of schooling. Even boys' education was weak at this period.[66]

So-called English Schools had been set up throughout Wales for the education of lower-middle-class boys. These were usually private schools, which charged fairly large fees. Lloyd George's father, William George, had just started an "English School for Scientific and Commercial Education" on Upper Market Street in Haverfordwest. He had trained at a normal school. Like Sarah Lewis, he offered a wide range of subjects: geography (physical and political), history of England and Wales, elements of geometry, mensuration, and algebra.[67] This boys' school, like the girls' school in which Royer was teaching, lasted only a few years, showing how ephemeral these unendowed private schools were.

The *Haverfordwest Telegraph* regularly recorded the speeches and activities of the liberal Dissenters. Until 1854 there had been a close connection with Bristol by regular steamboat, which was somewhat reduced by the coming of the railroad. Some of the liberal Dissenters reported on in the new paper may have found their models in activist Bristol Unitarians like James Martineau and Mary Carpenter, the sister of the physiologist and Unitarian William B. Carpenter. Mary Carpenter had recently led a crusade on behalf of the Ragged Schools, which were designed to teach poor children and reform those "going to the bad," an effort singled out for praise in the *Haverfordwest Telegraph*.[68] She was soon to be joined in her efforts by the future journalist and antivivisectionist Frances Power Cobbe. The Unitarian milieu in Bristol fostered literary women like Elizabeth Gaskell, whose novels and *Life of*

Charlotte Brontë had such an impact on mid-Victorian readers. For Dissenting families the visits of the American preacher W. H. Channing, nephew of the important Unitarian Ellery Channing, to Bristol must have been important. His book on the writings and letters of Margaret Fuller, which he edited together with Ralph Waldo Emerson, had just appeared, and this and other biographies of Margaret Fuller were being read with tears and appreciation by intelligent young women.[69] Many liberal journals were quoted in such a way that they could have served as important examples for Royer, among them the *Westminster Review,* which Marian Evans (George Eliot), translator of Strauss's *Life of Jesus,* had begun to edit with John Chapman. The activity of women was reported not only on behalf of the improvement of the education of the poor but also of the slaves in the United States, stimulated by the publication of Harriet Beecher Stowe's *Uncle Tom's Cabin.*[70]

In August 1854, a discussion from the Dissenting paper *The Leader* was reprinted in the *Haverfordwest Telegraph,* explaining the objections of Dissenters to public education of their children. They feared state education would conceal a religious dogma to which they did not subscribe. This objection had gained enormous popular support throughout Britain and led to the Dissenters Clause in the Education Bill. The interest in widespread education of people of all classes was demonstrated in the local paper with a report of 15 October 1854 on Frederick D. Maurice's lecture at the opening of the Working Men's College in Red Lion Square.[71] John Ruskin taught art at the college, while other lecturers offered information on machinery, geometry, Shakespeare, philosophy, and other subjects. In England, Maurice had an enormous impact on women interested in education, such as Emily Davies (the founder of Girton) and Cheltenham's Miss Beale.[72] When Maurice declared that "what was suitable for the education of boys was not suitable for men," Royer may have well thought—as she later expressed in Lausanne—that the entire education of women was also in need of a radical overhaul.

Royer's task was to learn English as well as teach French, music, and possibly mathematics. Always a hard worker and an omnivorous reader, she must have devoured the books available to her either through "Potter's reading room" or the Literary and Scientific Society. Even if she had done no more than read the local papers, she would have absorbed an enormous amount of information about English and European liberal attitudes. In that year of mastering a new language, she may have absorbed a radical liberal tone from articles in the *Haverfordwest Telegraph,* which advocated intellectual dissent. She could well have taken as a model for herself the letters to the editor, which formed a regular feature, giving voice to issues of public concern, from angry responses to unfavorable reviews of lectures or the closing off of popular throughways to local liberals' concern for adequate sewerage systems. Certainly, in later years, Royer was willing to use letters to editors of journals as a method of expressing her own dissent. The *Haverfordwest Telegraph* for the year of 1854 contains information on many of the topics that Royer would later deal with in books, articles, and finally as a regular contributor to the feminist paper *La Fronde.*

The Crimean War had just begun, and the new paper covered the war in detail, placing the French with the English news at the top of the column. Royer may have felt some satisfaction at seeing the French warmly commended for finally agreeing to form a military alliance with the English. Over the year, more and more war news filled the paper, including a regular map of the Crimea illustrating the location of battles fought. Florence Nightingale's new nursing organization was celebrated. Towards the end of the year, letters from young soldiers at the front began to be printed in the paper. In later years, Royer would deplore wars between civilized nations, declaring herself a pacifist. The *Haverfordwest Telegraph,* while not going so far, gave support for a peace meeting in the nearby town of Neath (led in all probability by the local Quakers). This meeting was interrupted and violently disrupted by some "respectable" locals who saw this as an unpatriotic attitude during the foreign excursion in the Crimea. Apparently, according to later reports, a brass band was used to disrupt the meeting. The *Telegraph* obtained a public apology for this disruption.

Revolutionaries like the Hungarian Kossuth and the Italian Garibaldi were applauded in the *Telegraph.* Sympathy was expressed for Garibaldi, who was reported to be ill with a fever from a bad leg. Kossuth's speech at Saint Martin's Hall in London on the anniversary of the Polish insurrection of 1830 was reported at length. Perhaps Royer's first interest in the Italian revolution, which she used as the general setting of her novel, came from this source. Certainly, around the same time, young women trained in Dissenting circles were responding with enthusiasm to Mazzini's vision of Young Italy. Bessie Rayner Parkes, a young Unitarian woman, wrote to her friend Barbara Smith (later, Bodichon), "Oh Barbara, have you seen Mazzini? With his fiery ashen face—I never saw such another—I am going to buy his first lecture on Italy."[73]

The widespread British interest in popular science was thoroughly illustrated in the new town paper. Royer, who later would write of the significance of matriarchal societies in the social life of insects, may have brooded in particular over the reported competition between the queen bee and her young rival, printed as one of the "Literary Excerpts" from Wood's *Bees.*[74] A selection that may have had a more direct impact on Royer's development was an excerpt from the biography of a mathematical genius. A poor boy, George Wilson, was sponsored by the French-born scientist Gaullaudet, in Philadelphia. He learned science, teaching himself through library books. He soon revealed himself to be a mathematical prodigy, winning fame by competing for prizes offered by the Royal Society and the Académie des Sciences.[75] That one could establish oneself as a scientist by such means may have struck Clémence, who was soon to follow the same course, first studying in a library and then competing for prizes offered by scientific societies.[76] Clémence Royer, as she developed her own ideas, may have taken to heart a reported quotation by Sydney Smith, which appeared in the paper: "I solemnly declare that but for the love of knowledge I should consider the life of the meanest hedger and ditcher as preferable to that of the greatest and richest man here present, for the fire of our minds is like the fire which the Persians burn in the mountains—it flames night and day and is immortal and not to be quenched."[77] Royer's own life was to testify to the truth of this statement.

Clémence Royer must have responded profoundly to differences between Haverfordwest and the Parisian environment with which she was most familiar. We know from her later autobiographical reminiscences that she adopted a "Unitarianism" along the lines of Ellery Channing soon after this period, although her initial reaction was to find Protestanism no less "ridiculous" a religion than her waning Catholicism.[78] To find a culture based on dissent and questioning suited the young woman who found herself so often in disagreement with authority.

The "culture shock" of her experiences in Wales may have encompassed other less salutary elements, bringing to the forefront a far darker side of her adolescence and enabling Royer to focus on her own mental development as she wrote about these and other issues, stirring painful memories. These issues provide the framework for the next chapter, which presents the possibility that Royer's novel yields insights into aspects of her life not available from the "surface narratives" of her autobiographical writings, letters, or other sources.

CHAPTER 2

The Question of Abuse and a Mission to Fulfill

One specific event that may have significantly affected the young French teacher and further weakened her respect for the power and integrity of the Catholic Church was a scandal reported at length in the local paper in Wales. Royer may have already experienced prejudice in the town against Catholics, who were seen as poor and alien, Irish, or foreign. There was no Roman Catholic church in Haverfordwest; Milford Haven's Catholic chapel catered primarily to poor fishermen. Everywhere she turned she must have had the sense of her religion as an ancient one now in decay. Within the town limits lay the ruins of an old Augustinian priory referred to as the priory of the "Black Canons," of which only an arch remained. She had written to her mother describing how "each Sunday she would take long solitary walks to the beautiful historic ruins around her, sometimes down to the seaside."[1]

From the end of September through October 1854, the reported rape of a poor Haverfordwest serving girl by a Catholic priest was regularly carried in the *Haverfordwest Telegraph* and the *Pembrokeshire Herald.*[2] By this time, Royer had been teaching for eight months or so in the town and must have been well aware of the local scandals. A fourteen-year-old Irish girl named Mary Sullivan, who worked part time in a local pub, brought an accusation of "violent assault and rape" against Patrick Kelly, a Milford Haven priest. He was duly arrested and held in the old dungeon of the castle, which served as the local jail.

Father Kelly had been relieved of all his sacred duties at the church as early as August, though whether this was because of his drinking or for other reasons was not clear. The priest had repeatedly sent Mary Sullivan for more whiskey until finally he locked her into a room and "pushed her down." Afterwards, when the girl asked him for a benediction, his curses astonished and upset her far more than the rape. The fact that she was intensely upset more by his wishing her "to the devil" than by his sexual assault counted against her in the court of law. Following the first hearing, the priest—always referred to as "Mr."—was discharged. Following an uproar, the case was heard again; but this time the whitewash was completed by testimony that Mary Sullivan had a bad character.

There was some conflicting testimony at the second hearing presented by the local doctors. One doctor (the fashionable surgeon Heslop), testified that she did seem to have recently been "interfered with." Examining her on Monday, a day after the incident, he supported the girl's testimony that she had had forcible intercourse, though he added that he could not, of course, tell if she had consented. The prison physician John Brown then examined her on Wednesday, three days later, and insisted that no evidence of rape could be found. Her young age does not seem to have been taken into account, for the possibility of statutory rape was not considered. Mary Sullivan had run to complain to two women who also worked at the inn, but they also gave conflicting testimony about whether she had cried—or cried sufficiently, in the court's opinion. The judges seem to have been concerned that she had not displayed the expected reaction to rape. The fact that her indignation was greater at the blasphemy committed by the priest than at the sexual act was even used as evidence that she had consented.

The priest was freed after this second hearing, although the *Haverfordwest Telegraph* felt that the case should have gone to trial and not been decided by the local magistrates. The Dissenting paper expressed its opinion of the case, showing some sympathy for the girl. This evoked the anger of the priest, who expressed his indignation, believing that he had been completely exonerated. The tenor of the testimony and the *Telegraph's* description of the priest's casual behavior—he consumed biscuits and quantities of snuff throughout the six hours of the testimony—leaves the impression that the priest was blasphemous and self-indulgent, whether or not he was a criminal.

A month of comments and discussion of such reports is likely to have had some effect on a young Frenchwoman brought up to venerate nuns and priests. She had, after all, adopted an almost puritanical martyrdom during her early adolescence and had even refused to attend the theater, because she felt this was not acceptable behavior. Was her later sense of betrayal by the church fueled by this trial? She could not have failed to hear the priest regularly castigated for his unseemly, if not criminal, behavior. We do not know what other memories these events may have evoked. Her later comment that the church "had darkened her childhood" expresses a developing rage at the church that seems to go beyond religious doubt or a retrospective anger at her convent school.[3] At the very least she must have felt a sense of humiliation at the castigation of a representative of her childhood religion, coupled with regular critical comments in the *Haverfordwest Telegraph* in reference to the Jesuits.

Clémence Royer was to integrate those comments into her own writing.

Her depiction of a wily and cruel Jesuit teacher in her novel *Les Jumeaux d'Hellas,* written only four years later,[4] may reflect a comment by Hannay, whose *Lectures on Byron* were printed in the Haverfordwest paper: the way to corrupt a youth would be to hand him, Hannay said, not Byron's scandalous poem *Don Juan* but a Jesuit text on moral questions.[5] Royer's indictment of the Jesuit priest in her novel extended to his moral responsibility not for the act of rape as such but for its retrospective validation, which has a certain continuity with Kelly's subsequent cursing of his victim.

There were other French writers who would come to feminism through indignation over the seduction of young women by members of the priesthood. Léon Richer, later a feminist leader, first came to public notice in France through his criticism of the inequitable treatment in the seduction of a young parishioner by a French provincial curé. While the curé was simply transferred to another area, the girl was sent to prison.[6] The power of this kind of event to rouse not only anger but an entire movement should not be underestimated. In Manchester, the great novelist Elizabeth Gaskell, like Josephine Butler later in the century, spoke out on behalf of unfortunate women who had become prostitutes through early experiences of seduction. Maria Deraismes, one of Léon Richer's associates, who later became a friend of Royer, became involved in the attempt to reform prostitution, expressing great sympathy for the women who had to turn to this profession for economic reasons.[7] Royer would soon depict her young heroine Lucie and her mother as sharing this concern in their work with former prostitutes.[8]

Royer wrote home to her mother about her impressions of her surroundings in a vivid manner, and these letters were passed around or read aloud to groups of friends.[9] Like many a diarist and letter writer of the period she was practicing her future craft. Although none of these letters has survived, and few comments survive reflecting directly upon her experiences in Haverfordwest, she did describe the area in detail in her novel *Les Jumeaux d'Hellas,* written only three years after she left Wales.[10]

Already, there are indications that a series of more or less transparent autobiographical references occur in Royer's novel: aspects of the characterization of the Jesuit teacher, aspects of the heroine's concern for "fallen women," and aspects of the description of landscape hint at the probability that she drew heavily and in a variety of ways upon personal experience in writing her one and only novel. This is an appropriate point to consider *Les Jumeaux* in detail, as a source for her experiences. Admittedly this is a risky strategy, since many novelists deplore the attempt to mine literary works for information about the writer's life. Nevertheless, it is not uncommon, especially in an early work, for the novelist to draw heavily from autobiography. In Royer's case this possibility is strengthened by her lifelong tendency in public talks as well as in her writings to wander off into what was or had recently been of concern to her in her life, as we shall see. This suggests that we may, with caution, read some sections of the novel as a direct reflection of her personal experience, amplifying and occasionally even suggesting elements that are missing in her adolescent history. More generally, we shall find that the novel helps us understand her attitudes towards women, love, marriage, and the bearing of children outside marriage. Her novel provides the clearest guide to her thinking of this early period. It also amplifies for us other aspects of her thought, from concepts of social rebellion to the role of law in establishing women's rights, her view of the Catholic Church, and her image of science.

The title of the novel, Les Jumeaux d'Hellas, can be translated as "Hellas's Twins" (in reference to the search by two twin brothers for their unknown father, a Greek hero named Hellas) or "Greek Twins," Hellas being a common poetic term for Greece. A first version, nothing of which survives, was composed in 1858; the surviving, much revised, second version was published in 1864.[11] The novel, in spite of some delightful passages and some bold aims, is rather wooden in conception. Two volumes, a thousand pages, in length, its second volume is far better written and indeed might make a respectable novel on its own, since many plot details are sufficiently explained in the last five hundred pages. Royer's story follows the conventions of French theater rather than those of the novel. At times the plot creaks along like a rather old stage vehicle, as individuals come and go in groups of two and three, according to good stage practice. Much of the action is reported in retrospect in correspondence between characters. Very little of it has vividly painted scenes or characters, possibly reflecting a combination of Royer's physical nearsightedness and the often deliberate vagueness of theatrical form.

Where influences can be detected they include Mme de Staël's *Corinne,* Bulwer-Lytton's *Last Days of Pompeii,* some novels of Alexandre Dumas, the French theatrical tradition, and perhaps Italian opera. In her preface to the printed version of the novel, Royer also cites two Chateaubriand novels: *René* and *Martyrs,* four of George Sand's novels, *Lélia, Jacques, La Mare au diable,* and *Marquis de Villemer,* and two novels by Voltaire to illustrate the widely different styles used by the same novelist, who creates something new with each novel.[12] We have seen the admiration that Royer had as a young girl for the popular actress Rachel. The parts that she had seen her perform, Jeanne d'Arc, Corinne, Phèdre, and others all called for the type of tragic and accusing speech with which Royer has liberally salted her text. Royer adopted the convention often used in the eighteenth-century novel as well as those in the first half of the nineteenth century, utilizing the exchange of letters as a means of conveying the plot. Here it is primarily the two protagonists, their mother, their mother's sister, and close female friends who write to each other, describing recent or long past events. Very rarely do the events take place before our eyes.

The story purports to tell the adventures of the Mondoni twins, bastard sons of the wife of the king of Naples by a Greek revolutionary hero, and is set in no specified historical time. The twins appear to represent alternative life choices or dispositions towards activity (represented by one twin, Matteo) or passivity (represented by the other, Stefano). One of the twins is an avowed debaucher, who rejects his religion and sees science as an alternative belief, the other is a monastic and devoted student of the Jesuits, given to mysticism and visions. In another sense they are also the male and female elements of a single, perhaps divided, personality. Some of Royer's later anger against the tendency of scientists to create dichotomies of male and female equated with active and passive characteristics stemmed from her realization, in this novel, that men and women contained both elements of action and inaction.

The doubling of the protagonists is matched by the women of the previous generation. The twins' mother and their aunt are the daughters of the emperor of Austria. Each has had to make a choice between accepting a safe, conservative marriage to the king of Naples or following her heart and staying with her first lover. The twins' mother, Amalia, has chosen to be a queen, has been deprived of her first two children, and is unhappy in her marriage. She has rejected marriage to the Greek revolutionary Hellas, who is the twins' real, though not legal, father. Amalia's sister, Joanna, has chosen exile in Switzerland, leading an idyllic life for some years with her lover, the Polish count Orlowski (former friend and co-conspirator of Hellas), whom she then marries. However, he dies not many years later. Joanna then devotes her life to saving "fallen women," like some of Elizabeth Gaskell's heroines.[13]

Much of the plot concerns the king's fear of the bastard sons, who are legally his since they were born during the marriage to his wife, Amalia, but who have been brought up in ignorance of their birth. As babies they were carried away and raised in Lausanne by Joanna along with her own beautiful daughter, Lucie. At ten they were removed from her care by the conniving Jesuit Ricci, who at the king's behest has concocted a scheme to neutralize them both either by introducing them to a life of meaningless pleasure or through binding them to the authority of the church. Matteo can be more easily induced to enter on a life of debauchery; Stefano is drawn to the church. Since the twins have taken an oath to make the same decision, that is, either to enter the priesthood or reject Catholicism, this presents a problem for Ricci. The king becomes apprehensive, as he believes the twins have learned of their parentage, and he considers them a threat to his throne.

Stefano, sensitive and almost hysterical, is overcome by his religious mysticism. He becomes delirious and experiences a hallucination in which he sees the queen of Naples, whom he adores from afar not knowing she is his mother. As he lapses into a coma, he is almost poisoned by a stereotypically evil court doctor, who, as the doctor at his birth, seems to have no qualms about killing him. Stefano is saved by the quick thinking of a friend of the queen, Mathilde, countess of Pembroke, the attractive wife of the malicious English ambassador Lord Howard. She knocks away the fatal potion and spirits the comatose young man to England in a coach. Lady Howard is thought to be having an affair with Stefano, and a sensational divorce case follows. She retires to her Welsh castle by the sea, refusing the young man's offer of marriage when he recovers, a gesture he makes not out of love but with the intent of restoring the countess's honor.

The plot now thickens to the consistency of potato soup. Both Stefano and Matteo are in love with their cousin Lucie, with whom they were raised. Matteo, however, now reveals to Stefano that he once raped his cousin, wrongly believing that she betrayed him with his dissolute companion Fabio. Stefano has fallen madly in love with Lucie, who tells him the sad tale of Matteo's rape. When he asks her to marry him, although she loves him, she insists that he first adopt her belief in a nature-based Deism. By this time, Stefano has discovered from Fabio that his Jesuit teacher, Ricci, was the cause of the betrayal of the innocent Lucie and that Ricci had warned Matteo not to marry her after the rape, since she was now a fallen woman. Ricci was, therefore, the root cause of Matteo's debauchery and his rejection of real love.

Stefano keeps vigil by the deathbed of Queen Amalia, whose true identity as his mother has only been recently revealed to him. He erupts in a great outburst against his mentor Ricci, finally putting an end to his passivity and rejecting both his teacher and his Catholicism. In the process he defends his mother, whom he believes has made only the error of failing to follow her heart rather than her duty. Stefano, like Matteo, now supports the principle of instinctual love over that of formal marriage, claiming that he and his brother are the mother's true children, while the legal children are the bastards. In anger, Ricci fulfills a previous order of the king of Naples to have Stefano thrown into the bizarrely named Château d'Oeuf and tortured.[14]

Meanwhile Matteo has been wandering through Europe and the Near East, having decided to abandon his former sybaritic life; he is being followed secretly by his former mistress, Léona, who has renounced her life as celebrated actress and courtesan and adopted the costume and the name of a boy, Chryses. Matteo, when he finally encounters her, does not recognize his mistress, believing her to be her younger brother. She, too, is closely related to the twins, a first cousin on the father's side, since her Greek mother was their father's sister. She is also the daughter of Greek heroes, and her motivation to protect Matteo seems to be a mixture of love, family feeling, and revolutionary idealism. When Léona encounters another of her former lovers, the cardinal Barbeschi, he gives up his religion and his cardinal's robes (but not his ideals) to follow her in turn.

The overburdened plot now meanders towards politics. Matteo is contacted by a secret society who see in him an opportunity for revolution at the moment of his mother's death and his father's abdication in favor of a half brother. Partly in order to free Stefano, he joins a revolutionary band led by a presumed bandit, Gioachino, leader of a (masonic) society and a master of disguises, who seems to represent Garibaldi in the novel. The defrocked cardinal joins the revolt against the kingdom of Naples. Although the revolutionaries want to use the Mondoni twins as a rallying point for their forces, Matteo insists firstly that his brother Stefano as elder twin should be the ruler, and secondly that neither of them will accept a hereditary rulership. Instead he proposes a republic whose new code will establish two principles: "Every man owes obedience only to the chief whom he has freely elected as such" and: "Every child must know the father and mother who has given him birth. The search for paternity is the first moral duty. Civil law only consecrates heredity in the maternal line."[15] Among the aims of the projected new republican government is the declaration of the right of women to raise their own children, to give them their own names, and to declare the true father of their children, rights that will incidentally vindicate the twins' mother and aunt. A triumvirate is set up comprising Barbeschi and the twins, along with a cabinet of three of the surviving women of the story, Mathilde Howard (the English countess, who seems to have re-entered the story in order to join the revolution), Lucie, and Lucie's mother Joanna (the twins' aunt). Chryses (Léona) serves as the secretary to the triumvirate. Although it appears at first as though the revolt has succeeded and the new republic been declared, the people become uneasy at the new "monstrous" rights given to women and the public denigration of the presumed miracles of the church. The doubtful populace turns against the revolutionaries and aids the armies of the king.

The Jesuit Ricci, now dressed as a soldier as befits his participation in the "army of God," enters with a group of soldiers. He aims his gun at his former pupil Stefano, who has been saved from the dungeon but is still weak and incapacitated. Mathilde, who is devoted to Stefano, saves him for the second time by taking the shot in her own breast. Dying, she reveals her suppressed love. Lucie, calling Ricci "a murderer and calumniator of women," grabs a sword and kills him, saying that he "must die at the hand of a woman."[16] An alarm is sounded, which brings the revolutionary leader Gioachino to their aid. He realizes that they are losing the battle for Naples and readies a boat for their escape. Chryses, wounded while protecting Joanna, is discovered by Joanna to be a woman when she tends her wounds. Finally Matteo recognizes the supposed boy as his lost, but still beloved, Léona and offers to marry her.[17]

The gods, probably feeling the curtain must come down, now lend a hand: a volcano erupts just as Mathilde is being buried by the doleful six at Pompeii. A crater erupts simultaneously near the coast of Naples, and a third on the other mountainside, burying Naples in lava in a brief Bulwer-Lytton-esque recapitulation. The triumvirate and the three remaining women, spared from this horror, depart for the Orient feeling that the time has not yet come for wide-ranging reforms in Europe, which, says Matteo, are more easily instilled in younger peoples. They leave the peasant revolutionary leader Gioachino behind to carry the revolution to Rome.

Royer was a little dismayed that those characters she had described with the greatest enjoyment were not those that her readers liked most. The weaker sister, Queen Amalia, mother of the twins, was preferred to the strong-minded, rational sister, Joanna, Lucie's mother. Léona, actress and courtesan, was admired more than virtuous (and wronged) Lucie. "The hetaerae are so much à la mode," Royer noted with regret.[18] Perhaps she was pleased that Matteo was preferred to Stefano, since it is Matteo who is the lover of science, although it is he who rapes her heroine, Lucie. Royer thought Matteo's rationality was appreciated without the expected criticism of his bad behavior because there was, despite her challenges to such assumptions, a different social standard of conduct for men and women.

Royer asks in her preface if writers "have put so much love into books because there isn't much of it any longer in life." But although she thinks a book should be entertaining and emotionally moving, she believes that the principal aim of a book should be to make one think. Speaking of her characters, she says: "None of them is completely false or true, it appears to me. None of them is completely my organ, and I make myself responsible for none of the doctrines they uphold in toto. Almost all are in advance of the present century; but to my point of view they ought to go further still."[19]

The often bizarre plot is not the real story so much as an elaborate frame upon which Royer hangs material she feels to be of great urgency: her intense feelings of betrayal by the Catholic Church, her love of science and learning, and her belief in the rights of women. Each of these discussions is detailed at great length, and they constitute the central core of what she wants to say. She addresses her readers in the opening pages of the preface:"I want first of all to declare to you, reader, that this book is that of a woman rebel [*une rebelle*]—a rebel who wants to be a rebel, who is more so in her thought than in her actions, and who will appear rather less so in these pages than she is by conviction and by will."[20] She adds, "They claim that a novel ought not to be a work of advocacy. Is it necessary that the poet make himself into a painter, who represents things but does not judge them? For my part, at the risk of not being proclaimed a poet, I prefer to think, to judge, to say what I believe as I think it, rather than to make my pen a simple brush, however rich the palette might be in which I dip my colors."[21]

However, she almost compromises this clarity of purpose by overburdening the story with a kaleidoscope of events. Frequently, unlike a modern soap opera, she fails to establish a convincing sense of time and place. For example, Royer admits in her preface that she had not seen Naples when she wrote her novel. We rarely have a sense of setting, such as details of a building or a room, and descriptions of the major figures are often sketchy. They have no specific clothing, except for their disguises during the revolution; we do not know whether the men are tall or short, dark or fair, although the women are better described. In the main the characters simply talk or write to, or rather "at," each other. Royer comments in her preface: "The characters which I present to you, reader, are not portraits. I even avow that their originals will be for the most part impossible to find."[22] She argues that, as in a Perrault fairy tale, she is justified in placing her characters outside of a specified time and place but with a real base on which she has designed "ideal traits."

A major question raised at this point is: how real a base? For there are certain startlingly clear exceptions to the general air of "never-never land." We have already noted the realism attaching to aspects of the characterization of Father Ricci and aspects of Lucie's and her mother's involvement with the welfare of "fallen women." Other exceptions to the air of unreality are landscapes with which Royer was familiar. She describes in an exceptionally vivid manner the landscape around Haverfordwest, including the brooding, overhanging Norman castle (used in the novel as the home of Mathilde Howard, countess of Pembroke), the old priory ruins, and the caves by the sea along the coast near Milford Haven, where Lady Howard walks and then hides herself away to meditate. The other vivid landscape is of Lausanne, where Lucie and her mother live, and the landscape (unspecified, but possibly also Lausanne) in which Matteo wanders as he writes his "Album of a Traveler."[23] In this last section she invokes nature and science in a manner that makes them seem like excerpts from a different book. They may have been taken from her own notebook when she first arrived in Switzerland, since the observations detail climbing mountains, isolation, and an initial enthusiastic response to science.[24]

These and certain other passages make it tempting to assert that, in general, those passages having a "ring of truth" contain specific autobiographical reference to Clémence Royer's life. These are varied in scope and content: the denunciation of the courtesan life by the actress Léona (probably inspired by Rachel's theatrical speeches), Lucie's appeal for a Deistic religion (reflecting Royer's new beliefs), Joanna and Count Orlowski's vows of eternal love (which resonate with Royer's love affair with Pascal Duprat), Stefano's angry denunciation of his Jesuit teacher, Ricci (reflecting Royer's angry response to her church), or the final scene of violence in which women as well as men battle (possibly echoing her mother's heroic view of her assistance in her husband's rebellion). Many of these points of reference will be enlarged upon in the following sections.

The principal passage relevant here is an account by the young heroine Lucie of her rape by her cousin Matteo. If a change in voice and tone from histrionics and stage voices to descriptions of real human pain can be taken as an indication that there is a direct autobiographical reference, then the striking realism of this particular episode raises disturbing questions about Clémence's past.

Lucie, like Clémence, has lost her father in her late teens. Like Clémence, she has a mother who gives her daughter an unusual amount of independence. The mother has carefully instructed the daughter about puberty and given her some idea of sexual desire. "For more than a year you had already armed my innocence against surprises of the senses. You had instructed me in the rites of love, you told me of the duties of the wife and how by a divine law of nature they must succeed those of the daughter. I was prudent because I knew the danger. Your wise counsel taught me to judge men without receiving the sad lessons of experience and deception."[25] Like Clémence Royer, at that age she is a naive but socially concerned young woman. Both mother and daughter are involved in an enterprise to save and protect unfortunate "fallen women," as Elizabeth Gaskell and Josephine Butler were doing in England. Lucie's cousin Matteo, a brilliant and wealthy young man, loves and desires Lucie. "I received him with affection, with confidence, freely, like a brother, since you treated him as a son," Lucie later admits to her mother.[26] Lucie feels a growing love for her cousin but hesitates to tell him before she is sure of his love for her. A false friend, Fabio, tells the cousin that Lucie has granted sexual favors to him, which changes Matteo's behavior towards Lucie. He begins to treat her with an insulting familiarity and then, when she rejects him, he frightens her with a declaration of passionate desire.

Lucie grows afraid of her cousin and refuses to see him. Trapped into meeting him by a letter purportedly from a woman needing her help, but in fact written by Fabio, she agrees to go to an abandoned pavilion. There her cousin meets her, enraged by his conviction that she has come to meet his friend. He forces her to have sex with him. Lucie, describing the scene to her mother, tells her,

> I was lost. I swear to you that I struggled with all my power. Did I cry out? I no longer know. I did not even care; I defended myself with desperation as if I were dealing with a wild beast. I did not lower myself to plead. No, I was exalted by indignation, by anger. . . . I bit his hands; my resistance only exasperated him. In one of my movements I struck my neck against the wood, and whether from pain, fatigue, or shock, I lost consciousness. If I succumbed, vanquished, I have no knowledge of it. . . . When I came to my senses, my clothes were disordered. I was overwhelmed, my legs were bruised, I could hardly get up. What had I become during that time between the hands of my wicked corrupter? I had no memory of it. I had become a woman, certainly, I understood that from sensations, instincts, unknown to me before that. But I remained ignorant of any voluptuous feelings. More dead than alive I dragged myself to the house. When you returned, you found me speechless with a painful illness that caused me to lose my memory for a month. I couldn't even remember the affront I had received or what had caused it. Only after a long convalescence did I recall the events with shame and intolerable pain.[27]

Upon her recovery, when the memory of the rape returns, Lucie hides it from her mother, feeling that it will do no good to tell anyone, after she is certain she isn't pregnant. The "violent act performed as though on a dead woman" fails to result in pregnancy. Her cousin may think he has dishonored her, she sobs, but in her own mind she rejects that description. She runs through the possible ways she might act. If she accuses him of rape, she knows she will be made to share his guilt. Had her father been alive, he could have challenged him to a duel, but he might have been killed. Any court case would be a cause of family shame. There were no witnesses. Matteo, who had been received in her mother's home, would have brought up the name of the false friend. "The lawyers would simply cover your daughter with their obscene raillery, with impure blasphemy."[28] If she were to win the court case and he were forced to marry her, she would have to carry the name of a man she considered a criminal and "grant willingly what he had taken only through an abuse of force. I would prefer a thousand deaths."[29]

She concludes that it would be better to keep the sorrow to herself rather than burden her mother with something for which she felt there was no redress. To her the rape was doubly horrible because her cousin had been her first love. She feels she had completely mistaken his character and experiences the tragedy of the loss of love as well as pride. An illuminating scene describes Lucie's reaction some time after her rape. She has lost the liveliness of her earlier girlhood. She has quite suddenly lost her beauty and grace.

> She became dreamy, sad, although always gentle and good. She sought only solitude and silence. She spent long hours in study, although before she had shared in the cares of the world. Her speech was slower, the sound of her voice graver, her accent more penetrating. . . . She sang but for her own hearing, and her songs made those who chanced to hear them weep. They seemed . . . cries of sorrow coming from the depth of her soul. . . . Her life unfolded between charitable concerns and mental occupations. Painting, music, reading, the study of nature were her habitual and exclusive distractions.[30]

Lucie turns to teaching as a way of relieving her deep depression.

In a further interweaving of art and the life of Royer and her colleagues in Wales, Lucie starts a girls' school after a period of isolation and study. She discovers that she is a marvelous teacher. "Her persuasive and gentle eloquence ran like a valley stream, refreshing and fertilizing the banks through which it runs, depositing the germs of a strong and virile morality in the hearts of her young students."[31] She cannot, however, shake off the sense of deep depression. "But what secret discouragement, what mysterious pain was hidden at the bottom of the soul of that woman, so richly, so powerfully endowed?"[32] The answer in Lucie's case is, of course, the humiliation of rape.

Some years later, Matteo visits her home, "pride on his face, a smile on his lips, the artisan of all the evils of my life."[33] Lucie freezes and walks out of the room without greeting him. The mother, knowing nothing yet about the rape, welcomes her sister's son. When he makes insulting suggestions about Lucie's ability to "love everyone, even those who don't deserve it," the mother is alarmed. Later, her mother, pressing her about her avoidance of her formerly beloved cousin and about his odd behavior, hears her daughter's sad story.

Lucie assures her, "I don't blame you at all, Mother, for the principles by which you raised me, for the independence which you allowed me. Far from that."[34] She adds sadly that when young women are raised in such a manner, young men need to be instructed how to restrain their passions and develop a sense of duty about the rights of women. "Otherwise without defense, without help, without protection, whatever the customs, whatever the laws, we are subject to their brutal will and exposed to worldly opinion, which makes us responsible for the faults that they alone committed."[35] These sentiments are repeated by Royer many years later in her suppressed discussion on women in society given before the Société d'Anthropologie in 1874.[36]

The mother is appalled that she has received Matteo into her house. "For that alone I blame you," she tells her daughter. Her silence has led the young man to insult her daughter to her face, mistaking the mother's ignorance for cowardice. She is distraught and asks her to explain why she failed to share her sorrow with her mother. The girl weeps profusely and explains that her silence was instinctive. For too many generations women have been taught to believe that rape was shameful, the fault of the victim. Even though she felt she had acted correctly, she could not overcome the feeling of shame. A year ago, if she had tried to tell her mother, she wouldn't have been able to speak. "I have often reflected on this strange psychological phenomenon; I have asked science for the solution."[37]

The mother, a kind woman, reassures her daughter of her pride and belief in her child. "No, your life is not bruised by an infamous love."[38] She can still have a radiant life and a happy marriage. Rejecting the cousin who attacked her, she eventually marries his twin, a more passive young man, after she insists on his accepting her Deistic beliefs.[39] One curious complication of the story is the manner in which Ricci, the Jesuit priest, advises his pupil Matteo not to marry the cousin he raped.

This last detail recalls Father Kelly's renunciation of the girl he raped, but the possibility that this story reflects similar abuse in Royer's own life remains. The realism is remarkable, especially in a depiction of rape by a nineteenth-century woman. Here the emotional consequences of rape, the sequence of anger, silence, pain, and the sense of self-denigration and betrayal are clearly laid out. One should not forget that at twenty Royer said in her poem about ideals that "struggle only produces renewed ardor," a comment repeated in Lucie's story of the rape in which she depicts vividly the "renewed ardor" of Matteo as she struggles with him. In the novel there is no permanent social damage to the rape victim. Lucie does, indeed, make a happy marriage with the twin of her rapist, while her rapist bitterly repents his act. By comparison with the seduction of Dickens's little Emily in *David Copperfield,* which leads to Emily's abandonment and death in a hospital for the poor, Royer's simpler story seems the more unusual and psychologically truer.

What accounts for this sense of reality? Had she perhaps gleaned enough from the reports concerning the case of Mary Sullivan or from accounts being written by contemporary women on the reform of "fallen" women to be able to depict the course of physical and psychological events with such power? Or could the only source of such accuracy have been personal experience? The known facts of her life yield no further clues.

Whether or not Royer had an unhappy sexual experience as a young woman, she rejected the possibility of marriage. Unlike many contemporary French women, Royer did not need to marry to gain social independence and she was aware that marriage could result in the loss of her legal and economic rights. In Britain she must have encountered many unmarried women who were teachers, social reformers, and writers content with their situation. In France, however, middle-class single women could not go out in the evening respectably or dine alone in public.[40] Royer would add later that middle-class women in her society were seen as social failures if they never married.[41] Although after her thirties, she found the title "Mademoiselle" to be demeaning, regretting that this appeared on her Darwin translation, she continued to distrust marriage as an institution.

Caution regarding the consequences of unfortunate marriages is reflected in the novel in yet another episode with a factual reference point in the mid-1850s. One of Royer's heroines, Lady Mathilde Howard, is portrayed, as we noted, as an aristocrat from Pembroke, the countyseat of Haverfordwest. Lady Howard, countess of Pembroke, lives in a castle overlooking the town, reminiscent of the manner in which the old Norman castle, ancient home of the duke of Pembroke, sat above the town of Haverfordwest. Mathilde is wrongly accused by her husband of adultery. After a sensational divorce trial, freed from her husband and exonerated by the English queen, she rides her horse along the seaside and sits in caves by the ocean in Pembroke, just across the bay from Milford Haven. She writes:

> I believed I still heard the faraway echo of a noise of arms and battles and saw the heralds of armies and valets pass in its courts. I asked then if women and daughters of our old Norman grandmothers suffered as we did, if the service of love of their cavaliers was more gentle than our troublesome love, if their tears moistened the linen of their long sleeves as often as the wools of our embroideries? Were they more free than we to choose a husband?[42]

Like Lucie, Lady Howard responds to her personal difficulties by setting up a girls' school. She founds it in Carew (in the county of Pembroke, like Haverfordwest), but she finds to her sorrow that the girls, previously affectionate and devoted to her, have become reserved and hesitant after the notoriety of her divorce. She writes to a friend: "These girls had loved me. You understand my agony, Amalia, when, appearing among them after the insults that I had submitted to, I no longer found among them the same frank welcome and affectionate respect. Their bearing towards me was troubled, and their responses were constrained and embarrassed."[43]

The character of Lady Howard may have been based on Caroline Norton, who was a beautiful and powerful aristocratic woman as well as a highly talented writer of the 1840s and 1850s. Her divorce was a *cause célèbre* of the 1850s. Norton served as hostess for important parliamentary figures in the 1830s and was close to more than one prime minister. George Meredith was later to use her as a model for his character Diana in his novel *Diana of the Crossways.* Norton's husband had wrongly sued her for divorce and had taken custody of her young children. He had also successfully claimed her mother's legacy along with the income derived from her books. Her agitation before the courts resulted in a partial victory in the Infant Children's Custody Bill. In 1854 and 1855 she brought a series of legal proceedings to prove her rights to her own money. In an appeal to Queen Victoria in 1855, she made her famous statement: "I have no rights, I have only wrongs."[44]

In 1854 the young feminist Unitarian Barbara Smith (later Bodichon), influenced by her friends who were supporting Caroline Norton's petition, printed an influential pamphlet deploring the lack of women's rights.[45] Smith then organized the first women's committee to agitate on this topic. In 1857 Parliament passed the Married Women's Property Act to protect the separate property of married women from their husbands.[46] Royer, interested in women's rights throughout her life, seems to have responded to these events, and she was later to write for Bodichon's journal.[47] Her interest in women's rights is already evident in *Les Jumeaux,* in which she includes rights for women as well as for men in the constitution of the revolutionary republic.[48]

George Eliot (Marian Evans) was a friend of Bodichon and was spending the spring of 1855 in the company of her lover, George Henry Lewes, close by in Tenby, writing the first of her acclaimed novels, *Scenes of a Clerical Life.* It is regrettable that Royer and Evans never met, although they might have had little in common at the time. Royer's interest in biblical criticism echoes Evans's interest in translating Strauss. Royer's later decision to live with Pascal Duprat was not unlike that of Marian Evans, whose decision to live with Lewes, a man bound by a totally failed marriage, was intimately connected with her intellectual and artistic development. This parallels Royer's association with Duprat. Royer, however, still had some distance to go to "recreate" herself.

Although she could not have helped being influenced by what she read and saw in England, Royer never formally adopted Protestantism. She later reported that "there I knew Protestants in their own homes and did not judge them less ridiculous than the Catholics."[49] But in conflict with this claim was an earlier biographical statement that she had around this time adopted "the Unitary Christianity of Channing" (Unitarianism), which gives some color to the long-lasting influence upon her of the Dissenting culture in Haverfordwest.[50]

At the end of her contract, which probably ran for the full year until the end of the spring term 1855, Royer returned to France. Her next position that summer took her as a substitute teacher to the beautiful city of Touraine with its famous Renaissance châteaux. The school was situated in an old château in which Jeanne d'Arc was said to have stopped on her return from Chinon, overlooking the village of Beauvais, in which the Maid of Orléans had been born. The connection with the Maid of Orléans was significant to her, since she had always identified herself with this rebellious heroine. In addition, the new biography of Jeanne d'Arc by the historian Michelet, whom she had long admired, must have intensified this identification.[51]

She soon discovered there a complete eighteenth-century library, long neglected, which like a true bookworm she proceeded to devour. Her reaction after first reading Voltaire, Rousseau, Diderot, and the other Encyclopedists was a feeling of true illumination coupled with a profound anger and indignation against her teachers.[52] She felt deceived by having been forbidden those great writings, and this sense of deception focused on the Catholic Church, which she thought had sought to ram dogma down her throat instead. The love of science, with which the *Encyclopédie* was filled, she later claimed, inspired her to study and understand nature. Although she did not say so explicitly, she must have absorbed a great deal of the popular interest in science to which British culture had exposed her. She read the Enlightenment thinkers with a prepared mind. Attending Sunday mass given by the local village curé in the tiny Renaissance chapel, a requirement for a schoolmistress, she began to debate with herself whether it was appropriate to attend mass if one no longer believed.[53] Although she had stopped attending mass regularly as early as her twentieth year, she did not find it so easy to relinquish the social expectations associated with religion.

During the early part of the summer of 1856 she was teaching in another château, which overlooked the village of Beauvais, Jeanne d'Arc's birthplace. This visit, coupled with her recent stay in the Touraine château, also associated with the French heroine, provoked what she termed a "mystical crisis . . . the last echo of my convent education," resonating with her childhood identification with the Maid of Orléans. "These two circumstances made all sorts of heroic ideas gallop through my head."[54] This time she focused her anger on the Catholic Church while for the next few months she tried to resolve her doubts.

As she recounted the subsequent events, sometime during the winter she entered the confessional of a priest she did not know and insisted that the priest help her. If he failed to give her an answer, she threatened to leave her teaching position, take up her pen as a sword, and make war against the church. This alarmed the priest enough to take on the burden of her reconversion. He urged her, as Pascal had suggested, to practice her religion in order to believe gradually in her faith again. The priest gave her books to read, including one he had written on the conversion of Veuillot. When she read the quotation from Pascal, "One believes what one wants to believe," she sent the book back with a note in which she insisted one does not believe what one wants, one must want what one believes. "Your book is immoral; I have done with it," she proclaimed.[55] Later she added that at that point she hated the church, which had "lied to my childhood and darkened my youth."[56] Ten years of studying nature would pass, she added, before she gave up Deism and "arrived at absolute negation."[57]

A deep ambivalence towards the church is illustrated by her characterization of priests in *Les Jumeaux*. There are some contradictions: the cardinal Barbeschi, like Matteo a former lover of Léona, becomes a revolutionary leader who, instead of opposing Matteo (with whom he would seem to have a natural rivalry), becomes his associate. Royer seems to have included a converted member of the Catholic Church to indicate that Catholic leaders do not have to be villains like the Jesuit Ricci. To illustrate the hypocrisy of the claimed celibacy of the church, both the cardinal and the Jesuit have affairs with women. Ricci maintains a household with a married woman, and his children are born under the protection of the complacent husband and take the husband's name. In spite of or perhaps because of this, Ricci seems to have no sympathy for the position of the Mondoni twins, who are born in a similar situation, to a married woman. Hypocrisy in her church, the contrast between the ideals that the priests held out to others and some of the revelations of their own behavior continued to trouble Royer for some years.

For Royer, this moment of rejection of her church was associated in her mind with her father's truthful speech before his judges. She, like her father, had been raised "in the cult of loyalty and truth."[58] Her mystical crisis led her to believe that she had a mission in life to "illuminate humanity" and deliver it from the lies and errors by which she felt she had been "abused," a word that carries the same double meaning in French as in English.[59] Although she described her reaction as anger directed against her teachers, she may also have been in revolt against her emotional loneliness, first experienced when she was isolated as a foreigner in Britain, then as a substitute teacher in France. She may have been unwilling to adjust to a life that repeated the convent experience that had shaken her self-confidence as an adolescent.

Given that teaching was seen by Royer as a way of relieving depression caused by severe emotional turmoil, it is not evident why a renewed emotional crisis should have driven her out of the profession, nor is it evident why Royer's response should have been so absolute. Yet that initial abandonment of her position was the end of her teaching career. Her decision was sudden and total in spite of the many years she had spent in qualifying herself. Why then did she make no further attempts to teach within the French system? A good part of the explanation may be provided by the article written by Julie-Victoire Daubié on girls' secondary education just ten years later.[60]

Daubié describes the setting up of the examinations that Royer had taken under the Second Republic to qualify as a secondary-school teacher. Only a few years after these examinations and qualifications were established, their value was debased, although the certificates awarded were seen as near equivalents for women of the *baccalauréat,* which was awarded to young men finishing the *lycée.* According to Daubié, the holders of these prestigious qualifications were thrown into total confusion by the change of government when a law passed at the beginning of the Second Empire in 1850 placed primary instruction under the control of the church. Although this did not at first apply to girls' boarding schools at the secondary level, it led to another law passed at the end of 1853 that formally abolished female secondary schools and teaching by lay teachers and eliminated the very examinations that Royer had so proudly passed. Her high qualifications had, in effect, become worthless.

Royer, along with her fellow lay teachers and heads of boarding schools, found themselves in a difficult economic position, feelingly described by Daubié. The secondary-school lay teacher with certificates from the Paris municipal government found herself competing unsuccessfully with primary-school teachers holding a certificate from the Sorbonne and with unpaid nuns who taught in richly endowed convent schools. With the exception of a few wealthy provincial schools, the lay boarding schools found themselves pushed to the wall in competition with the convent schools. Daubié describes with some emotion the head teachers who found themselves forced to turn their high-minded teaching position into a money-making proposition in order to eke out a living.

The new laws, urged by the Catholic Church, which had reasons for wanting to retain control of the education of girls and women, produced increasingly severe effects in 1854, the year when Royer returned from Britain. The result was that all secondary-school teachers who held these certificates found themselves, like Royer, economically and perhaps emotionally betrayed by their church in a very real sense.

It is in the context of the role played by the church that Royer speaks of being "abused"—rather than, for example, in reference to any specific physical incident. This makes the question of rape more complex. She may have undergone a sexual ordeal at about the age of nineteen or twenty at the period when the final loss of her father's protection left her exposed to the attentions of some unscrupulous relative or acquaintance. However, the accusation of "abuse" Royer levels against her church has a different foundation in fact, referring back five or ten years to her depressions and traumas concerning sin as an early adolescent. Her age at that time was almost exactly that of the rape victim Mary Sullivan in Haverfordwest, bringing the story line behind this chapter almost full circle. Clémence Royer, like Mary Sullivan, reacted much more vehemently to the spiritual maltreatment than to any physical maltreatment she may have suffered. In the end, of course, these two elements cannot be disentangled, and it is significant that Royer uses a word as strong as "abuse" in speaking of the role of the church in her development. She suggests a kind of rape of the mind, a betrayal of emotional trust, and of trust in the concept of truth, for which the church seeks to claim a monopoly. Royer appears to have felt betrayed most acutely in the realm of education. She realized these issues clearly during the period of 1854 to 1856, when she inserted in her autobiography a paragraph explaining her reaction: "In recognizing the falsity of the education she had been given, she was seized with an ardent rancor against the teachers who had betrayed her childhood and failed to shake her reason. She thought that her sad experience would serve to enlighten humanity and deliver it from the errors in which she had been maintained and the lies with which she had been abused."[61] The interwoven themes of this chapter provide a partial explanation of the absoluteness and suddenness of her abandonment of her teaching career in the light of the newly enforced grip of the church on the secondary-education process in France.

Whatever the source of Royer's sense of betrayal, whether physical humiliation, a threat to her future livelihood, or simply a religious and emotional crisis, Royer now acted like a woman with a mission to accomplish. Like Jeanne d'Arc, she set off alone, breaking all her ties to family and friends. In June 1856 she "burned her bridges behind her so that she could not return."[62] She left most of her clothing as well, taking with her the proceeds from the small inheritance from her father. She had sold the property he left her and realized about Fr 7,000. Like her father almost exactly twenty years before, she traveled through Lyon to Lausanne, to her first remembered childhood home. Her first biographer adds that when she passed through Lyon, she was so impressed by the misery of the people she encountered who had just been made homeless by a disastrous flood, that she gave part of her little patrimony away to the poor.[63] Royer's own account is less romantic. She states simply that she calculated she had enough to live on for a few years if she lived simply.[64] She was gripped by the desire to understand the fundamental core of her discarded religion and the new science that she had only sampled; what she would gain from her experiences in Lausanne would more than repay her.

Chapter 3

Mind and Love Awaken: Royer in Switzerland

Clémence Royer arrived in Lausanne in June 1856, bringing nothing except what she was wearing and her small inheritance. This pretty city, built on a steep hill overlooking Lake Léman and the mountains, had been celebrated in the literature of the past century. Rousseau had described his lovers embracing along the lake's shores, Byron and Shelley were inspired to write and live near the lake in the 1820s. "Mon Repos," where Voltaire's theatrical pieces had been performed, stood a little way outside the city center. Gibbon had written *The Decline and Fall of the Roman Empire* in the city; the great French critics Benjamin Constant and Charles Augustin Sainte-Beuve had more recently sung its praises.[1]

The walk from the railroad station into the center of town must have been a difficult one for a nineteenth-century woman dressed in long skirts. The street wound at a steep incline past stores and hotels to the top. Yet the walk was worth the effort, since the view from the medieval Romanesque cathedral, which stood in the center of the old city, was a breathtaking one. Victor Hugo had celebrated the city as "coiffed with the cathedral like a tiara. . . . I was on the esplanade of the church before the portal. As though at the head of the city . . . I saw the lake above the roofs, the mountains above the lake, the clouds above the mountains, and the stars above the clouds. A staircase on which my thoughts ascend step by step, expanding at each level."[2]

At first Royer stayed at a small hotel not far from the railroad station and tried to earn a living from ornamental needlework. Shortly after she arrived, Royer calculated that if she lived simply enough she could support herself for at least two years on her inheritance. Since she had brought few clothes with her, she determined to dress like a peasant, adopting the distinctive straw hat and attractive dress of the Lausanne peasant girl. She established herself in a little room in the home of Vaudoise peasants in a chalet called Praz-Perey in Cully, near the Savoy Mountains, about ten kilometers from Lausanne. The room's furniture consisted of no more than a bed, a chair, a table, and in the winter a stove, but the room cost her only Fr 20 a month. Everything else she owned could fit into a small suitcase.[3]

Isolated in her mountain retreat, at first she must have felt like her hero Matteo. She would soon describe his thoughts in her novel: "I am going, but what do I leave behind? Everywhere I am a stranger. My house is that of the voyager who pays every morning for the evening's hospitality. My inheritance is credit with the banker. I have on this earth no furrow that I could labor upon and say, 'This is mine.' "[4] She turned instead to the world of the intellect, where she always felt at home.

One of the delights of Lausanne was its public library. It was a two-hour walk each way to Lausanne, but fortunately the lending library would send her as many books as she wished by post. When the weather was fine, she returned the books herself, even through the snow. She worked first on biblical criticism and then on scientific texts, formulating the ideas upon which she would eventually lecture.

From her window, she looked out upon the Alps bordering Lake Léman, still the only landscape that visually impressed her. While she read or wrote, she watched the mountains change color every hour. This sense of beauty seemed to become combined with the new philosophy she was developing. She was convinced, as she later said, "that truth existed and that it was accessible to man" (or rather, in this case, to woman). She would argue in later analyses of the sense of beauty that truth was built into the "molecular constitution of the universe" much in the way that she thought music and geometry harmonized with the nervous system.[5]

She began by studying German texts on the origins of Christianity but, with her habitual self-confidence, she soon decided that her own logic extended beyond those writers. She then considered a variety of philosophical systems, but, she later insisted, she found faults in each. She disliked Kant almost from the beginning and rejected the utopian social systems of Fourier and Saint-Simon as impractical.[6] Wanting to find a more "positive" truth, one she could believe in, she began to read scientific texts, beginning with the eighteenth-century writers who had so fired her imagination. Possibly annoyed by the adulation of Rousseau in Lausanne, where people came to follow the footsteps of the lovers in *La Nouvelle Héloïse,* she strongly objected to Rousseau's patronizing attitude towards women. She suggested more than once that one should chose as a guide not Rousseau but Diderot and Voltaire.

As she began to read about science, she made it a rule to neglect technical details that would "clutter up her mind" and "which today encumber the intelligence of our university students." She was looking for a doctrine she could live by, she said, not trying to qualify herself as a professional. Retrospectively she described her intellectual progress through science in this manner, speaking of herself in the third person:

> First completing her work on physics [she had heard Becquerel's public lectures in Paris and had written a discussion of atomic theory], she then ran through the very incomplete laws of chemistry, the great truths acquired by astronomy, the hypotheses of the physical structure of the globe, the great facts of geology and paleontology, illuminated by the science of currently living organisms and by general laws of biology. Finally she passed to the history of humanity. The history of primitive peoples especially attracted her attention: the great problem was to explain the passage from animal to man, whose appearance on earth prehistoric anthropology had pushed back to a period before our geological epoch.[7]

Is this an accurate description of her intellectual progress? Some evidence exists from the list of books she took out of the Lausanne library, as compiled by her first biographer, Albert Milice, in the 1920s from the library records. Of course this list does not include books she read sitting in the library, as she began to do in 1857. She proceeded to speculate upon the atomic nature of the universe. Later she described these first ideas as having come to her in Switzerland, "when I lived all alone in a peasant chalet with my books, facing nature."[8] In 1858, she tried to develop an atomic theory in a memoir on Maine de Biran with the intention of submitting it for a scientific prize competition.[9] A few years later, she considered a theory of fluid and expansible atoms; she hesitated upon being told that her interpretation violated Newtonian physics. She returned to the problem of matter again in 1869 in her book on the evolution of human society, and between 1880 and 1900 she revived her early interest in physics and chemistry, expanding upon her earlier ideas.[10]

In her almost monastic retreat she began to consider issues of time and space and mathematical abstractions as they could be applied to the natural world around her. She incorporated some of these observations into her "Album of a Traveler," the scientific part of her novel.[11] "A brook runs along the plain; what gracious meandering designs. I approach and follow it. These turnings are angular with bends along dry, unequal, abrupt banks. I approach more closely. No, I was mistaken, these lines are formed from multiple sinuosities, the angles are gentled into curves, and these granules trace spheres. An infinite variety of directions links these thousands of fractuosities."[12]

The insight that coastlines are composed of many broken "fractuosities," as she called these segments, almost anticipates the recent mathematical "fractals" of Benoit Mandelbrot. "Let us look through my magnifying glass. These curves are formed by right angles; each molecule has its angles and its faces—and can I ever get to the end of this? Who will succeed in knowing the form of the atom or the generative line of being?"[13] Clémence Royer was one of the exceptional women in the nineteenth century who enjoyed the intellectual pleasure to be found in mathematical games and concepts. In her novel, she invoked mathematical forms as though she were invoking deities:

> Cold and regular figures of geometry, are you the innate revelation of laws that rule worlds and serve to limit the elementary dust particles that compose them? Are you the amplification of the real, the birth of the human spirit, which is incapable of conceiving the infinite variety of designs of the great architect? Or are you on the contrary idealized forms, symmetry, regularity, absolute beauty, the model that nature realizes only imperfectly? Are you in the end only, as others have said, a form of thought, a condition of the perception of things, without reality in the things themselves, a phenomenon, an appearance?[14]

She invoked time and space in the same manner:

> You, the laws of time and space, are sovereign and regulating. Nothing escapes your universal empire. You alone are truly inviolable laws. You regulate man, who knows you as well as the nonliving molecule, which knows you not. The world machine, in order to function in its movements, its attractions, its forces, through the immense extent of time without end, does not in the least wait for Laplace to measure it or Newton to weigh it or Galileo to see it through his telescope glass.[15]

Although it may be an apocryphal story that Margaret Fuller ever declaimed, "I accept the universe," Clémence Royer came close to saying precisely this in her meditation on the fact that one can escape space but not time. "The law of time and succession, a law of grandeur, a relation of container to contained, rules my thought as well as matter and dominates my liberty. I submit to it, I accept it, and, as the law of my being, I adore it."[16] With a sensitive awareness of the psychological impact of mood on perception, she describes a sequence of changes she observed as she looked at nature in the course of a steep climb up the side of a mountain. She explored her psychological changes, describing the feeling of desolation as she gasped for breath on the way up and her awareness of dying plants and animals around her. After reaching the summit of the mountain, a feeling of exaltation transformed the same path on the way down, when all nature seemed beautiful and in harmony.[17]

Working alone and in isolation for those first two years, she was aware of the problems of solitude. She must have experienced a sense of being bottled up without anyone with whom to discuss her ideas. In her novel she explains the consequences of isolated contemplation. Human beings need to share their ideas and their "interior emotions." As she explains in a passage that discusses her invocation of abstract ideas:

> Thought needs to translate itself into a language, otherwise, vague and floating, it hampers and fatigues the brain that holds it captive. A man

> [*sic*] feels pressed to say what he feels, what he proves. In this way, he shares with other men his interior emotions, his gentle or painful sensations. Lacking human beings, he invokes objects, or he speaks to himself and has a conversation with his own intelligence, interrogating it and responding to it in turn.[18]

Perhaps recalling her own periods of mysticism, she describes the effect of damming up this running stream of thought that "cannot accumulate in the reservoir of memory without losing its clarity. It condenses and sometimes is corrupted; its elements disintegrate and become impure and unhealthy."[19] The "resulting fermentation" produces increasingly vivid, but less real, images. If nothing serves to release these "retained images," they eventually escape "with more violence the longer they are retained." This explosion of ideas she saw as the source of powerful, but false, ideas. "Isn't that the secret of the force of those unhappy geniuses who are enlarged and deformed by the obstacles that they ought to have conquered, who have given such a powerful form to somewhat false ideas?"[20]

Seeking communication with family and friends, Royer sent word to her mother to let her know she had gone to Lausanne. Her mother and her family friends, looking for a reasonable explanation for the young woman's sudden abandonment of her former life, thought she must have suffered some mental disturbance; perhaps she had gone mad. Through diplomatic channels, the local police were contacted. As she recorded the event, "One day she saw the district policeman [préfet] of Cully approach the chalet with the intent of finding out some information about her mental state. She received him herself, and soon, conquered by her answers, astonished by her knowledge and her mind, he recognized that her mental state left nothing to be desired and said that few people had a mind like it."[21] The local police may have been satisfied as to her sanity but, nevertheless, they also noted her eccentric clothing and life style, as a Paris police dossier disclosed many years later.[22]

Clémence Royer was fortunate in the city she had selected as a base for her self-education. Most importantly, Switzerland had a history of encouraging intellectual women. Madame de Staël, the author of *Corinne,* which had so moved Clémence, had grown up just across the lake. Twenty years before, when the critic and novelist Sainte-Beuve taught at the Académie de Lausanne, another brilliant woman, Marie Forel, and her friends had formed an admiring circle around him. This female audience was responsible for Sainte-Beuve's great success in Lausanne. He, like Royer, had been moved by both the scenery and the literary history of the area and had written a poem that celebrated "the secret joy of the lake seen from the garden, the great flaming mountains of Savoy crouched facing it."[23]

One of the women who came to hear Sainte-Beuve, Caroline Olivier, put him in touch with the future theologian Charles Secretan, then a young poet, who exchanged verses with him. Olivier, Marie Forel, and other members of the circle of women who had attended Sainte-Beuve's lectures on the literary history of Port-Royal presented him with a watch and their heartfelt thanks.[24] Marie Forel may have been inspired by Sainte-Beuve's long critical essay on Alexandre Vinet, for she continued the task of editing the works of Vinet with Sainte-Beuve's friend Secretan, celebrating the Swiss Protestant theologian and literary critic, who had written on Pascal and on French seventeenth-century literature.[25] Madame Forel, actively wrestling with difficult editorial problems, was to prove to be an important link between Royer and the intellectual circles of Lausanne. Equally importantly, the Forel family had close links to scientific as well as literary groups, and a nephew later became a devoted follower of Darwin.[26]

Royer continued to be isolated after she moved down from the mountains to Lausanne and relocated close to the public library and the Académie de Lausanne.[27] In 1858, during her second winter, she began to work daily at the library, still dressed in her distinctive clothing, where some individuals became curious about her newly adopted Indian dress and her peasant hat.[28] When a large public lecture was given by the Swedish novelist Frederika Bremer, who had traveled to the United States five years before, Royer was in the audience. Bremer spoke not only of her own work but of those women's issues that had begun to interest her. She emphasized the important role of women in the United States, and commented at length about the significant position of women lecturers there.[29]

Bremer's book on her trip to the United States, published in 1853, describes both men and women she encountered. The impact of individuals like Dorothea Dix, Julia Howe, and the still green memory of Margaret Fuller remained with her. A recent commentator has observed that, although Bremer felt respect for "masculine ambition" and masculine knowledge and advocated improved access to formal education for women, "she never lost that which may be called the 'difference of view'—a feminine heritage and a feminine perspective."[30]

Royer, seizing the opportunity presented by a heightened interest in lectures developed and presented by women, proposed her own course of lectures in 1858. She first suggested a series of four lessons on logic for women; she excluded men, partly because Lausanne was a University town and she did not want to be heckled by students.[31] The lectures were very successful and may have put her in touch with Marie Forel, who shared Royer's enthusiasm for biblical criticism and French literature.

Not only did Royer have access to a fine public library in Lausanne, but she was in a city noted for its publishing and printing houses and with an excellent academy that, although it emphasized training for the Protestant ministry, opened its large public lectures to women. The Académie de Lausanne (later the university) provided teaching opportunities to some of the exiled

French freethinkers and republicans whom Royer was soon to know intimately.

The leading member of this group was a former deputy of the Second Republic, Pascal Duprat. He taught political science at the Académie de Lausanne and edited two journals. The first was a literary journal, published in Brussels, which published a wide variety of noted writers of the day. A second journal edited by Duprat, *Le Nouvel Économiste,* was published in Lausanne, emphasizing social science and economics.[32]

Whether Royer first met Duprat through the intellectual circle around Marie Forel, or whether Duprat first noticed her at the library in her peasant dress and spoke kindly to her, or whether she met him at a public lecture at the Lausanne academy is not noted. She knew that he was the publisher of an important local journal and soon gained enough courage to go to his home and ask him to advertise and promote a second, longer course of lectures, on "The Philosophy of Nature." She planned to hold the second lecture course, like the first, exclusively for women. Eventually, she later explained, her Lamarckian and anticlerical explanations for natural origins frightened off the women at the same time that they attracted more male auditors.[33]

In 1858, Duprat lived in a beautiful home by Lake Léman. Here Clémence Royer met for the first and only time Duprat's wife, who, understandably, became her lifelong enemy. Royer described this woman as a "constant whirlwind."[34] She was, Royer noted, very pretty, but much pleasanter to men than to women, almost seductive in her manner. The wife may have seen in this intense young woman a possible rival, or perhaps she did not take her seriously. In any case she seems to have treated Royer quite rudely. Perhaps the wife spoke sharply to Duprat as well, since it was immediately obvious to Royer that theirs was an unhappy marriage, "an ill-assorted nest," as she described it later. One imagines Duprat surprised and then pleased to have this intense young woman whom he had met only briefly come to talk to him. He not only agreed to advertise her lectures, but printed the introduction to her course both in his journal and as a separate pamphlet.

Undoubtedly she was impressed by this man who was to be the one love of her life, the father of her son, and her constant companion from 1865 until his death twenty years later. Did they become lovers soon after their meeting? One biographer, who speaks with authority about Duprat, has made the flat statement that she became Duprat's mistress in 1859, which would have been within a year of their first meeting.[35] Royer herself implied to a close friend that they delayed a total sexual involvement until they agreed to live together permanently.[36]

Pascal Duprat, now nearly forgotten as one of the figures of the Second and Third Republics, deserves more than a cursory mention. He was born in Hagetmau in the department of Landes on 24 March 1815. Raised in the Pyrenees, it is not surprising that he oriented himself towards the south, to Spain and to the northern coast of Algeria. Like many young people in that area he spoke Spanish. First, however, he went to Germany to study in Heidelberg, where he obtained his degrees. He then went to teach history in the new French colony of Algeria, where he wrote a book on the history of ancient and modern African coastal races in 1845.[37] Soon after he returned to Paris, joining the group around William Edwards debating racial theories in the Société Ethnologique, and began to work as a journalist. Taking his book on Algeria in hand, he went to meet the great scientist François Arago, who also had ties to the region of the French Pyrenees. As director of the Paris Observatory, Arago was head of an intellectual center to which provincial young men of talent were welcomed.[38] According to Royer, several figures who would become important in the politics of 1848, including Duprat, were regular visitors to Arago's home. His younger brother, Étienne Arago, close in age to Duprat, was to become Duprat's close associate in the Constituent Assembly during the Second Republic.[39]

Duprat also was a regular habitué of the republican and Saint-Simonist circle surrounding Pierre Leroux and George Sand, which included the idiosyncratic theologian and poet Abbé Félicité Lamennais, the abolitionist Victor Schloecher, and Marie d'Agoult, who, like her friend George Sand, published novels under a man's name, writing as Daniel Stern. Here Duprat also encountered the brilliant Italian historian Giuseppe Ferrari, whose articles he later published and whom he would meet again in Italy.[40] Duprat collaborated on a number of journals, such as *La Reforme, Le Droit,* and Leroux's journal, the *Revue Indépendante.* He founded, with Lamennais, who had become an ardent republican, *Le Peuple Constituant,* a journal that celebrated the beginning of the Second Republic.

Duprat was elected as a deputy from Landes to the Constituent Assembly, where he worked in close association with François and Étienne Arago and Lamennais. Although not a major member of this circle, he was nevertheless a significant one. Duprat deplored the closing of the workers' ateliers, which led to riots throughout Paris, but he supported the moderates against the socialists. He endorsed General Cavaignac's repressive actions against the socialist uprising both in the assembly and in his journal. He had the unfortunate "honor" of proposing the 1849 law declaring a state of siege against social unrest, which was used with such bloody effectiveness by the general. The same law would be used again with disastrous results to shoot and exile many men and women during the Paris Commune some twenty years later.

Reelected to the Legislative Assembly and linked by some with the socialist Ledru Rollin, he was later commended for "opposing the Mountain" (the extreme Left). Yet by the end of July 1848 his journal, *Le Peuple Constituant,* was suppressed by the Cavaignac government in spite of its moderate tone. He vehemently opposed the subsequent events that led to Louis Napoleon's coup d'état. Not surprisingly, he was proscribed under Louis Napoleon's presidency and by the empire that grew out of it and was thrown into jail; after he was released, he went first to England, and then to Belgium. In Liège, in 1852, he published an indictment of Louis Napoleon and his government, *Les Tables de proscription de Louis Bonaparte et ses complices.* He followed this with an analysis of the function of the state in modern society.[41] The same year he married his mistress, who had given birth to a daughter, "having nothing but his name to offer her," according to Royer. His new wife remained in Paris at the home of the aunt who had raised her, while Duprat in exile "most often dined on the proceeds from a book he was able to sell during the day." Once again, he started a journal in Brussels, *La Libre Recherche,* which gained some success as a literary and political journal.[42] Upon the collapse of this journal, he went to Switzerland to teach at the Académie de Lausanne where he edited two other journals, *La Revue Philosophique et Littéraire* (1856) and an economics journal, *Le Nouvel Economiste* (1856).[43] Duprat's wife and child joined him in Lausanne not long before Royer arrived.

It was at this point in his life, when Duprat was juggling two journals and teaching in Lausanne, that Royer first met him. He was forty-four, almost exactly fifteen years older than Royer. He was unusually tall, while she was very small. All his life he wore his black hair full and long, flowing to his shoulders in the style of the 1840s, and sported a long, drooping moustache. She was struck by his sparkling and incisive mind, with its touch of irony. He had a marvelous memory and a gift for languages. (He knew Arabic, Spanish, and German and easily picked up Italian.) An eloquent speaker, he was "captivating," as she put it, "even more in intimate conversation" than when addressing a large group.[44] She suggested in the preface to her first edition of Darwin, three years after meeting Duprat, that mammalian females are "attracted by the strongest voices or charmed by those singers least fatigued during the reproductive phase."[45] Duprat's "songs" were of the 1848 revolution, which had so inspired her ten years before, and the intellectual and literary world of France and Europe, with which he was closely connected. He made a profound impression on her. At about the same time, the writer Marie d'Agoult wrote to her friends from Paris, recommending Duprat's literary journal and praising Duprat's southern effervescence, the liveliness of his mind, and the courage with which he endured both adversity and poverty in exile.[46]

For Royer, the opportunity to open her mind and heart to Pascal Duprat apparently relieved the growing intellectual and emotional pressure she had felt working in isolation. In her novel, she contrasted unhappy, bottled-up geniuses with a description that might well be of Duprat. "Those thinkers, light in spirit perhaps because they have been happier, those open minds that one sees float over all problems as if they flowed from the tip of a wing perhaps owe their harmonious equilibrium to friendly circumstances that permit them to open the treasure of their thought with tranquil facility to everyone, everywhere."[47] She contrasted the energetic, overreaching mind with this happier, patient thinker. "The first are often swept away by great faults and by irreparable heartbreak. People who meet them only see one face of the statue half veiled like ancient Isis. The second, less eloquent because they are less convinced, are less creative but more critical, less absolute but often truer; they are more prudent guides and more surely illuminate. Following them, one marches, although with small steps, following the others, one leaps and falls."[48] The description of an open and harmonious mind also seems an accurate description of Duprat's literary style, which was light and conversational.

Royer was inspired by Duprat not only to lecture and to read but to write, with the immediate reward of publication. At that first meeting he suggested she write a novel, promising her publication in his Brussels literary journal.[49] For this last suggestion, he may have been influenced by materials from her notebooks. The section of her novel entitled "Album of a Traveler," from which I have quoted extensively, shows every sign of being just such a notebook, full of fascinating insights into psychology and the responses of a young mind first encountering science. Impressed by Duprat's interest, she reacted to his suggestion like a command. She began work immediately. "I promised to bring it to him in three months, during which I did not see him again. But three months later I brought it to him. I had worked fourteen hours a day to keep my word."[50] When she returned with the novel, he took it without explaining to her that his literary journal was bankrupt. It would be published only five years later, following heavy revisions.

The fact that we have only the second version means that we cannot know which parts she added after her relationship with Duprat became established. Her friends also may have wondered. Ghénia Avril de Sainte Croix, to whom she wrote the only detailed description of her lifelong love affair with Duprat, apparently suggested that strong statements in her novel about the primacy of love over legal marriage may have stirred Duprat's love. She denied it, adding that he never read it until it was published, since he had handed it back to her three years later in the same unopened folder in which she had given it to him. She added that she had heavily re-written before it was published, since the following year (1859) Garibaldi completely overturned Naples, the "theater for my drama."[51]

Royer did not offer a clue to either her friend or to her readers as to which material dated from 1858 and which from 1864. She denied any influence of Duprat on the novel, a claim that could only be true of the first version. It is possible to guess at the development of her thought by unraveling different threads within the novel.

Some influences of George Sand's belief in the supremacy of love over social formalities can be found in her novel. In a chapter entitled "Héloïse and Abélard" a touching scene occurs between two lovers. Count Orlowski, a

Polish revolutionary in exile, has been tutoring Joanna, the young daughter of the archduke of Austria. Having fallen in love with the count, she refuses to marry the king of Naples, whom her father has chosen as her husband. She is placed in an isolated cell by her father, who hopes she will change her mind. Here her lover manages to meet her. As each makes a vow of eternal love to the other, Orlowski says to the heroine, "This is the marriage of our souls, of our lives, of our wills. What links a heart is not at all vain human formalities, it is a vow, a promise, the given word: it is more yet, the first caress of love on the face and on the lips of a beloved . . . Swear to me to be my companion, my wife, let my lips print on yours the sacred seal of hymen." He then swears by the eternal heavens to be faithful to her until death or until she releases him from his vow. She makes the same vow, "invoking nature and its creative and conserving powers," and they embrace as a ray of light enters the window and illuminates them. The young man breaks off the embrace "with an effort whose energy I admired, wrenching himself from my arms that had entwined around him in spite of myself. 'Enough, enough,' said he, pale and trembling. 'I would have succumbed, and the time has not come when you could be a mother before men.' " Vowing his love, he escapes, pushing her away as she cries out, "You are leaving me," in some dismay. The woman, describing this scene many years later to her daughter, adds, "It seemed to me that we had become a single being who could not be separated into two parts without lacerations."[52]

Although these are not unfamiliar scenes for a Romantic novel, the details Royer added are suggestive. The "monastic cell" in which it occurs matches the description she had given of her small room in Cully. The two characters renounce their positions and run away to live near Lake Léman in happiness and unity, underscoring the likelihood that this represents Royer's view of the crucial love scene between herself and Duprat near that same lake.

At the end of her life, Royer admitted that one of the major flaws of the novel was that she had written it twice. Although she may not have realized it, the real flaw lies in her failure to integrate its conflicting stories and styles, as discussed in chapter 2. The final version was a thousand pages; one assumes the first version was about half that length. It is worth noting that the eventual publisher in 1864 was the prestigious firm of Lecroix and Verboeckhoven in Brussels, which had published Victor Hugo's *Les Misérables* only two years before her novel appeared.[53]

Whatever Duprat thought of her novel, he was amazed at her energy. He asked for her assistance on his journal. She began to write unsigned reviews and to collaborate without pay on his surviving journal *Le Nouvel Économiste.* Soon after their second meeting, he moved with his family to the shore of Lake Neuchâtel, returning to Lausanne only twice a month to put out his journal. When she began her series of lectures for women on natural philosophy in the winter of 1859–1860, Duprat's Lausanne publisher in 1859 printed Royer's first signed piece, her "Introduction to the Philosophy of Women," which had been the opening lecture of her second course on philosophy.[54]

This lecture for women is the only existing example of the early writing of Clémence Royer on science, if we exclude the "Album of a Traveler." It dramatically illustrates the remarkable response of a woman encountering scientific ideas for the first time. While it stresses the importance of science for women, it also recounts the sense of liberation that both science and philosophy had brought to her. Her first impulse was to share that sense of liberation with an audience of women.

She began by insisting that woman should not imitate men, since "we have, as women, our own particular genius and we should guard it with care."[55] Servile imitation of men by women was to be avoided in science as well as in art and literature. "It isn't a new science that I must find. Science is at its core as much a unity as the truth it seeks; it will not differ within itself. What I must find is a form, a feminine expression of science. This is a new art that I have to create." Women had to make science the underpinning for their lives rather than adopt the contradictory ideas of men. "That supremacy of reason that they [men] presume over us is more affirmed than proved." In response to Proudhon, who had attacked the right of women to function as independent intellects, she suggested that "the freedom of thought that men claim for themselves they have dared to contest for us."[56]

Royer felt that it was important not to confound scientific means with the aims of science. She began by asking why philosophy should have been the exclusive domain of men. "Why should women be forbidden to know science, truth, wisdom, or goodness? And how can one love what one is prevented from knowing?"[57] Philosophy had once meant both science and wisdom and had become divided into theoretical and practical science, which she hoped to reunite.

She described truth as a marble statue, depicted by the Greeks as "austere and correct" without the seductive aspects of poetry. "Finally, let us use the word, science has remained imprinted with a virile character. . . . If I could be the Pygmalion to that statue, if I could make it speak and speak a language intelligible to all . . . That is what I shall attempt to the limit of my ability."[58]

Burdened with Greek and Latin terms, science appeared as something frightening to women, who were not educated in ancient languages. The terminology had acted on women like "scarecrows set in the field to frighten the birds." She spoke from personal experience, describing her first reaction to scientific language: "I, myself, was for a time greatly afraid of science. I found it to have a tedious and boring appearance about which I have already spoken to you. Given this impression, I persuaded myself that it was useless to me." But after some helpful explanations "the night of my mind" was illuminated. The scientists had "surrounded the field of science with a thorny hedge, but beyond it was full of flowers."[59]

Her description continued as though she were describing the prince in the fairy tale "Sleeping Beauty." "From that moment I resolved to break through the enclosure or to jump over it, if possible. I have entered that field, and I have gathered a bouquet of flowers. This bouquet I am offering to you." Royer invited her audience to discover the new knowledge. "For you, mesdames, what have you to fear from phantoms? Approach, touch, they won't bite you."[60]

In a phrase that hints unconsciously at the seductive qualities she attributed to this new mode of thinking, she added: "It is greatly to be desired that women give themselves to science, that they give themselves with pleasure, with taste, with love, finally with philosophy. The difference in the language of ideas and opinions between the two sexes renders them in some way strangers to each other, divides them, disunites them not only in society but even in the family, to the point that they will not meet each other any more except like, if one may say so, some kind of herd animal in the stable."[61]

The different education of men and women had resulted in men's education for the head, women's for the heart; the result was a caricature in which both sexes lost. Science was needed within the family in order that women pass the knowledge on to their children. "I'll say more. As long as science remains so exclusively in men's hands, it will never descend into the depths of the family and society. It will remain on the surface, like an ice crust below which water remains at an invariable temperature. . . . If, on the contrary, women seize control of science, they will soon radiate it out around them with that sympathetic expansion that so essentially distinguishes their nature."[62]

In an age in which so many of the women served science as popularizers this would not have been a foreign sentiment. One wonders if Clémence Royer had encountered in her teaching in Britain some of the charming series of books for children on science such as the late-eighteenth-century works of Priscilla Wakefield. A more recent example of a woman popularizer, who had lived in Geneva, was the Englishwoman Jane Haldimand Marcet, whose popular books included *Conversations on Chemistry, Conversations on Natural Philosophy,* and a more recent book, *Willy's Railroads,* which were all published anonymously. She had been in close contact with many of the literary and scientific families in Geneva, including the botanists De Candolle, both father and son, and the Pictet family. Madame Marcet had divided her life between London and Geneva; she had died in Geneva, at the advanced age of ninety, a few years after Royer arrived in Switzerland and the very year that Royer published her first lecture.[63]

Royer expressed surprise that the men of her day should evidence so much "fatigue, ennui, moral doubt." She did not explain in her lecture that she herself had just passed through a period of religious doubt. Perhaps in reaction to her previous unhappiness, she depicted a feminist science and philosophy as "affirmative and above all practical"; it would "keep among us a special character, a feminine character. . . . We are better made for action than thinking about it; doubt kills us; we have an ardent impatience to affirm, to conclude, to attain the serenity of certainty."[64]

It was easier, she explained, to give her listeners an overview of science in some hours of lectures than to explain any one science in detail, for the detailed knowledge of any one science could take a lifetime. On the other hand, she criticized scientific specialization, which she saw as an error that she would continue to denounce throughout her life. Scientists, such as chemists and physicists in their minute analyses, were like someone examining "all the atoms of sand in a pyramid" and explained all phenomena in terms of their own speciality. German scientists were especially guilty of this, they had also made the additional error of splitting science into two parts: theoretical and practical. Adopting a vivid kitchen metaphor, she termed this "deboning the world," dividing it into "living palpitating flesh" on one side and exposed skeletons on the other.[65] Both aspects of thought were part of a living whole; neither could survive unless they remained united. This holistic approach to problems prefigures her later monism. She praised the mathematical basis of science, which she thought had put philosophy on a secure base. A feminist philosophy needed to "gather together all the evidence that science possesses."

Royer's course, open only to women, continued from 1859 to 1860. Soon she would be lecturing to a wider audience. By 1860, Duprat had moved again, this time to Geneva, presumably because his wife wanted her daughter to have a proper First Communion in the large city. His journal moved with him, and he began to rely on other assistants. Nevertheless, Royer's work on the journal continued, in spite of her later claims to the contrary.[66] Her extensive reading continued, now as part of her preparation for her articles for the *Nouvel Économiste.* In late 1860 and early 1861, she worked for a while in Geneva, making a name for herself as a thoughtful reviewer. Requiring ready access to books, Royer wrote to the Bibliothèque Publique et Universitaire in Geneva, objecting to their policy of restricting borrowers to a single book at a time. She asked for four or more at a time, if possible. She had to review all the available books on Eastern antiquity and needed to scan a great many books quickly rather than read any one book in detail.[67]

At the end of 1860, Duprat left Switzerland, this time without his family, fleeing to Italy where he hoped to make some money as well as to escape his wife's debts and, possibly, his own unwise railroad speculations.[68] He still met Royer, however, on his trips through Switzerland every summer; she had established a pattern of lecturing outside Switzerland in the fall, returning to Lausanne in the summer. In the spring of 1861, Royer returned to Paris for the first time since her departure, giving a lecture before a "small nucleus of those opposed to the Empire."[69] One of those who attended, at the urging of her friends, was Marie d'Agoult, a brilliant and delightful aristocratic woman who had dedicated herself to republican ideals since 1848 and who held the only republican salon in Paris. She noted in her journal in June 1861 that she had been invited to attend a lecture by a "demoiselle Augusta Royer" from Lausanne, who, "without being pretty, had a striking appearance, was very resolute and erudite." D'Agoult noted also that the literary critic Ronchard had termed her a mathematician and that Royer had been recommended by Duprat to one of his scientific friends to explain a mathematical discovery.[70]

The Countess Marie d'Agoult (born Marie de Flavigny) had been the lover of the great pianist and composer Liszt, with whom she had two children. She was also an old friend and associate of George Sand and a novelist in her own right, publishing under the pseudonym of Daniel Stern. Marie d'Agoult had left her husband, her firstborn daughter, and a glittering aristocratic life for life as a famous musician's mistress. Her economic independence gave her a social freedom that Royer never knew. After she and Liszt separated, she returned to Paris and faced down a disapproving society, creating her own environment among the freethinking republican intellectuals, journalists, and politicians of the Second Republic. Under the Empire, her salon served as a focus for those republicans who had escaped proscription.[71]

Both because of d'Agoult's life and her political beliefs, she sympathized with Royer's dilemma. Her own memoirs illustrate in a dramatic manner the same concerns of a young woman finding her way intellectually through literature and politics, after briefly toying with the church as a possibility while attending a convent school (the great aristocratic convent school of Paris, Sacré-Coeur). She, like Royer, had passed through the same intellectual process from mystical believer to anticleric, from royalist to republican. As an adolescent, d'Agoult had been a favorite of the Bourbon dauphine. After her marriage to Comte d'Agoult, she continued for some time to entertain friends who, like Royer's father, were anxious to see the July monarchy of Louis-Phillipe overthrown. Like the Royers, both father and daughter, her ideas of honor were based on a personal commitment to truth rather than to social norms.

D'Agoult would have sympathized as well with Royer's decision to cut all bonds and live publicly with a man she loved and with whom she was allied, although in d'Agoult's case public hostility was cushioned by wealth, social position, and a previous marriage. Marie d'Agoult had been a friend of Abbé Lamennais, with whom Duprat had published his newspaper in the days of the Second Republic. She had known Pascal Duprat from the period of the 1848 revolution and had read some of her essays on republicanism to him. She later published in, and her novels were reviewed by, his Brussels journals.[72]

Royer corresponded with Marie d'Agoult from their first meeting in 1861, writing long and intense letters about her experiences and detailing social and philosophical ideas she was in the process of developing. By the end of May 1862, she sent to her the articles she had written for the *Journal des Économistes,* which Marie d'Agoult found "full of ideas."[73] Royer's production of intellectual work over the next few years was quite incredible. The stimulus may have been not only the passion for her work, but her newly awakened sexuality. Her almost epigrammatic remark reflects this: "Without passion, there is no action, without action, no thought."[74] The unleashing of her emotions had sparked her intellectual life as well, and she recognized that fact.

When the canton of Vaud, of which Lausanne is the capital, established a prize for a reconsideration of the income tax, the Academy of Lausanne, in 1860, set up a conference on this topic with the support of Duprat and his journal. They brought together major French-speaking notables interested in economics and political science. Among them were Joseph Garnier, editor in chief of the *Journal des Économistes.* The publisher of that important liberal journal was Gilbert-Urbain Guillaumin, who also attended the conference. His publishing firm was to play a significant part in Royer's life by producing and advertising her first two books, her prize-winning book on taxation, and her translation of Charles Darwin's *Origin of Species.*[75]

Royer attended the economics conference, reviewing it for Duprat's journal. She was one of the women noticed by Joseph Garnier in his own extensive review of this conference for the *Journal des Économistes.* Garnier reported at length on Duprat's role as organizer of this conference, giving a brief résumé of his life as a man dedicated to economics and political economy. Royer was introduced to Garnier by Duprat as "Madame Royer," and Garnier expressed his admiration of her excellent journalistic pieces. The following month Garnier praised the ability of women to work sucessfully in the field of economics, giving Royer as the most recent example of intelligent women publishing in this field and describing her as "one of the principal collaborators of the *Nouvel Économiste,* which M. Pascal Duprat publishes in Geneva, whose fine appreciations and just criticisms are remarkable in all respects."[76]

The conference had followed closely on a competition sponsored by the canton of Vaud for the best essay on the income tax. Almost certainly at the urging of Duprat, Royer took a group of books on economics back to her retreat in Cully and wrote her own contribution for the competition in two volumes. She was awarded the second prize, the first prize going to an essay by the great social theorist Proudhon. Juliette Adam, who had written a clever answer to Proudhon's attack on woman's position in society, reported that Royer's letter to Marie d'Agoult on the occasion of her prize added a postscript meant for Juliette: "Will you share the news with your very young friend, Mme La Messine [Adam's married name at the time], that she must rejoice about this if not for me at least against Proudhon."[77] Royer's prize-winning volumes, describing the history as well as the practice of income tax, were published as *Théorie de l'impôt ou la dîme sociale* by Guillaumin.[78]

Beginning with a series of definitions of taxation, or "impôt," she quoted Montesquieu, Adam Smith, John Stuart Mill, Turgot, Mirabeau, de

Girardin, and finally Pascal Duprat, who had given his own definition during the Conferences sur l'impôt at Lausanne in 1860. Adopting Duprat's definition with some modifications, she specified that this included services that the individual had received or would receive from the community. This restitution of advances from previous generations on behalf of future generations was an obligatory and personal requirement for each individual "to the current measure of his faculties. It must be sufficient to maintain the social state in the degree of civilization that it has attained and to permit it to continue to progress." Royer also developed a new term, "dîme sociale," derived from "dîme royale," a term that indicated a tithing paid to the king as a percentage of income. She considered income tax as a form of social tithing.[79]

Royer's book on the income tax is interesting even today because of her insistence on the economic role of women in society. In a section on the necessity to tax the idle, she produced a long statement on women's social roles. "From this obligation to work we in no way exclude women. Each of them must have an accredited profession to safeguard her dignity in case of need or in case of reversal of the wheel of fortune."[80]

Yet Royer appears to contradict herself by extolling the role of mother (*mère de la famille*) above all other professions. Motherhood was a social duty for which women needed an education. "Becoming a mother was the professor's chair, for which a preparatory education was required."[81] Mothers had the right and the duty to teach their children, but they needed training for this. This maternal education represented the professional capital on which she must pay interest. In preparation she could teach orphans or the children of incapacitated women, or she could produce, write, work, be an artist or tradeswoman. Even the wife of Mohammed, Royer remarked, had led a busy life. In past eras, only the woman merchant enjoyed civil rights, while both noble and servile women were under feudal Roman law.

As soon as a woman becomes a mother, "her truest work, her greatest, most important work, is the education of her children." This is work, Royer added, which costs her nothing, produces nothing for her own benefit but is completely for the profit of society, "for which she prepares new useful citizens." It is, therefore, a sufficient contribution to society. "No man pays the state anything comparable unless he gives his life on the battlefield." Echoing Emile de Girardin, she added that maternity was the "military service of women."[82] If she relinquished part of this obligation, refusing the task of education, for instance, by sending her children to be educated in public schools, then she would owe a tax.

She recognized that not all women were capable of properly educating their children, in which case it was preferable that they earn a salary to pay for those women who had special aptitudes to teach. The role of mother alone, if a woman remained idle, would not be enough to exempt her from tax. She had to discharge her obligation with some kind of labor. Although she had been told that a married woman who has to watch over a household is certainly not idle, Royer questioned whether this was a productive role. She doubted that it was real work to advise a cook or command a chambermaid or to pay out of her husband's account "bad servants, who were often unintelligent, unfaithful, or negligent." On the other hand, if she was a real administrator, she should be regarded as someone who needed some formal training. A wife, however, who acted as her husband's assistant, as bookkeeper, clerk, secretary, and aide, as well as fulfilling the roles of "mother and wife, educator and economist," should be freed of any contribution to the state. "Her life is full, full of free devotion. She gives everything, one cannot ask more from her."[83] Again she invoked the image of a soldier during a battle. For her system of taxation, not maternity but what she termed "a complete kind of maternity, as a sacred role" could exempt a woman from any professional costs: "This will be the only free profession."[84] After the children have left her house to follow skills whose acquisition she has supervised, she would continue to be exempt from tax like a retired military man.

While a woman was teaching her young children or in case of illness, she could have one domestic to help her, without paying any additional tax. Otherwise, all additional servants should be considered luxuries. Where a wife was only "a useless plaything in the house of a legal lover," she fulfilled no social role. In a cry against luxury, reinforced by her own austere life, she added: "Give women as much luxury as they wish but do not let them be idle. Luxury by itself makes dolls of them. Luxury with work will make them into living women knowing how to associate beauty and elegance with utility."[85]

She believed that women were under an obligation to produce children that continued throughout their lives and could not be avoided because of trivial apprehensions. Of course this was a barbaric requirement as they aged. After fifty for women and after sixty for men, the idleness tax should not apply. Ten years later, the old man of seventy and the old woman of sixty-two should be considered as having passed their productive period. If they continued to work "with trembling hands or a debilitated mind," society should let them keep the entire profit of their declining years: "These citizens have paid their debt." Personal taxes should always be elastic according to the individual case and apply only to the "individual in possession of all his faculties."[86]

The book on taxation first made her name known outside Switzerland. As she explained in her autobiography: "The fact [that she had won a prize and published a work on economics] appeared so original that the press grabbed hold of it. From that time on, the name of Clémence Royer traveled beyond Switzerland and became European. They knew nothing else about her, not even her nationality. Successively they made her Swiss, Belgian, or French according to the country through which they saw her pass."[87]

As a direct consequence of the recognition of her book on economics, she was presented at a meeting of the French Société d'Économie Politique in

1862 as a "young and knowledgeable author" by Joseph Garnier, secretary of the society.[88] This society has been described as a laissez-faire group of French economists who conceived of themselves as embattled against the institutional and mental residue of the *ancien régime*.[89] Many of the members either were or soon became members of the Académie des Sciences Morales et Politiques. They promoted political economy as an important aspect of individual liberty, as Royer was to do throughout her life. In 1862, both Jules Simon and the publisher Guillaumin were members of Garnier's society; by 1868, Duprat was also a member.

In Royer's one speech before this political science society she spoke of the need for women to work if they did not wish to marry or could not marry someone of their own choosing. She added, "It is good for women to read all, know all. Moreover it is only her ignorance that will be dangerous. We are no longer living in a time when Virtue is believed to be able to march only with a blindfold over her eyes. If she can march with her eyes open, she will march in a straight line."[90] The society, in spite of the urging by Garnier to admit women, failed to do so, possibly frightened off by Royer's comments. Royer was admitted only posthumously.[91]

From 1862 on Royer regularly reviewed books and reported on social science meetings for the *Journal des Économistes*. Her interests moved between economics and science. In the early 1860s she attended the European congress of the Association des Sciences Sociales, which met every summer somewhere in Belgium, Switzerland, or Holland. This allowed her to participate in a professional association and also to meet Duprat on a regular basis outside Switzerland. Now widely known, she lectured on science throughout Switzerland and traveled to Morges to lecture on a section of her course on psychology. "This time I admitted men. Charles Secretan came there from Neuchâtel, and Pastor [Ernest] Naville from Geneva. . . . Some societies of public utility called me to give lectures in Neuchâtel, in Locle, in Chaux de Fond, and in Yvedon. Then I went on to give lectures in Geneva."[92] Her autobiography continues: "In opposition to the full triumph of the school of Cuvier, she declared the evolutionary theory of Lamarck to be true, to which Charles Darwin was going to bring new proofs in his book *The Origin of Species* in 1860."[93]

Royer insisted later that it was her support of Lamarck and of evolution that made her female audience flee in 1860, not her discussion of the Bible.[94] However, Royer also attacked religious interpretations of nature. Ernest Naville, the Genevan Protestant theologian, found her so irritating in her style of argumentation that he told her she was "the only woman whom he had ever wanted to beat." That may have been from fatigue and frustration, since, as Royer explained, "I had beaten him dialectically in an eight-hour discussion until two in the morning."[95] The encounter took place at the home of Madame Forel, described by Royer as "a woman of spirit." Later, Naville would attempt to "beat her" intellectually again when he came to discuss the eugenics arguments in the preface to her translation of Darwin's *Origin of Species.*[96] This young woman interested in economics, physics, mathematics, and psychology (but as theoretical, not experimental sciences) took on the rather formidable task of producing the first French translation of Darwin's book and consequently made a lasting name for herself. Her efforts resulted in both favorable and unfavorable responses from casual readers, scientists, and Darwin himself.

CHAPTER 4

"True Science": Translating Darwin, Seeking a New Life

Lecturing in Geneva, Royer may have first heard of Darwin's new work on evolution through the review of *The Origin of Species* written by the Geneva-based Swiss scientist F. Jules Pictet in 1860. Pictet was one of the first to receive a copy of the *Origin of Species* directly from Darwin. He had discussed it favorably in the Genevan review *Bibliothèque Universelle.*[1] The following year there was an even more thoughtful and enthusiastic review by René-Edouard Claparède in the *Revue Germanique.*[2] In a later autobiographical statement Royer described her motivation to translate Darwin in the following terms: "It was then [after lecturing in Geneva] that I translated the *Origin of Species* of Ch. Darwin, which had appeared in England, during the same winter in which I had affirmed in my course the doctrine of Lamarck. If I translated Darwin, it was because he had brought new proofs to the support of my thesis."[3]

In Geneva she had opportunities to meet the scientists clustered around Carl Vogt and the Natural History Museum. Vogt had long been interested in evolutionary theory. He had translated Chambers's *Vestiges of Creation* into German fourteen years earlier. He would soon correspond regularly with Charles Darwin and later arranged French translations of Darwin's books *Variation of Animals and Plants under Domestication* and *Descent of Man* by J. J. Moulinié, a Geneva-based naturalist.[4] In 1862, he had begun to write his anthropological book *Lectures on Man,* deriving human beings from a number of parallel lines of evolution from different species of apes.[5] Royer met René-Édouard Claparède, who was making a name for himself as a remarkable researcher in invertebrate physiology and who admitted to a strong initial admiration for her as an individual.

It is not clear precisely how the arrangement for Royer to translate Darwin was made, but the fact that she had a close relationship with a French publisher was strongly in her favor. In many ways she must have seemed to be a logical choice. She had adequate English skills and had read both Lyell's *Principles of Geology* and Lamarck's *Zoological Philosophy.* More significant was her knowledge of Malthus and other economists, on which Darwin's basic mechanism, natural selection, was based, a point she would emphasize in her preface to the translation. "It is especially in its moral and humanitarian consequences that the theory of Darwin is so fecund. Never has anything so vast been conceived of in natural history. One could say that this is the universal synthesis of economic laws, the social science par excellence, the code of living beings for all races and all times."[6]

In her autobiography Royer speaks of the opposition of the Swiss churches as having fired her desire to do the translation. As she explains it: "This boldness in a woman who dared to contradict the naturalists of the time was discussed throughout all the Swiss sects. It was like a kick against the formulas of the believers. It was in response to their criticism that Clémence Royer translated the work of Ch. Darwin and wrote at the head of her translation the preface that made so much noise in France some years later."[7] Her preface, written in a strongly confrontational style, reads, indeed, like a "kick against the believers."

It was no secret that Darwin was keen to obtain a French translation. He had negotiated unsuccessfully with Louise Belloc, who had translated Maria Edgeworth novels and Harriet Beecher Stowe's novel *Uncle Tom's Cabin* into delightful French.[8] Belloc's interest was not really in the *Origin* but in Darwin's earlier, popular book, *Voyage of the Beagle.* Even this she found too difficult because of its scientific language and withdrew her offer. She later published only a brief translation of a section from Darwin's description of coral islands.

In early 1860, Darwin had been approached by a Frenchman, Pierre Talandier, who was teaching at the Royal Military School at Sandhurst and was eager to produce a translation. After lengthy negotiations, none of the large French scientific publishing houses such as J. B. Baillière, Hachette, or Masson agreed to publish it, rejecting it with "contempt," as Darwin wrote to Armand de Quatrefages, possibly because the translator, Pierre Talandier, had close ties to the socialists Louis Blanc and Alexander Herzen, both in exile in England at this time.[9]

Darwin had close ties to Geneva through his wife's aunt, Jane Allen Sismondi, the widow of the economist Sismondi. Although she had died in 1853, several years before Royer appeared on the Swiss scene, some of her old friends might have heard of this bright young woman who lectured on Lamarck and Lyell, on Malthus and Ricardo and who had made a reputation by challenging established authorities. Some former colleagues of Sismondi in the field of economics might have noted the name Royer was making for herself in economics and read her regular reviews on a wide range of topics for the *Nouvel Économiste.*[10] Sismondi and his wife had been part of the lively literary and scientific circle that included the botanist Augustin Pyramus de Candolle and his son Alphonse, the paleontologist Pictet, and the science popularizer Jane Marcet. Royer, as noted below, had carefully cited Pictet's 1860 review of Darwin's *Origin of Species.* However the connection came about, by 10 September 1861 Darwin had asked his English publisher Murray to send a copy of the third edition of the *Origin* to "Mlle Clémence-Auguste Royer; she has arranged with a publisher for a French translation."[11] The publisher was Guillaumin, who had published Royer's book on taxation. Since his publishing house did not specialize in scientific books, he joined with the Parisian scientific and medical publisher Victor Masson (who had rejected the Talandier translation) to put out the edition. In spite of the joint publication by both houses, as long as the Royer edition appeared it would be Guillaumin and not Masson's publishing house who would regularly advertise the edition for sale.[12]

When Royer agreed to translate Darwin's *Origin of Species,* Edouard Claparède offered his services to assist her to understand the technicalities of biological science. Claparède had had a thorough training in natural history and physiology in Germany. He had studied for a number of years with Johannes Müller in Berlin in the 1850s and had met many of the famous scientists there, including the great physiologists Dubois-Reymond and Rudolphe Wagner. He was a fellow student of Ernst Haeckel, later the strongest Darwinian in Germany, and their friendship continued when Claparède returned to Switzerland. Claparède was an excellent scientist; he specialized in insect physiology, and in his short life became a lecturer at the University of Geneva and published a large number of well-received papers.[13] Physically ill, he found Royer difficult to deal with because she insisted on her own interpretations of Darwin. She added not only extensive footnotes but a startling anticlerical preface that suggested that Darwinian evolution had implications for human society as well as for the rest of the natural world.

Clémence Royer challenged not only Catholicism but all revealed religion in the opening phrase of her preface to the *Origin.* To religious scientists it must have been startling, to say the least. "Yes, I believe in revelation, but it is the permanent revelation of man to man by himself." She singled out the audience of Swiss Protestants who had challenged her—"Calvinist Rome"—rather than the scientific readers of Darwin. Was it her attack against Christianity or against orthodox science that was uppermost in her mind? Later she would affirm more than once that she was searching for support of Lamarckian evolution when she first translated Darwin.[14]

Royer's preface drew attention to the plain quality of Darwin's style, which included arguments both for and against his theory, with the balance coming down on his side. "You will search in vain here for those phrases for effect that inflate the style of so many writers as certain pigeons inflate their empty crop."[15] Her explanation for agreeing to the translation of the *Origin* was "not because it was amusing," but because "it is important to study it and know it." The translation had been too long delayed, and she saw it as a duty towards "true science" (*le vrai science*). Darwin's book had been "badly understood, badly judged, without doubt because it was not read," an error that she hoped to rectify with her translation.[16]

She apologized for her lack of scientific knowledge: "I regret my insufficiency for such a task that a more specialized scientist would have fulfilled better in details."[17] However, she had no doubt that she had understood what Darwin intended as a whole, even where she had not explained his ideas well. She felt a real "solidarity" with Darwin. Had she not tried to discuss evolution in her own course of natural philosophy just the previous winter? Had she not encountered the same kind of opposition among the Swiss Protestants that Darwin had encountered among the English? She had been sent caricatures describing her simian ancestry as well as anonymous letters threatening her with the horrors of hell. She recalled in her preface the Oxford meeting of the British Association in 1861, in which Thomas Henry Huxley responded to the jeering tone of Bishop Samuel Wilberforce. If she adopted an inappropriate tone of raillery, she commented, she should be excused, since "an Oxford bishop has provided me with the example."[18]

For the lengthy notes with which she had laden Darwin's text she excused herself with the argument that she was addressing the general public rather than scientists, because she felt this book was so "full of information" that it should have a wider readership. At the same time she realized that she, far more than Darwin, could be criticized for having "dared hypotheses" in those notes. Her excuse for this extension of Darwin's ideas was her belief that hypotheses are always in the mind of the scientist in the process of observation, long before a law is formulated.[19] What compounded the issue was that she appended a table at the end of the book to guide the reader not through Darwin's arguments—as it at first appears—but to her own notes commenting on Darwin's ideas.[20]

Discussing the Swiss response to Darwin, she complimented the learned paleontologist Jules Pictet, who had published a review of the book in 1860 in his journal *Bibliothèque Universelle*.[21] Since he had earlier opposed evolutionary ideas, it was sufficient, Royer observed, that his review should be "affirmative without formal negation." He was "an adversary very close to being reconciled, a rebel half-converted but vacillating between his old opinions and the new idea." As for Pictet's other objections to Darwin, "M. Darwin has sufficiently refuted [these] in his third edition."[22]

Royer seems to have been unaware of Claparède's deep discomfort with her additions. In her preface, she warmly commended Claparède in spite of his Genevan background, which, like Jules Pictet, made him subject to "Calvinist Rome." In his review Claparède, far more openly than Pictet, "rendered full justice to Darwin's work in a lucid and complete exposition of his theory. . . . " She cited his judgment that the new theory "has the advantage of being more in harmony with the habitual procedures of nature than its rival" and quoted a comment, also from his review of the *Origin of Species,* that was endlessly echoed by the French transformists, including Paul Broca, "It is better to be a perfected ape than a degenerated Adam."[23]

Royer's preface also included a lengthy description of the consequences of Darwinian evolution for human beings. In a section that gained her instant notoriety she made the first eugenic suggestions about the consequences of natural selection. Noting an "exaggeration of that pity, . . . that fraternal song, in which our Christian era has always sought the ideal of social virtue," she argued that the human race was "aggravating and multiplying the evils that it pretends to remedy." She added that, through an excess of devotion, human beings regularly "sacrifice what is strong to the weak, the good to the bad . . . beings well-endowed in mind and body to vicious and malingering individuals." An ill-considered protection of the weak, the infirm, the incurables, and the wicked had resulted in "the evils with which they are tainted tending to perpetuate themselves indefinitely."[24] In this first edition of her French translation, she posed the issue in a manner that seemed to imply the need to eliminate such individuals. The preservation of "beings incapable of living by themselves" weighed heavily "on the arms of the strong." "These unfortunates tend to take the place of three healthy individuals who could have produced far more happiness than they consume." She asked dramatically: "Has no one seriously considered this?" Within five years, she would back away from the implications of her remarks.[25]

The effect of marriage and mating selections on human society and particularly on women she extended and maintained throughout her life. Through the selection of partners on the basis of passivity and beauty, men had weakened human development. Women tended to pass these characteristics on to their daughters, but were saved by the mental and physical strength that they inherited from their paternal ancestors. She believed that this must be changed: "One must conclude that, in order to hasten the progress of the race in all senses, it will become necessary to ask for woman a part of what has been asked for man, that is, strength united to beauty, intelligence united to gentleness, and for man, a little idealism united to vigor of mind and body."[26]

Royer finished her translation in late spring, and when the book appeared in early June, she eagerly went to urge her friend Marie d'Agoult to share her pleasure in the translation. Marie d'Agoult remarked in her journal not on Darwin's science but on Royer's challenge to religion. "Her preface is extremely remarkable and, as far as I have read, of great courage. She speaks as if Catholicism was a political party and Christianity a dangerous error for the human species that must be uprooted and destroyed."[27]

Darwin received his copy of the preface about the same time, and his first response to Royer's translation was a mixture of amusement and surprise. He wrote to the American botanist Asa Gray, who was warmly seconding his theories in the United States, "I received 2 or 3 days ago a French translation of the *Origin* by a Madlle [*sic*] Royer who must be one of the cleverest and oddest women in Europe: is ardent Deist and hates Christianity and declares that natural selection and the struggle for life will explain all morality, nature of man, politicks etc etc!!! She makes some very curious and good hits and says she will publish a book on these subjects and a strange production it will be."[28] At the end of her life, Royer reported to one of her friends that when Darwin wrote to her to thank her for her translation, he remarked that if he had dared to say what she had said in her preface he would have been "a lost man" (*un homme perdu*).[29]

Darwin, on reading further in Royer's translation, regretted that she did not know more natural history.[30] By September of 1862, Darwin wrote to thank Claparède both for his excellent review of Darwinism in the *Revue Germanique* in 1861 and for his help on the French translation. Claparède replied with gratitude, speaking of the love with which he had written about Darwinism, which he believed to be the greatest scientific idea of his time. He had tried, he added, to "examine your ideas without passion, leaving all enthusiasm at the door."[31]

Claparède spoke with embarrassment to Darwin about the assistance that he had given Royer. "I would have preferred that you had remained ignorant of this detail, because I must tell you that I regretted to see your book translated by this person, for whom in other respects I profess a great deal of esteem. Her translation is heavy, undigested at times, incorrect, and the notes that accompany it will certainly not at all be to your taste."[32] He had tried to use all of his influence over Royer to make her limit herself to the "simple role of translator," but in vain. He had managed to get her to suppress "without exception" all the notes he considered absurd and nonscientific. "In retaliation she printed a very large number [of other notes], the major part of which she had never submitted to me."[33]

His view of how women ought to behave colored his reaction as strongly as the way in which she handled the translation. He had married only a year before he began to work with Royer on this translation, and the contrast between his young wife and Royer may have exacerbated his uneasiness. In explanation he declared that "Mlle Royer is a singular person whose attractions are in no way those of her sex." He spoke of her "half-masculine education" and her devotion to an "exclusively deductive philosophical school." "She had thought in translating your work to introduce some corrections on her own authority, corrections that would have strangely and disagreeably surprised you."[34] He had been able to dissuade her only by pointing out that she would be treating the author in an "indelicate manner" if she persisted.

From Claparède's viewpoint, the corrections she wished to make were interesting only to the extent that they showed how much "a mind like Mlle Royer's is opposed to the advance of natural sciences." He gave two examples: In Darwin's chapter "Instinct," which appeared as chapter 7 in the first through the third English edition, Royer had replaced the term "three-sided pyramid" (for the base of the honeycomb cells) by the term "hexagonal pyramid," because she believed bees could not terminate a hexagonal form except by a hexagonal point.[35] "The idea had never occurred to her to take a look at a honeycomb before introducing such a major modification," he said, speaking as a scientist with extensive experimental and observational training.[36]

A second example Claparède produced of Royer's misunderstandings was that Royer had "thought of nothing better than to make all electric fish descend from a common ancestor having an electric organ. Since she had no notions of zoology nor of comparative anatomy, I had a great deal of trouble getting her to understand that you would have had your reasons not to suggest such a simple idea. I finally succeeded in convincing her for good or ill by a description of the electric organs of the torpedo, the electric eel, the malapteure, and the mornay eel and the nerves that serve them, that these organs, although identical from the point of view of tissues, are certainly not at all morphologically homologous."[37]

If Claparède sounded intellectually uncomfortable, it is important to recall that he was physically unwell. Royer had received her copy of the *Origin* to translate by September 1861. Claparède mentioned in his letter to Darwin that he had been in discomfort following typhoid fever for seven or eight months, a period of time that overlapped with his assistance on the translation. In fact, he was seriously ill not just with typhoid fever but with the heart and kidney problems that had troubled him since his youth and that would eventually kill him ten years later. He was also preparing for new teaching responsibilities at the University of Geneva, which began in 1862. Within a very short time, he had to take regular leaves of absence from the university for health reasons, although he continued to produce an amazing number of scientific articles.[38] Although he did not mention it in his letter, another source of discomfort for Claparède must have been a religious one. His brother Theodore was not only an evangelical preacher but a famous historian of Swiss Protestantism.

Claparède's reaction colored Darwin's perception of both Royer and the French translation, and Darwin began to worry that her preface was affecting acceptance of his ideas in France. Immediately after he received Claparède's letter, Darwin wrote to Joseph Hooker, repeating some of Claparède's comments about Royer and adding: "Almost everywhere in the *Origin* when I express great doubts she appends a note explaining the difficulty or saying there is none whatever! It is really curious to know what conceited people there are in the world."[39] In anticipation of her translation, Darwin had sent her a presentation copy of his book on the coadaptation of orchids and insects, published in early May 1862.[40] This was the first and last such copy he would send her.

Given that Royer's publisher Guillaumin was a close friend, associate, and colleague of Joseph Garnier, president of the Société d'Économie Politique, it is not surprising that Garnier was one of the earliest reviewers of the translation of *The Origin of Species* into French. He pointed out Royer's discussion of the importance of Malthus in Darwin's development of the concept of natural selection, signaling her "condemnation of the consequences that Malthus drew for the human species."[41] Royer, unlike Malthus, considered excess population as a positive motor for human as well as animal and plant evolution.

Royer's major writings during the early sixties outside of her Darwin preface were squarely in the field of economics and political science, and she sent her publications on to her good friend Marie d'Agoult, who expressed her appreciation of them.[42] Among her regular articles for the *Journal des Économistes* appeared an extensive description of the first meeting of the International Association of Social Sciences at Brussels in late September 1862.[43] This proved to be the most thorough description of these congresses carried by the journal. Most of the founding members of the association were significant in republican politics over the next few decades. Many became major figures within the Académie des Sciences Morales et Politiques, the social science wing of the Institute of France. Not only Duprat, Garnier, and the future press baron Emile de Girardin attended these congresses, but also Jules Simon, who later became an important political figure and general secretary of the Académie des Sciences Morales et Politiques. Royer's report included extensive excerpts of her own public comments on income tax reform.[44]

Royer's growing fame gave her the income and the freedom to travel. She found she could earn a living lecturing to small audiences interested in economic theory, women's rights, and Darwinism. The hottest topic of the day, of course, was Darwinism, and she was uniquely situated to speak authoritatively on this subject in front of eager audiences in Brussels and Italy as well as in Switzerland.

Royer spent the winter of 1862/1863 speaking and lecturing in Belgium and in Holland. It was at that time that she appears to have attended the celebration in honor of Victor Hugo's novel Les Misérables. During the winter of 1863/1864 she remained in Brussels where she worked with the publishers on her "transformed" novel published finally in the spring of 1864. The novel was not permitted to be sold in France because of its strongly anticlerical tone and possibly because of its advocacy of sexual and family relationships based on love and mutual commitment alone. According to Royer, it was placed on the Index and excluded from France during the Empire. It was, however, reviewed by a number of journals, including the *Revue Germanique* and *Le*

Temps, at the urging of Marie d'Agoult, who had close connections to the publishers.[45] Even with this support, the reviewer for *Revue Germanique,* while admitting that Royer was a writer with a serious reputation in science and other fields, found many flaws as she moved into a "new terrain." "Nothing is stranger," he commented, "than the fable imagined by the author to put her characters into play. There are a series of unlikelihoods." As for the characters, he added, "they are pure abstractions, their passions have no reality, they do not exist, they signify." To illustrate, he enumerates the characters: "There is a repentant courtisan, a repentant cardinal, two repentant libertines, a brigand, and an unrepentant Jesuit." He adds that "the author is always ready to forget her fable to philosophize, and if finally there is a denouement, one could almost say that is not her fault." But he admits with some fairness, "Without doubt there is more than one beautiful page to detach from the novel of Mlle Royer, but these are by the way." At the end of the review he commended the poetry and prose of the 126 pages that formed the "Album of a Traveler." These, he added, were "imprinted by a sadness that comes from the heart."[46] Curiously, he overlooked Royer's discussion of women and the underlying feminist themes discussed in chapter 2. Many years later Royer estimated that she had earned only Fr 1,600 from the sale of her novel.[47]

During this period, Royer also continued to see Duprat at the International Congress of Social Sciences held in different Swiss cities every summer. She often supported Duprat's point of view at these meetings, giving his and her own comments an important place in her reviews of the congress for the *Journal des Économistes.* While reviewing the 1863 congress in Gand, she reported a long discussion during the congress on the question of whether or not one could impose moral criteria upon art. Pascal Duprat, she noted, "victoriously established the fact that there was no direct link between the public or private weaknesses of a great man and the good or bad influences he had on his own era, citing the names Bacon, Seneca, Raphael. . . . " Royer entered the discussion with a comment that sounds like a personal defense of Duprat: "Judge their works, their influence. That is your right and your duty, and on that you—and we more than you—are severe. But respect the man." To do otherwise was to "resurrect the Inquisition," since there could be "no absolute criteria of morality of works of art." No one had a right to analyze the conscience or the private life of a man of genius with the intent of making a moral judgment. "Everyone tends to call good what he permits himself and bad what he avoids."[48]

One cannot help but wonder if the friends of this couple were amused to hear such an ardent defense of moral utility endorsed by the two lovers. In a later session Duprat, backing away from a purely relativistic view of the morality of the artist, insisted that art was not just "a voluptuousness of the spirit" but must instruct as well, a comment certainly reflected in Royer's novel.[49] Royer's discussion of morality was her first discussion of the "moral law," on which she believed science was based, depending upon a relative social good and the usefulness for the species that practiced it. Although she outlined this moral law for the congress, she expanded this concept and its biological constraints twenty years later.[50] By 1863, as her fame spread out beyond Switzerland, she began to travel again not only to lecture but to study in Germany. She was struck unpleasantly by what she saw as the rude behavior of students in Heidelberg, who played games of chance and denied any knowledge of the location of the university library. Attacked by a depression that might have resulted from her intense work the previous year or from Duprat's continuing stay in Italy, she wrote to Marie d'Agoult, expressing her feeling of isolation and comparing a woman's existence to that of a traveler crossing a glacier, an image that evokes her first childhood experience of exile. She concluded that if she was going to remain alone it was preferable to follow her own course rather than find herself "jostling with crowds of strangers."[51] Her depression increased somewhat. She was in the process of rethinking the problems that faced a woman forging a unique path through her life; in a letter to Marie d'Agoult in October 1863 she recognized that being a woman meant that the realm of the possible was quite limited: "You have had the same experience as I had, Madame, that the advantage and disadvantage of being a woman always narrows any possible spheres for us."[52]

In the same year, she also contributed an article on the legal position of Swiss women to the feminist English journal *The English Woman's Journal* that emphasized her debate with herself over the legal position of unmarried mothers.[53] This journal was started by a group of energetic and socially committed women friends who called themselves the Langham Place Group and included the famous feminists Barbara Smith Bodichon, Bessie Parkes, and Emily Davies. The group also sponsored an organization that undertook to find work for women.[54] One wonders if Royer's energetic intellectual activities, which seemed somewhat eccentric in the French and Roman Swiss environment would have appeared more acceptable in the English context, where unmarried women commonly carried out both intellectual and social missions. However, her choice to live with a married man would most certainly have produced the same kind of social ostracism that George Eliot was experiencing at that time.

Royer's piece "Women in French Switzerland; The Laws Relating to Them" included in its original form not only an account of the legal position of daughters and married women, but also that of unmarried mothers. Royer had been struck by the way in which Swiss political freedoms did not translate into rights for women. For example, regarding a husband's obligation to protect his wife, Royer asked, "Will [the husband] protect her against himself? And who will oblige him to protect her against others if he does not choose to do it? Who will prove that he has not done it? How far is this protection to extend? Who regulates it? Where is the penal sanction that menaces him if he breaks the law? There is nothing of the kind, and without this the law is without effect."[55]

The editors, Emily Davies and Bessie Parkes, chose not to print the final section on unmarried mothers (*filles mères*), perhaps because Royer had emphasized her belief in the right of women to bear children outside of marriage. Instead, they briefly summarized the eliminated conclusion, commenting that "on the whole the laws appear to be more favorable to women who have transgressed against morality than to lawful wives and mothers." The editors added that "while the children of married woman are by law exclusively under the father's control, the mother whose children are illegitimate is by law their sole guardian, although in many cases the father is obliged to contribute to their maintenance." These Englishwomen were struck by the apparent greater protection for the unmarried than the married woman, should she find herself with an abusive partner. They commented on a similarly unfair aspect of English law that also appeared to protect the "immoral more than the moral citizen."[56]

Royer's article, especially the suppressed section on unmarried mothers, indicates the degree to which she was concerned on a personal level about legal rights, should she decide to set up an independent household with Duprat or have a child outside marriage. As we have noted in a number of other situations, her objective discussions often reflected her immediate concerns. It is only because of the existence of this article that one can project a growing decision to form a companionate marriage with Duprat as early as 1863.

Duprat had come from a Saint-Simonist milieu that in the late 1840s had advocated free unions, and his marriage had begun as one. For a man, the choice was far simpler than for a young middle-class woman. Royer had been conventionally raised, in spite of her mother's independent attitude and the freedom she had been given as a young woman. Although Royer's father and mother had made a similar choice to form a free union before her birth, Captain Royer's position as an unmarried man meant that there was a future possibility of marriage to regularize the situation. The mother's situation was, therefore, not strictly comparable to that of the daughter. Royer never advocated free love in the sense of uncommitted and indiscriminate lovemaking, since she adhered to a strict code of monogamy for women and men unless the parties failed to meet their social obligations. She regarded her union with Duprat as a lifelong commitment, not a temporary one.

Clemence Royer would soon make the decision to remain with Duprat and to bear and raise his child. She did so proudly, although she was to suffer socially from the consequences of what was in those days a difficult, even courageous, act for a woman who had neither wealth nor aristocratic position to cushion her. The ambiguous position in which she found herself caused her later argument for "natural morality" to subject her to attack more than once. She had decided to put her "life in accord with her convictions."[57]

Italy, where Duprat had established himself, especially attracted her, and she soon began to give a series of lectures on Darwinism throughout that country.[58] Marie d'Agoult helped her by writing to her friends in Italy to arrange lectures for her.[59] The Italian women must have received her lectures warmly, since later she mentioned that her only jewel was a brooch given to her by the women of Milan.[60]

Duprat's choice of Turin as a place to settle may have been influenced by the presence of his old friend Giuseppe Ferrari, whom he had known in Paris during the Second Republic. Ferrari had returned to Italy and entered politics, sitting on the extreme left as a radical republican in the Parliament of the Risorgimento, then located in Turin. He also held a chair without pay at the university that allowed him to combine his interests in academic affairs with support of democratic reforms. Duprat may have obtained assistance from Ferrari in establishing a journal at Turin, *La Novella Italia.* Like Ferrari, Duprat taught at the University of Turin, probably as a lecturer on political economy.[61]

Although Duprat had sought an escape from his marriage in Turin, his unhappy wife chose to follow him there. She had left Geneva for Paris in 1861, "fleeing her creditors" according to Royer, having bought Fr 1,500 worth of linen on the pretext of an upcoming marriage of her fourteen-year-old daughter. She solicited financial support from both Duprat's friends and enemies in Paris. Interestingly enough, Duprat's wife was able to obtain a tobacco license from the government, which was commonly granted to widows of soldiers or minor government officials. Royer hinted in a later letter to a friend that Duprat's wife had also winked at a relationship between her daughter and a young officer. The last straw, as far as Duprat was concerned, was his wife's attempts to get him to return to Paris and support the Second Empire by dangling before him the promise of a ministerial position.[62]

Duprat indignantly showed Royer letters from his wife, describing her maneuvers and assuring Royer that he was doing everything possible to "break this burdensome tie." It would not prove easy to be rid of a wife in a period before divorce. At the very moment when Duprat decided to "take his liberty," his "legal proprietor," as Royer referred to his wife, came to Turin to live with Duprat, placing the daughter in a local boarding school. Within three months, she returned to Paris once again, removing the daughter from school on the pretext of another marriage that never occurred.[63]

Perhaps it was at this point that Royer, during one of her periodic trips back to Paris, met Juliette Adam at the home of Marie d'Agoult, whose intellectual and political salon offered a friendly environment for republicans during the Second Empire. In her later memoirs Adam reported that d'Agoult read aloud long scientific and philosophical letters written by Royer to her. While d'Agoult expressed her admiration, Adam seems to have cared little about these topics and ridiculed both the serious tone and the science-based philosophy expressed in these letters.[64] Juliette Adam—who had published her famous anti-Proudhon book under her maiden name, Juliette Lamber[t]—was introduced to Royer as Madame La Messine, then her married name. The two women superficially appeared to share many interests: their feminist commitment, a strong dislike of Proudhon, their devotion to republican politics, and a lively personal devotion to particular republican leaders. Personally they could not have been more dissimilar. Juliette Adam was a conventionally attractive, young married woman who dressed in the fashion of her day and relished small talk, gossip, and mild flirtations. Royer was direct and intense, with few "feminine" charms. Her look, as she was introduced to Adam, was searching and appraising. The slight frown of her myopia must have given her a more forbidding appearance. Adam read it as disapproval and never forgot or forgave.[65]

As Adam described the scene of this meeting, Royer wanted to talk to her about Adam's book on Proudhon and suggested they move to a quite corner to talk privately about the subject. Adam was not in the mood for piercing feminist analyses. She had just been having a delightful time flirting with Edmond Texier, another republican and journalist, who accompanied them into a corner. As Adam reports, he acted protectively towards her, "as though I were running a serious danger, which gave me a mad desire to laugh." When Royer quizzed her about her feminist ideas, Adam responded rather flippantly, prompting the indignant response from Royer as she got to her feet: "Madame, you lack criteria." Adam's response, which she later admitted was ill advised, was to rise in turn and to address Royer, very pointedly, as "Mademoiselle," calling attention to her unmarried status. Knowing that Royer had obtained highly esteemed teaching certificates, she added that her own "license," although "very inferior to yours, has little weight but at least has the advantage of not making anyone else desperate." Her remark, intended to wound, as she admitted in her later memoirs, was a deliberate reference to Royer's liaison with Duprat. As Adam put it, "Duprat's wife was screaming about Royer all over Paris." Adam realized by Royer's shocked response and immediate withdrawal that she had made an enemy for life, further aggravated by the amused retelling of the story as lively gossip by her friend Texier.[66]

Royer seems to have expected to find a real intellectual in Juliette Lambert, like the other feminist writer on Proudhon, Jenny d'Héricourt, also a habitué of Marie d'Agoult's salon. Royer long after extolled the piercing intelligence of d'Héricourt's feminist analysis, whereas Adam had a difficult relationship with this feminist and saw her, as she did Royer, as a rival.[67]

In 1864 Pascal Duprat began another journal in Turin, this time emphasizing economics and statistics, with an Italian colleague, A. Gicca. This was reviewed by Maurice Block in the *Journal des Économistes* as "a very well done résumé of official Italian documents, both statistical as well as legislative." Block wished the new publication well. "Further, the name of Pascal

Duprat is too well known to the reader to make it necessary to add anything more."[68] Like many of Duprat's enterprises it did not survive long but reappeared a few years later in Florence under Gicca's editorship, with Duprat listed only as a founding editor.[69]

Where Duprat was, Royer followed. Her friends in the Société d'Économie Politique at the end of 1864 commented that Royer was "currently in Turin after having made "a biting analysis of the Franco-Italian convention."[70] Florence had just been made the capital, and the legislature had moved there, leaving the city of Turin in a poor economic state. Royer evaluated the potential of Turin as a future industrial city, recommending that the city fathers study the means by which Turin could become in a few years the "Lyon of Italy."[71] The reviewer in the *Journal des Économistes* applauded her suggestions.

The best-known photograph of Royer derives from this period, taken by the great photographer of the period, Félix Nadar, who with his brother took many of the most vivid portraits of celebrities of the time (fig. 3). He was soon to be celebrated as a balloonist during the Franco-Prussian war. In the photograph, Royer sits looking straight at the camera. Her brows come together, probably because of her myopia, but her eyes are wide open, and her firm jaw yields in a slight smile as she leans her elbow on a table, showing off the Breton lace at the sleeve of her satin dress. Her hair is severely parted but ends in fashionable corkscrew curls.[72]

In the only explicit description she ever gave of her relationship with Duprat, Royer explained to a friend that "I found Pascal again in Italy, where I gave conferences in Turin, Milan, Genoa, Naples, and Florence."[73] Here she had lectured on Darwinism before audiences stimulated by the recent publication of an Italian edition of the *Origin of Species* and the lectures of Filippo de Filippi. A friend and former colleague of Carl Vogt, Gabriel de Mortillet, had also moved to Italy and would soon advertise Royer's lectures in his new archaeological journal, *Matériaux pour l'Histoire de l'Homme.*[74]

In 1865 Duprat journeyed to Florence from Turin for the Dante festival, which celebrated the six hundredth year of the great writer's birth. The Dante festival included many special exhibits and spectacles. Royer may also have traveled to Florence to see another old friend, Marie d'Agoult, whose daughter Blandine was then living in Florence and on the verge of her marriage to Émile de Girardin, the son of an exiled republican politician and later an important press baron. In the *Revue Germanique,* a journal created and sponsored by her, Marie d'Agoult published a famous series of articles on Dante and Goethe, in the same issue in which Duprat published articles on Italian politics.[75]

Royer met Duprat under these unusually festive circumstances in Florence, undoubtedly a welcome relief from their continual lecturing, writing, and intellectual preoccupations. Sometime during the Dante festival, the two lovers, perhaps at the urging of their mutual friends, considered living together on a more permanent basis, forming a companionate marriage, since they could not form a legal one. "I hesitated still and returned to Paris," Royer later confided.[76] By August 1865, Royer had made her decision. The two arranged to meet at the Congress of Social Sciences in Berne with the express intention "no longer to leave each other" and to travel as a couple from Berne directly to Italy. According to Royer, Duprat had just delivered a brilliant reply to Jules Simon on the subject of compulsory education.[77] At this meeting, Royer attacked needless luxury, citing the expenditure of money by women on fashionable clothing and giving as an example the purchase by one woman of a dress costing Fr 1,500. Some of the men in the session questioned her flat condemnation, replying that this price would not be an extravagance for some households. Royer, incensed, no doubt, by Duprat's reports of his wife's extravagances and because of her own frugal life style, insisted on the point.[78]

The two lovers left their baggage together in one room while they took a last excursion with the rest of the congress members around Berne. On returning to their room, Duprat was arrested for debt, since Duprat's "political adversaries" had obtained the notes of credit from Duprat's unpaid debts in Geneva. Since one could be thrown into prison for debt, his debtors found it "amusing" to have him arrested in front of the full congress. "Their pleasure was augmented by finding my suitcases in his room," Royer reported. They insisted that Royer pay the debt, which amounted to Fr 3,000, but she had no such sum, having never had that much money in her possession at one time. "Some mutual friends, who had just left the congress, were still at Lausanne. I wrote to them about the situation, and they came to release the prisoner."[79]

Duprat and Royer found themselves free to leave Berne but without any resources to travel on to Italy. Royer commented, "The moment was badly chosen to realize our project for a common life."[80] She felt herself compromised and wanted the situation resolved. They went instead to Paris, where Pascal Duprat, proscribed by the Empire, could have been arrested. Royer had a small apartment there, and Duprat remained hidden for three months, doubtless as wary of his legal wife as of the Empire. The two lovers worked hard on books to earn some money for their travel. Duprat wrote a charming little book on the Enlightenment and the *Encyclopédistes,* the Enlightenment figures surrounding Diderot, so dear to Royer's own heart.[81] Royer took the opportunity to prepare a second French edition of Charles Darwin's *Origin of Species.*[82]

For this second edition of her Darwin translation, both Charles Darwin and Royer took some trouble to make improvements. Among other changes, Darwin suggested a closer translation of his subtitle, eliminating her phrase "laws of progress."[83] Royer also agreed to change her translation of natural selection from "élection naturelle," to "sélection naturelle" since the term had been widely adopted by friends and enemies alike, although, she pointed out, the term "sélection" was not a French term.[84] "Élection," however, had overtones of conscious choice, and the term had been strongly attacked by Pierre Flourens, secretary of the Académie des Sciences, in a polemical book written in opposition to Darwin in 1864.[85] Royer felt that the term could be supported by analogy with the chemical term "elective affinities."[86] Royer had simply adopted the term "élection naturelle" from Claparède. One might add that the term "artificial selection" for animal breeding had been translated many years earlier as "élection artificielle" by the early writer on heredity, Prosper Lucas.[87]

Darwin's later dissatisfaction with his French translator was aggravated by his annoyance with the increasingly elaborate notes with which she supplemented his text, whereas she kept insisting that she had written her notes to facilitate understanding by the nonscientist and to improve the accuracy of his science. Darwin did not eliminate these notes in the second edition, though he may have reduced their length. At least one example exists of his removal of an extended note. In the first edition of her translation, Royer inserted a note comparing animal breeding practices to the strict marriage laws governing Hindu castes. For her second edition, she expanded this with a list of references to the Hindu "Laws of Manu," adding that natural selection (she uses her earlier term *élection naturelle*) was embodied in these laws, producing human differentiation and "transforming the instincts, habits, and physical characters of the Indo-Germanic race" (fig. 4). Darwin removed this addition but placed her note for future reference in his notebooks along with a partial translation of the note by his wife, Emma.[88] He also corrected some major errors, although these are not noted, and Royer incorporated changes he had made in his second German edition, each of which is signaled by a note. He was quite ill during the period in which he worked on the second French edition and had to postpone his review of her work from early April to June 1865.[89] When he took it up again, his wife, Emma Darwin, reported to her daughter Henrietta Darwin's unhappiness with "the Verdammte Mlle Royer whose errors are endless."[90] Nevertheless, he appears to have written in an encouraging manner to Royer, as she reported in her new foreword.[91]

Darwin, she explained, had asked her to correct certain errors "that had slipped into my first edition," and she had carefully obliged. She also took his advice and that of other "competent men"—not identified here, but possibly including the naturalist Armand de Quatrefages—in editing her notes. Royer defensively suggested that Darwin's own notes and other textual modifications had weakened the flow of his original argument.

She replied to the accusation made by "an adversary in Switzerland"—possibly Claparède, whose remarks may have reached her ears—that Darwin himself was "frightened by the boldness of our preface." She assured her readers that she had received letters from Darwin in which he had written that "we had, more than other critics or translators, understood the general spirit of his doctrine."[92] She recognized that some individuals had blanched at the suggestion that Darwinism raised questions about "excessive" private and public welfare, referring obliquely to her own extension of the implicit eugenic possibilities in Darwinism. She had been criticized for the implication that saving lives by modern medicine was not in the interest of the human race. But, she protested, this was a common point of discussion among political economists. She had merely brought in a new point of view, without necessarily endorsing the conclusions implied by the questions. "Although Darwin may have feared for a moment that our temerity would weaken the success of his ideas, we have reason to believe that [he is] for the moment completely reassured on that account." She suggested rather coyly that, not wishing to compromise him against his will, "we do not affirm here that he dares to think nearly everything that we have dared to say."[93] However, she quietly made her own changes to her preface to the first edition, which was reprinted in the second edition, modifying the severity of her eugenic statements.[94]

Royer also complained in her new foreword about the nasty comments she had received from the Catholic press, which had resorted to "truncated citations, insulting epithets, and jokes of doubtful taste." She added, "We knew in advance that any woman who dares to act, speak, or even think without taking the advice of a spiritual director either from Rome or Geneva, cannot fail to raise religious anger."[95] On this topic and on topics attacking freethinkers, both churches, she argued, were in surprising accord.

Influenced by Duprat's work on the Encyclopedistes while she was working on her new Darwin edition, as well as her own earlier admiration for those figures, she invoked the names of the great Enlightenment writers Diderot, Voltaire, and d'Alembert, remarking that the enemies of these men were now forgotten. She spoke of her pride in seeing her name linked as a freethinker with the great thinkers of the previous century, who had shown so much courage, and she was proud to see ideas she had advocated becoming widespread. However, she denied that she belonged to any philosophical school. Although having been called a Fourierist, Saint-Simonist, and Comtean, she proclaimed her independence. "We recognize no master." Her desire to support Darwin's theory came simply through her love of truth. Nor had she hesitated to "keep her independence," even as regarded Darwin himself, as she believed her notes made amply clear.[96]

Just before Royer left for Italy at the end of December, she sent two copies of her second edition and a short note to Paul Broca, general secretary of the Anthropological Society of Paris, asking him to keep one copy for himself in recognition of her high esteem for him and to present the other to the Société d'Anthropologie at the next meeting. She regretted that the statutes of the society appeared to prevent her election as a member, and she spoke of her unhappiness at the "harsh exclusion with which its statutes strike a mind like mine, unhappily joined to a feminine form."[97] She had intended writing to him about possible membership before the previous meeting of the society, "but multiple concerns about an upcoming departure prevented me."[98]

Broca was not pleased to find that Royer had singled out his society in her new foreword to the Darwin edition. She had hailed the Société d'Anthropologie de Paris, "so scientific and so active," as being the one place in France where "the theory of Darwin reigns, so to speak, without contest among the most influential and the most competent members."[99] Broca, for political as well as intellectual reasons, wanted to disassociate himself from this claim. He insisted to Carl Vogt that very few members of the society were in fact Darwinists, "in spite of what Mme Royer said in her second edition."[100] As a polygenist, a believer in multiple origins for the human species, he insisted he could not be counted among the Darwinists, of which there were no more than about nineteen in the whole society.

One must add in Royer's defense that Broca's claim was a bit disingenuous, since the "few" were to be found in the central bureau of the society. They included Eugène Dally, Gabriel de Mortillet, Charles Letourneau, and Camille Dareste. Broca himself had just declared that a new human fossil, "the Naulette jaw," had provided the first solid evidence for Darwin's theory.[101]

Royer's sin in both Darwin's and modern eyes may not have been her advocacy of free thought but her insistence on her role as not only an advocate but a critic of Darwin's evolutionary ideas. Mistaking her role as translator, she associated herself so closely with the work she was translating that it was hard for her to tease apart her very different ideas of progressive evolution from those of Darwin, as evident in the analytical table she attached to her first edition but removed from the second. Darwin complained about this conceit. It was a trait Darwin himself was singularly lacking. We shall discuss at the end of chapter 5 the consequences of her later frontal attack on pangenesis, Darwin's theory of inheritance.

Chapter 5

Motherhood, Social Theory, and Social Realities

With the money from their books, Duprat and Royer left together in December 1865 for Florence, settling there some months before their only son was born. Florence was beautiful and inexpensive and a center for exiles and European tourists. This choice seems to have been partly influenced by the move of the Italian capital to that city.[1] Duprat's friend Giuseppe Ferrari, whom he had known since the 1848 revolution, had followed the government there in 1864, while retaining his university seat in Turin. Ferrari's position on the influential High Council on Public Education meant that he could and did use his influence to get his friends academic chairs. He resigned his parliamentary seat over the accusation that he was trying to wangle a university chair for himself in Florence, but soon regained his seat in the parliament.[2] His influence may have obtained support for Duprat's publishing efforts and provided opportunities for him to lecture on political economy in Florence.

It is illuminating to read Alexandre Dumas's description of how well one could live on very little money in Florence twenty years earlier.[3] He described how the city was nearly deserted in the summer by travelers and natives, except for those poor Italians who had to remain. The wealthy aristocrats hid behind the cool walls of their palaces, emerging by carriage at four in the afternoon to promenade solemnly in the nearby woods. Even in the 1840s, from November until March the city filled with travelers from France, England, and Russia. By the 1850s, groups from these countries sought escape from an unpleasant climate or social and political persecution.

The English colony included the important presence of the poets Elizabeth Barrett Browning and Robert Browning, until her death in 1862, the painter Walter Savage Landor, the aging mathematician and scientific popularizer from England Mary Somerville, and between 1862 and 1867 the journalist, later anti-vivisectionist, Frances Power Cobbe.[4] Although this community would seem a natural one for Royer towards which to gravitate—especially since Cobbe had made a similar move to Unitarianism and was interested in both the writings of Darwin and Lyell—the English were more at ease with the Italian aristocrats than with the community of French and Russian freethinkers and republicans.

Maurice [Moritz] Schiff, a friend and colleague of Claparède and Carl Vogt, supported an intellectual circle dedicated to private discussions of science and revolution that must have seemed more suitable to Duprat and Royer. It welcomed women auditors in its discussions, including the brilliant young daughters of the Alexander Herzen family.[5] Royer may have made a contact with the Russian community through the Herzen family, which later had close links to her future colleague, the anthropologist Charles Letourneau. Some years later she regularly contributed articles to the Russian opposition newspaper *Goloss.*[6]

In Italy, many of the republican Italian and French thinkers were interested in the topic of Darwinian evolution, although many of them adhered to the polygenist view that human beings derived from multiple sources, as Carl Vogt believed in Geneva and Paul Broca maintained in France. One group in Turin centered around Jacob Moleschott and Filippo de Filippi. Moleschott, like Carl Vogt in Geneva was a "scientific materialist." He was a lecturer in the University of Turin and an active member of the Turin government.[7] De Filippi, a professor of zoology at the University of Turin, had just published a long discussion of the place of the human in nature, insisting that many new paleontological facts had been produced to support "the great general inductions of Darwin's theory," although he retained his religious beliefs and separated the "Human Kingdom" from other living organisms.[8]

The physiologist Schiff with his student Alexander Herzen Jr. recognized the importance of Darwin's work in the early 1860s.[9] Most importantly, there was Paolo Mantegazza, soon to be, like Royer, a member of the Société d'Anthropologie de Paris. He became an enthusiastic Darwinist, especially after the publication of Darwin's *The Descent of Man* and *Expression of the Emotions in Man and Animals* in the early 1870s, and corresponded with Darwin about the importance of these studies to his own work.[10] Over the next twenty years he would establish his name as a republican politician and anthropologist and develop a personal friendship with Paul Broca and Charles Letourneau.[11]

The Italian translators of Darwin, Giovanni Canestrini and Leonardo Salimbeni, were less friendly to Royer. They had deplored the errors of her French translation in a preface to the first Italian edition of the *Origin,* published in 1864, faulting it for being "in many points erroneous and generally too free and imprecise" and adding that in their own (short) preface they would refrain from adding "untimely annotations" to Darwin's theory.[12] The French translation, however, served as an important source for their own translation, and they preserved some of her word usages, and even her errors, as Pancaldi has shown.[13] Their translation was, therefore, probably made from French to Italian and not directly from the English.

In 1864, Frances Power Cobbe and her English and Italian friends began a campaign in Florence against Schiff's physiological experiments, which included vivisection. Cobbe, voicing her opposition to his physiological work, identified Schiff as a "red" republican. The Italian nobility joined her, for political as well as humanitarian reasons.[14] The nature of the debate, just before Royer and Duprat arrived, centered around Schiff's use of a number of species of animals in his laboratory. Among the English colony, even the aging Mary Somerville lent her name to the campaign against Schiff. She was joined by Walter Savage Landor, known best now for his portraits of noble dogs. He had been, in his earlier years, an enthusiastic believer in tyrannicide, but apparently drew the line at the willful deaths of dogs and cats.[15] Eventually such attacks would drive Schiff and his disciple, Alexander Herzen Jr., from Florence back to Geneva. Royer would soon make a subtle endorsement of Schiff against the antivivisectionists by citing his research in her book on human evolution, published a few years later.[16]

There were a number of republican and nationalist women's groups in Florence at the time,[17] but Royer may not have been in complete sympathy with them for political, religious, and personal reasons, complicated by an advanced pregnancy. Like the Italian republican women, Royer had depicted motherhood as equivalent to military service even before her own experience of childbirth. She thought that the state should honor women's fertility whether it resulted from a legal union or not. A woman should, in turn, recognize that her task was to give the state "citizens to defend it, to raise them seriously, strongly, sensibly as well as lovingly, to free herself from sectarian prejudices instead of inculcating them, and to instruct herself in order to direct their education."[18]

In Florence, a city in which Renaissance art and architecture was the most vital feature, even this nearsighted young woman who had claimed an immunity to art felt herself moved. For the first time Royer saw art as something of social importance. Surrounded by large and dramatic sculpture and enormous murals, she began to see painting and sculpture as another version of drama, depicting suffering and other human emotions. "Pity is a sentiment so profoundly, so anciently rooted in man that it has become for him the source of the most fecund of his aesthetic pleasures."[19] She had remarked on the boldness of early Renaissance art, which didn't scruple to visualize God's creation of the human race as similar to childbirth. She described one of the frescoes over the Campo Santo in Pisa, in which God was represented extracting Eve from Adam's opened side "like a midwife delivering a newborn foetus."[20]

In Florence Royer and Duprat's only son, René, was born on 12 March 1866.[21] Years later a biographer, who appears to have known the couple, commented on Royer's recollection of her life in Florence as a radiant period.[22] The lovers had rented a large room in the Villa Morelli, which Royer had divided into a multiplicity of smaller rooms by means of blue curtains. This turned one huge room into living room, bedroom, dining room, nursery, and a small place in which she could write. Royer was a devoted mother, and many observations about newborn and young children crept into her book on the origin of human society (*L'Origine de l'homme et des sociétés*) that she had begun to write.

She may have found childbirth quite traumatic and unexpected. Later she wrote, "Maternity! Do women even know what it is until they are wives? It is for them up to the day of delivery a terrible, unknown, frightening thing, since they simply know that it might result in their death."[23] Young women, she added, are so ignorant that, should she find herself taken by surprise by her labor and deliver her child alone, it would be "without even knowing that she must hasten to tie off the cord that attaches it to her entrails."[24] She deplored the lack of knowledge about the care of a newborn child. It must have troubled her that her son, recognized by his father by Italian law, which placed both parents on the birth certificate regardless of marital status, could never inherit from him because of the harsh discrimination of French law against illegitimate children.[25] A strong argument on behalf of women and illegitimate children was put forward in the Italian parliament in Florence at that time; a number of republicans spoke in support of women's rights, of the need to secure parental inheritance for illegitimate offspring, and of the legal right of children to investigate their paternity. It must have pleased her to hear arguments on behalf of women placed before the Italian parliament that echoed the laws proposed in her novel.[26]

Royer was surprised to find, contrary to what she had been led to believe, that the love between a man and woman might be strengthened when the woman became pregnant. Rousseau, she decided, must be wrong when he thought that in primitive times men and women met only to satisfy their appetites. On the contrary, she said, humanity was able to perpetuate itself only because of a passionate instinct "that attaches a man to the woman who carries in her womb the fruit of their union."[27] In turn, the pregnant woman will "follow him, help him, and even serve him rather than abandon him, whether from fear or affection." The two parents are also held together by the love for their children, for whom they have "an instinctive, natural, blind, and unreflecting love stronger than all their other passions, more violent than all their other appetites, more clairvoyant than all their other instincts."[28]

She contemplated human origins and simian ancestry as she observed the development of her young son. Watching her child grasp for things both as he tried to stand and as he developed intellectually, she argued that not only had the hand and the brain of humans developed together, but that both hand and brain could have developed only at the same time as the foot became adapted for walking.

She also argued that the father or some adult male was necessary for young mothers and children in the savage state, even more than in civilization. At least in the modern state it was possible for a widow to survive and raise young children. She visualized the unlikely survival of a young mother in the primitive world if abandoned alone in the wilderness with three or four young children trailing after her. Since the mother had to stay with them at night, possibly in some cave while wild beasts roamed outside, she would have to abandon them during the day to seek food. Her food could be taken from her by hundreds of rivals, anyone better armed than she, even by the man who had fathered the children. She considered the possibility of the survival of such a human family to be so absurd that it was not worth considering. The protection of the young family by a male was an absolute necessity, even if this protection was bought at the cost of paternal tyranny.[29]

Royer's comments on the acquisition of language appear to reflect her observations of her own child's development. Although the popular linguistic analysis of the time insisted that words were at first very specific and referred to local events and were then generalized, she thought children's language began more generally and was only slowly applied to specific cases. A child who said the word "dog" indicated only by voice inflection whether he meant "I like that dog" or "I am afraid of that dog." A child, she observed, often spoke for the pleasure of hearing himself talk, sometimes talking to himself for hours together "without attaching clear ideas about what he says; but always the accent of his voice, if not the sequence of his words, faithfully renders the state of his mind and the nature of his feelings and emotions, like expressive music."[30] She even argued from her experience and her observation of other European children that the change of hair color from blond to dark brown, as the child grew older, might indicate a descent from light-haired people.[31]

The aim of her new book went further than echoing her own insights. She wanted to draw out the consequences of human evolution from both Darwinian evolution and social science. She saw "intellectual and passionate activity" as a need for truth that required "scientific methods to be satisfied." This need had become as essential for civilized humanity as the need of the oyster to be "caressed by the sea twice a day."[32] However, objectivity in viewing the human being was hard to achieve, "because this is the only [situation] in which the thinking subject confronts the thinking object. . . . To study humanity best, it would be necessary to cease to belong to it."[33] She was soon to make a similar argument about the study of women.

Now the mother of a young infant, she soon found herself embroiled in a bitter exchange with a former acquaintance, the Swiss theologian and philosopher Ernest Naville, over the eugenic claims of her first Darwin preface.

Previously, objections had arisen primarily from Catholic clerics. A friend alerted her that an article by Naville, drawn from his course on moral philosophy at the University of Geneva, had appeared in the Swiss journal *Revue Chrétienne* in 1867, referring to Royer's Darwin preface without naming her.[34]

Naville began by a discussion of "ancient socialism," which wanted to "suppress the family" and which permitted the destruction of infants who "did not promise to be strong citizens." He continued: "A modern theory has furnished us the same instruction. This has been deduced from the system of Darwin, whom we in no way hold responsible for it. The preface of the French translation of the English naturalist's work informs us that the discovery of 'élection naturelle' changes the foundations of morality."[35] Noting rather indignantly that Royer—who was not directly identified by name—had placed the moral rule for the human being "on a level with that of the rabbit and the caterpillar," he added that, "the author, who does not recoil before the consequences of these ideas, insinuates that it would be opportune to care less for the sick in the hospitals and to allow a few more weak infants to die."[36] To illustrate his point he quoted sections from her first preface at length.

Royer was stung by this article. Having changed her mind about the elimination of the weak, and perhaps because of her heightened maternal feeling, she responded on 17 February 1867 with a letter to the editor of the *Revue Chrétienne,* which was subsequently published in that journal.[37] She quoted Naville's remarks and asked the readers to judge. She referred to the pages from her second "edition of 1865" [*sic*] for "those of your subscribers who do not feel disposed to accord to the Genevan apostle the infallibility that they so rightly refuse to popes."[38] She felt that Naville had quoted her unfairly by not using the latest version of her preface and asked, since Naville recoiled with such horror at these ideas about the cruelty of nature, why he did not recoil with an equal horror at "that dogma of predestination that refuses eternal life to a great majority of unhappy humans. . . . " She suggested that "this law of divine election" alone should "permit me to find that the law of natural election [natural selection] is incomparably gentler in spite of its very evident severities."[39] Echoing Huxley's words to Wilberforce, as she had in her preface to Darwin's *Origin,* she added that she regretted "to see men of such incontestable talent employ the resources of their ingenious mind to disfigure the thought of those who have consecrated their life to the search for truth, the most immortal of the gods."[40]

Naville's answer was short and to the point. He had just obtained the second French edition of Darwin and checked the passage of the preface that he had cited. Although the first preface was the only edition in print at the time he had given his lectures, he complimented her on the wise modifications made in her second edition. He reprinted at length the passage that had been omitted from the new version of her preface and in which she referred to "those beings, incapable of living on their own, weighing upon healthy arms as burdens to themselves and others, who take up more places in the sun than three well-constituted individuals." Interested readers, he added, might note variations she had introduced into her preface in the second edition, not only in the section he had cited but in the preceding pages, "in order to know the most recent expression of the ideas of the author."[41] He insisted that his judgment had been made on the first edition, not the second. It was an "inadmissible procedure" to judge his interpretation of a particular edition by studying "*another text*" (Naville's italics). He added with heavy sarcasm that he did not believe it appropriate to discuss in reply "predestination, theologians, apostles, the infallibility of the pope, and the friends of immortal truth."[42]

As far as Royer was concerned, this was not the end of the debate. She wrote a lengthy letter to Naville, never printed but preserved among Naville's papers.[43] This is a surprising letter from Royer because of its unusually aggressive tone. She repudiated any intention of expounding "a harsh social law" for the unfortunate and ill. She had consulted only the second edition of her preface in her earlier reply, she said, because she did not bring a copy of the first edition with her from Paris, "not presuming that you would search for an excuse within the slight differences of the two editions, which *differ only in form and not at all in content*" (italics mine).[44] If she had eliminated "one or two amplifications," these were only stylistic corrections and not fundamental points. She insisted that neither edition legitimated his interpretations. It was only fair, she thought, to refer to her most recent edition as her definitive opinion. She had not only the right but the duty to answer attacks when they concerned "the moral honor of the doctrine which they represent. . . . I can therefore only insist on the letter that you have asked me to suppress. If you regret seeing this develop into a personal debate, then you have no other choice than to confess to your readers that you have done me the wrong of not only having not read my second edition but of having not even read the first."[45] Had he only been repeating "the accusations of some unknown critic or of an obscure journalist perhaps whom I could have ignored or whose judgement I could have ignored," then his errors—or, as she said, "your sin"—might still be prejudiced, "but it would not be yours." Replying to Naville's comment of the "charitable sorrow" with which he viewed her remarks, she said that "I have for [your errors] an indulgence even more charitable. In my eyes a man can perhaps be guilty of making a mistake, [but] I am astonished to see a man of your intelligence and your knowledge in the ranks of the adversaries of free reason and unprejudiced science."

Royer then spoke of human intellectual varieties by which, she said, humanity "in its progressive evolution was represented." She compared Naville's dogma to "the blind violence of fixed and acquired instincts." He had acted "like an ant, defending the subterranean constructions of his republic thrown into peril by some indomitable enemy. . . ." Not only were religious passions instinctive but, like other passions, they could easily become excessive. She approved of the positive aspects of religious emotions, admitting them to be "powerful instincts designed to produce an equilibrium among other passions." As a sort of backhanded compliment to Naville, she expressed her belief that "the force of religious hereditary instinct so powerful in the old Genevan race will not go so far as to abort or falsify your moral judgment." She was willing to give him an opportunity to publicize his protest against the dogma of predestination by continuing her "struggle with the *Revue Chrétienne.*" Replying to his remark that she had adopted a doctrine that left her "no gentle illusions," she suggested that such a term ought not to be coming from the pen of "an orator of eternal life." "No illusions are without danger," she added. Even if they seemed comforting they could produce cruel deceptions. Shouldn't he be concerned that he, on his side, was propagating "deceptive illusions"? She ended her letter with a suggestion that the "wisest position" would be to establish a new morality by attempting to "establish on earth through our laws and our customs an image as close as possible to the justice that our conscience seeks to find." She would continue, she said, to search for a morality, based on science. Ending her letter with a paean to this future morality, she signed her letter only with her name without the usual polite closing salutation. Naville, not surprisingly, refused to continue the debate with this woman who was apparently more anxious to convert him than he was to convert her.[46]

Royer had adopted a rather strident tone in this letter. Why was she so unwilling to recognize her changed views about harsh social attitudes towards the weak and malformed? Perhaps she was reacting with some mild depression at finding herself tied down to a household and a young child. Considering the strong link between her experiences and her choice of topic, a piece she wrote for the *Revue Moderne* soon after her letter to Naville was published may be an indication of some strong emotional concerns. For a woman who had admitted to have a very limited response to art it was also an unusual subject. In "La Tristesse de l'art" she emphasizes that pity as well as sadness were motivating factors in artistic expression. Although the topic gives evidence of her reaction to the powerful Italian artistic environment, she expressed her fears that the excitation of pity and sorrow produced by art might result in a "sapping of the will."[47] She picked up this theme in her new book, expressing the fear that human beings forced to respond to imaginative images might find their ability to act compromised or weakened when they observed real social evils. "If all human pity is confined to compassion for imaginary evils that our artists present us, . . . humanity . . . dried at its source will not be long in falling into depression [*langueur*] and perishing."[48]

Royer was no longer a free agent, in spite of her earlier emphasis on the necessity of motherhood. But she could write, and she was soon projecting her own experience onto primitive society. In her book on human society, *L'Origine de l'homme et des sociétés,* she observed that women and men could share the same pursuits only when they had little to encumber them. Once women had to take care of the baggage, "light at first, then more and more heavy," and watch the provisions, the tools, and the utensils, a division of work occurred. Even if women were at first as strong and agile and capable for the hunt as men, "after being hampered by the duties of motherhood, in charge of her youngest children and the care of others, she became reduced to a fatally subordinate role . . . that is to say, the carrier of burdens in the migrations and the guardian of baggage in the encampments."[49] Royer exorcized some of these feelings of being burdened by motherhood in the book that she now began to write.

Royer vividly conveyed a sense of her changed social role in her discussion of changing male and female roles, as she had previously questioned the possibility of role reversals in articles on the fabled Amazons.[50] Her comments echo in an interesting manner her discussion of these roles in both her novel and in her Darwin prefaces, in which she extended Darwin's ideas of sexual selection that he had not yet fully detailed in his own book on human evolution, *The Descent of Man,* published in 1871.[51] Speaking of primitive man, she commented: "When the sexes are equal in strength, the choice is generally reciprocal, and one observes little difference with respect to the physical and intellectual attributes of male and female with respect to their clothing or their instincts. Rather, one observes that with equality of strength the advantage rests with the female. . . . The man who is quarrelsome and a warrior is in general stronger than the woman. One can induce from known facts that woman was always more or less dominated, taken or given, but always chosen with some discernment, and to this choice in sexual selection she owes the finesse and superiority of her form and her beauty. . . ." But she goes on to say that "if in certain races the type of man has progressed and become refined, polished, and gentled, it can be explained only by the greater or lesser liberty that women had in these races to chose the progenitor of their children."[52]

Admitting that in modern times the two sexes had to some extent different physical and mental aptitudes and functions, Royer insisted there was nothing fatal or absolute about this (390). It was even likely that in earlier periods the anthropoid male nursed the child also, although the mammary glands had become reabsorbed. She thought that the subordination of woman had become destructive to those human groups where it continued. "The current relationship of the sexes could alter more or less profoundly in the future to the point of becoming reversed under the influence of contrary laws," Royer remarked (390). She wondered whether it would be useful for men and women to reverse their social roles. Although uncertain what society would gain from this, she was intrigued by the possibility of a "more efficient use of human capital" that might result in the development of female genius. "There would be a chance for a human variety to be formed and to prosper . . . to realize at the top of the animal scale and in the sub-branch of mammals the same marvels of female genius that in no way astonish us among the insects and that we find completely natural among the bees and ants" (381). Royer's image of female genius inevitably evokes both her own discussion of women's genius in her first essay on science and the later fictionalization of a totally female society along the lines of insect society by Charlotte Perkins Gilman in her novel *Herland*.[53]

Rousseau had proposed that originally there was sexual promiscuity among humans. Royer denied this and argued that this occurred only with the arrival of civilization. It could not even be shown in animals, she argued, nor was it to be confused with periods of rut that resulted in fertilization.[54] Humans and other primates were not subject to periodic ruts but could conceive throughout the year, a phenomenon linked to female menstruation. "Excess of sexual ardor," on the other hand, resulted in sterility, as she and many medical men of her day believed prostitution demonstrated. Where promiscuity existed, as was reported in Oceania, she believed it occured under special circumstances, as a method of birth control in an area where otherwise there would be a superabundance of children (376–377). She was convinced that only a durable relationship between male and female could result in the successful raising of children.

Royer insisted that if the human species was to continue it had to rely upon solid instincts instead of some "vague and general sense of need to conserve the family." The human species, she argued, would have been quickly eliminated "if a sentiment as impetuous as a need did not push [the man] to unite himself to a companion and to feel himself inspired with an affection and a passion durable enough to continue after the birth of the children (383)."

Only by improving the social situation of women could one reduce the necessity for the traditional marriage. "The essential condition for equilibrium of a social state in which the father did not know his children and in which a mother alone could be charged with nourishing and protecting the children would be for women to be endowed with mental and physical faculties superior or at least equal to man so they would be capable of filling all the lucrative positions today reserved for men" (383).

She tried to analyze the differences in aptitude and function between "the two halves of humanity," man and woman. Her later claim that sexuality itself was a contingent part of reproduction echoed her claim that male dominance was a contingent law. "One could affirm today that the subjection of woman to man has become harmful in human societies in which it is perpetuated, [although] it was useful in the early development of human races." Any nation that would improve woman's position would experience a great social advantage. "People among whom woman recovers her liberty, her faculty to freely progress, will be carried forward in the vital struggle [*lutte vitale*] over all others to the extent of forcing them to reform their customs under pain of rapidly disappearing from the surface of the globe" (391).

Royer's view of the rise of society admits an initial patriarchal tyranny and reads like a description of her father during his paranoid period towards the end of his life. A former warrior turns his despotic and quarrelsome nature upon his wife and children. "We find in this [behavior] all the primitive elements of that paternal tyranny that—although beneficial relative to conditions of human life in the period when it developed—in later eras has retarded the progress of humanity. . . . The authority that the male exerts over the female quickly becomes abusive and is extended to the children. Once established over the child it tends to become invincible by virtue of the general law of instinctive and passionate accumulation and is perpetuated by the adult male" (549–550). Paternal tyranny continued in the form of the chief's authority and explained the rise of tyranny even in advanced societies. Later there was a growing reaction against social tyranny in all civilized cities, in which wives challenged their husbands' despotism, children questioned their parents, and young girls insisted on independence.

She reiterated her feeling that divorce was a necessity and that the mother must have rights over the child and the child's education. "Urban customs inevitably tend to make the conjugal union dissolvable and temporary, to make the rights of spouses equal before the law, to produce a predominance of maternal influence in the education of children. . . ." And the tendency is stronger, even irresistible, because it is manifested in spite of all laws, all contrary traditions" (516).

It is amazing that along with Royer's interest and involvement in the life of her developing child and the demands made upon her she continued to produce so much written material. Not only was Royer hard at work on her book on human and social origins, announced five years earlier in her first preface to her Darwin translation, but she collaborated on Charles Dollfus's journal *Revue Germanique,* later the *Revue Moderne,* for which Marie d'Agoult had been a financial underwriter.[55] She also served as one of the organizers of Charles Letourneau and Gabriel de Mortillet's scientific materialist journal *Pensée Nouvelle.*[56] She was to retain her close ties to both scientific positivists and the materialists who had formed a strong alliance within the Société d'Anthropologie.[57] She also finished a three-part analysis on Lamarck, one of the first attempts to systematically reconsider his evolutionary ideas. This appeared in 1868 and the beginning of 1869 in the scientific positivist journal *La Philosophie Positive,* edited by two important figures, the positivist Émile Littré and the crystallographer G. Wyrouboff.[58] In this three-part article, she countered the common misconception that Lamarck's theory proposed a direct transformation of one form into another. The problem, she explained, was that Lamarck used poor examples to illustrate his meaning, with the consequence that his concepts were ambiguous and therefore misunderstood. She deplored that he had not known the economic theorists of his time, especially Malthus, in order to give a basis to his theories, as Darwin had done.

Royer's interest in a materialist explanation of matter and life was highlighted in her book on human origins, *L'Origine de l'homme et des sociétés.* Published on 15 September 1869—because of some delay many copies bear a 1870 date—her book on human society placed Royer's concept of evolution on the firm basis of scientific materialism, although she was later to deny that she was a materialist. "If matter can move itself, act by itself, why could it not organize itself, live and think? The hypothesis of a creation *ex abrupto ex nihilo* [abruptly out of nothing] of each of its living forms was previously recognized impossible, contradictory, unimaginable. How could these forms then appear?" she asked. "Not only our ancient metaphysics, which has encumbered the avenues of human knowledge, but our physics itself has for a long time participated in our errors. Up until a recent epoch we have held as a scientific dogma—and all our elementary treatises, even the best, still carry it written on their first pages—that matter is inert, inactive, and immobile and that forces whose intensity we measure act on it from the outside. All our past errors in physiology derive from this first error."[59] Royer insisted on the inherent activity of matter. "Each of its atoms moves and moves other atoms by its endless reactions. The forces that we have believed to be outside it are in it, are inherent in it, being only the manifestation, quality, essence, and being of it. Force, mind, and life are of the same earthly substance; intelligence and thought are only phenomena, of the same kind as extension, impenetrability, and movement." She cited the experiments of Dr. Schiff that gave "the heat equivalence of the work of thought."[60]

Anticipating her later insistence on conciousness as a basic aspect of matter, she added: "Inorganic matter moves, acts, and from the moment that it is organized, it lives, it feels, it thinks. Let us investigate through what evolutionary phases it has passed to arrive at the production of this still imperfect instrument of knowledge that we call the human mind. Let us investigate how life has been able to appear upon our globe."[61] The debate between heterogenists and panspermists was insoluble, she declared, because it was posed in insoluble terms, since the current conditions on the earth were not the same meteorological, physical, chemical, or cosmic conditions that existed on the surface of the planet when life first appeared. In order to demonstrate this, she assumed an early period of the planet with an incandescent and hot core. She detailed geological sequences, beginning with a weak crust of lava, still burning, waves of minerals, oceans of liquefied minerals, an immense atmosphere surrounded by gases, with water vapors and all kinds of chemical elements combining and destroying each other. As the oceans appear, she assumes them to be saturated with salts and acids, which "produce and destroy a great many births and creations, finally resulting in warm waters, which, when electricity passes over them, produce a germ of life everywhere, an immense effluvia with vast organic crystallizations. . . . This was amorphous, hideous, but powerful. These were spheres and lines, links branching into links, a mad arborescence. It was organization searching form, life in quest of its law."[62]

When living organisms finally did arise, she wrote, echoing Robert Chambers's view of early life, "their birth was a spontaneous germination, their life a vegetative crystallization. Like mineral matter they had not learned yet to move."[63] She described these early prelife forms as "covering the oceans like a living crust. [They] soon began to lack space and nutrition and as a result disintegrated and were succeeded by other beings equally monstrous and ephemeral, existing only as floating cellular masses. The aggregations, once they are destroyed and disappear, appear no more."[64]

In the midst of these spontaneous attempts, which continue during an indefinite length of time until the atmosphere is "purified of its vapors and the seas of their acidity," Royer speculated, a very small number of germs begin "to realize the start of a vegetative regularity following an already defined plan, and these alone, operating according to a regular law, furnish the sources of all other beings, which generation upon generation are transformed and slowly progress by a series of successive and divergent variations until they have sent their last representative through the successive ages of our globe."[65]

She insisted on the multiplicity of early forms that entered into intense competition with each other, leaving perhaps six or seven prototypes that would evolve in a parallel manner.[66] Upon her return to France, she would soon find herself surrounded by members of the Société d'Anthropologie dedicated to the concept of the multiple origin of human races, who would endorse this kind of "polygenist evolution" stemming from an initial abiogenesis or at least from unorganized organic matter.[67] She would, however, be challenged by Armand de Quatrefages, who believed her description of life developing from multiple prototypes put her in conflict with Darwin.

Royer also maintained that "thought is virtually like life in every germ of being, however inferior it may be." She described these "thinking and living atoms," which became increasingly hierarchical and centralized "by progressively augmenting the intensity of their mental power and allowing it to pass from potential to action," an idea that echoes the scientific materialist belief in life as a form of energized matter.[68] She continued this analysis by a discussion of intelligence as an energized form of sensation, since thought, in her opinion, could not exist without passion. In a charming passage, she described the child in the womb as having only vague sensations and being kept from direct reactions to an environment that, after birth, causes pain but also allows children to develop their potential intelligence.[69] Many years later she would speak of the "egotistic atom," a variant of Haeckel's term "cell-soul,"[70] but even in this earlier period she emphasized an inherent psychological aspect of matter that might explain both differences and similarities between humans and animals.

The isolated human being never existed, she proclaimed, because it was not possible for human beings to survive outside collectivities, in hordes or tribes.[71] She relied on contemporary reports on the comparative abilities not only of humans and nonhumans but of "primitives" and Europeans, and drew on the work of John Lubbock, E. B. Tyler, and many others. She objected to Rousseau, whom she thought glorified the "natural man." Much of the beginning and final chapters of her book on human origins serve as a critique of Rousseau, so beloved of Ernest Naville and the other Genevan and Lausanne philosophers.[72]

Royer's particular quarrel with Rousseau derived from the misogyny of the great thinker. She and her feminist friends in Paris in the late 1850s had attacked Proudhon for similar reasons. All men might be equal in Rousseau's view, she noted, but women were meant to serve them as a sort of "animated womb." She added, "If woman has no right to this equality, to [Rousseau's] equivalence, it is because as a complement to man, pulled from his flank to serve him, to please him, to procreate for him, she is a sort of animated womb, an alternating germ destined to reproduce, having a purpose only in him. She must forever serve this master to whom she has been given by a primitive divine act to be used or abused at his will. That is what woman is for Rousseau in spite of some fugitive excesses of sentiment and poetic passion. . . ."[73]

She thought that social tyrannies derived from early patriarchal authority and advocated a development towards matriarchy. Socially she endorsed the initial liberty of individuals. Constant competition between them produced hierarchies and provided a wealth of different kinds of labor, a concept that she may have formed not only from her knowledge of the economists but from Spencer's view of increasing heterogeneity or specialization at both cellular and social levels.[74]

Happily, she added, the study of humanity was now based on science, which no longer included preconceptions but "real, visible, palpable facts, verifiable for all, which on every principal question lead every logical mind, free of prejudice, to the same solutions."[75] It was necessary to reconstruct the history of humanity in the primitive era in order "to formulate the law of its development."[76]

She tried to rethink Rousseau's view of the relationship of the two sexes. "Love is, therefore, far from being an invention of women, as Rousseau affirms, since from the first it has been used as often against them as for them. If it assures for all time the protection of a man's arms, it places [women] under his fist, which weighs on them with a weight so crushing that it can stop and arrest in them that development, that progress of the faculties, that has been demonstrated in such a remarkable fashion in man."[77]

Rousseau had also misjudged the role of science and art in society. "If Rousseau had, like his rivals, the Encyclopedists, been nourished from an early age on classical literature, if he had encountered Lucretius and Lucan,

Cicero and Tacitus, Montaigne and Descartes before the Bible, if he had belonged to the French bourgeoisie of the eighteenth century, which was aware of art, science, liberty, and progress, instead of coming from the bosom of Calvinist Geneva, his mind would have been different."[78] She ended her discussion of Rousseau with a paean to the nonequality of humans, which had produced "equality of liberty and progress by inequality."[79]

The destruction of privilege was not identical with Rousseau's (or Proudhon's) call for social equality, which she saw as opposed to both liberty and freedom of action. "What is this right? Is it savage equality, the specific equality of the animal, equality in poverty and abasement? Or is it only the initial equality of liberty, permitting each individual to develop his faculties to exercise his activity and his special aptitudes under the law of a free competition, giving each individual a right that is proportional to his strength . . . the liberty to become, according to his responsibility, what he has the strength to be?"[80]

The development of fixed social castes originated, she asserted, as a method of trying to insure that professional skills did not become washed out by the introduction of many new aptitudes. In a strongly Lamarckian appeal to heredity, she added that this protectionism within trades and guilds explained why in the past it was necessary to marry within closed castes. However, this created a problem. Intelligence, in order to progress, could not become routinized and instinctive. Occasional inventive intelligences had to arise within a caste. Her argument, she believed, supported the claim that natural human inequalities resulted in a division of labor. If at first only the castes of priest or shepherd existed, later it would become advantageous for society to add a warrior caste, as she supposed the "primitive Aryans" would have recognized. Warriors then took over as the dominant caste, but over time the priestly caste dominated in turn.[81]

While she recognized that castes might be useful at first for quickly accomplishing movement, they then become "a scourge that retards its development."[82] The Graeco-Roman world had broken down caste systems, but after the destruction of Rome the old caste system returned. Perhaps referring to Duprat's endorsement of revolution, she suggested that the French Revolution was always "the *Revolution* among all revolutions and reforms" because "on August fourth it finished what had already begun, to put an end to the old regime of privileged castes."[83]

Royer ended with an endorsement of colonization as a social good if it was disinterested and spread civilization, a common theme of the republican colonialists of her day. She attacked war between civilized nations as evil, since it destroyed important elements in society. The elimination of any human variety was evil in itself, except for "poorly endowed individuals or the destruction of inferior races that retard the average condition of the species to the harm of varieties superior in some way."[84] Even while extolling colonial wars, she hesitated to suggest that any human group should be eliminated. On the contrary, "other human varieties" might prove necessary for colonization. It might be advantageous that they "fulfill social functions of which our race is incapable." But, echoing Gobineau and Renan, she thought that, unless it served a specific purpose, the mixing of inferior and superior races was "immoral" since it could result in a lessening of a superior race, even more immoral than crossing a species line.[85] However, she did go on to decry wars as an example of the misuse of "the warrior instinct" used against humanity. Such "selective action" acted on unequal individuals in the same group and tended to make those individuals that were "retarded in the development of all their faculties" disappear. She may have rethought this attitude, as Clemenceau would do following the Franco-Prussian war, after hearing the arguments of Germans "drawn from a misreading of Darwin" that they had beaten the French because they were a superior race. This, said Clemenceau, had made him "look twice before turning towards a man or a civilisation and pronouncing: inferior man or civilisation."[86]

It might be possible, she suggested, to retain "inferior races" if only to "mix their blood with ours in a proportion just sufficient to give to the mixed race that results the physical qualities and faculties that we lack." However, echoing the fears of her time, she asserted that "the repugnance of mixing of blood is manifest in superior races and in females more than males."[87] Crosses that did exist, she stated, unless they were the result of violence, were of white men and black, Indian, or Australian women, but she did not mention the possibility of violence by white colonial men against these women. Royer extolled the intelligence of "a Descartes, a Newton, a Goethe, or a Lavoisier" as far superior to the intelligence of a Bushman or a Papuan. In her description of the tree of evolution, the white race was at the peak, overshadowing all other "inferior branches," much as Haeckel had recently drawn these trees.[88]

Nevertheless, she did not claim, as some of her contemporaries did, that some races were infertile when crossbreeding with each other. She recognized that existing races were fertile between themselves. Why were they not fertile when mating with the closest anthropoid apes? Because, she asserted, there had been a "prompt destruction of all the primitive forms of two-handed anthropoids who . . . might have remained fertile with them."[89] She hesitated before the possibility of modern civilized man interbreeding with "savage races," which might produce a retrograde race with diminished "intellectual reaction over instinctive faculties."[90]

In spite of a warning against those who had created "the mothers of dangerous utopias," she dreamed of the creation of a new human race with the same ambivalence that Tennyson expressed in his poem "Locksley Hall." She ended her book with an evocation of a future when, animal having given birth to man, man [*sic*] could "give birth to the divine race that will govern the earth with justice in joy and peace."[91] Royer was to expand her ideas further in

1870 upon her return to Paris, when she entered the Société d'Anthropologie de Paris.

Duprat, on his side, had begun to develop his former "1848" beliefs, which endorsed the role of revolution as a positive force in the life of societies. He wrote a book, *The Spirit of Revolutions* (*L'Esprit des révolutions),* prefacing it with a paragraph addressed to "La Jeunesse française."[92] This address, dated 19 February 1868, reads like a greeting to his nearly two-year-old son as well as a call to Young France.

> You will succeed in our struggles and you will continue our efforts for the freeing of humanity. The evil of the times will push you, perhaps, as it has us, into the melee of revolution, which is always full of perils. May you come out of it victorious and, following your victory to the applause of the world, found a government of total rights and liberties. If fortune vanquishes you, carry your wounds proudly. Never bend your head before despotism and always keep in your heart, as within an impregnable fortress, the sacred cult of justice.[93]

There is a tension between Royer and Duprat's support of political revolution (as long as it did not go too far) and the advocacy of colonial expansion. This is a tension to be found in many contemporary writers. Contradictions in the thinking of both Royer and Duprat were to be emphasized vividly during the period of the Paris Commune and the early years of the Third Republic.

Royer had a growing regret about the loss of her freedom to pass easily from one city or country to another. She was no longer free to lecture throughout Italy, nor could she follow Duprat when he left Florence at the end of 1868 to report on the Spanish revolution for the *Journal des Économistes.*[94] Duprat was exploring a new and exciting period in Europe. He had gone to Spain at the end of 1868 upon the outbreak of revolution there and had written an open letter to his friend Joseph Garnier at the *Journal des Économistes* that reflected a heightened enthusiasm about changes and possibilities. Whether the revolution was successful or aborted, he had no doubt about the future. He had seen in Italy, Hungary, Germany, "even in that England formerly so linked to its tradition: old Europe is going, it is dying."[95] Duprat had already returned briefly to Paris, to a liberalized France under the new prime minister Émile Ollivier. He had put up his name for election to the Chamber of Deputies in the spring of 1868 and again in November of that year, but neither campaign was successful.[96]

While Royer may have found the quiet period useful for finishing her articles and her book on human evolution, she clearly missed her former freedom. In the section of her book that discussed the changed life of woman hunters and warriors compelled to live a "pastoral" life among children and animals, she describes in vivid terms a woman's isolation and sedentary existence. In her new condition, she remarked, a woman had to assist and support her man instead of working as an equal with him.

> So the woman, the moment she is condemned to a life more sedentary than the man, starts to lose her strength and her agility and acquires more skill in those manual labors committed solely to her care. She loses all initiative, seeing her courage diminish, and her nomadic and warrior instincts disappear in a calmer, more retiring, more fearful life. [She lives] entirely on the defensive towards other species or tribes and in passive subordination to the man, whose plans or projects she must second, since her life and that of her children depend on his success. But she acquires in contrast more gentle and affectionate instincts in the exclusive society of her children or young animals, which she learns to tame. By transforming her hunting instincts into pastoral ones under the impulse of need . . . [she] sees in [these young animals] either a resource for the days of famine or a distraction in the long boredom of her enforced and often perilous solitude.[97]

For all her efforts to balance positive and negative features in such a life, the sense of loss of freedom is strong in this passage.

Royer's description of a woman left alone to guard a young child carried with it a quiet warning, which Duprat may have read and understood. In a later passage, describing the urbanized woman, she added: "The young girl who once has lived an individual life, who has known independence, has felt its responsibilities, will no longer be easily conquered, absorbed, dominated. She has a more or less lively sense of her rights and her dignity, and if the husband that she has freely chosen oppresses her, she will quit him for another."[98]

In late 1868 and early 1869, while finishing her new book on human social evolution, Royer began to consider a new edition of her Darwin translation in order to raise money for the household. She had not heard from Darwin for some years. He had turned to a Swiss translator for *Variation of Animals and Plants under Domestication* (1868) at Carl Vogt's suggestion. As she read that book, Royer reacted strongly against Darwin's new theory of heredity, pangenesis, described there.

Her negative reaction was strengthened because she had just written a lengthy analysis of what was right (and wrong) in Lamarck's theories.[99] She believed that Darwin exposed himself to the same kind of attack as Lamarck if he produced less rigorous theories. She decided to survey the French response to Darwin and to examine Darwin's new books more carefully before she produced her new translation. Unfortunately, she neglected to write directly to Darwin or to examine his more recent editions, a mistake Darwin would not overlook. How much of this was due to fact that her publisher Guillaumin was no longer alive to supervise the new translation?

In preparation for her third edition of Darwin, Clémence Royer purchased a copy of *Variation of Animals and Plants under Domestication* and went through it with some care to understand the manner in which Darwin had expanded his concept of natural selection.[100] She discarded her foreword to the second edition that had embarrassed Paul Broca but kept the modified version of her first preface, which she retained in subsequent editions. She added a new preface, however, which was to offend Darwin deeply.

Pangenesis had not won whole-hearted support among Darwin's closest associates, not even from his closest friend, Joseph Dalton Hooker.[101] Royer made the enormous error of deciding to make a criticism of this new theory the focal point of her preface. Darwin might have tolerated blasphemy against the church's authority, but he was uncomfortable with her blasphemy against this new and fragile child of his mind. Her decision to introduce this criticism may have been spurred by the arguments of the Italian scientist Federico Delpino, who used pangenesis as a focus for his discussion of vitalistic and teleological ideas in order to rule out materialism, or, as he put it, "monism."[102] Darwin reprinted Delpino's text in English and added his own commentary to it. He was pleased to have pangenesis appreciated by an Italian scientist even though Delpino rejected materialist interpretations of heredity that appeared to require infinite quantities of invisible matter. Darwin's support for Delpino may have been stimulated by his desire to demonstrate that vitalists like Delpino as well as materialists like Ludwig Buechner and Carl Vogt appreciated his ideas.

Royer had written extensively on Lamarck as a forerunner of Darwin. She now claimed that Darwin had fallen into the same trap as Lamarck by venturing out into false theories.[103] "Just as the false notions of Lamarck in physics and meteorology have too often furnished weapons to adversaries of the author of *Philosophie zoologique* that are more passionate than just, so Ch. Darwin's pangenesis has done wrong to his theory of transformation of species by natural selection." She added that readers might think twice about accepting Darwin's excellent evolutionary theory if he insisted on a bad hereditary theory. "There is no lack of those who conclude that the same human brain could scarcely elaborate logically on the basis of known facts such a grand doctrine and trace new roads in biological science while dreaming up an impossible and contradictory hypothesis on the special phenomena of heredity."

Royer went on to question Darwin's knowledge of modern chemistry and physics, saying that his new hypothesis "would make one suppose he is ignorant of the law of the conservation of energy, and Faraday, Wurtz, Mayer, and so many others might never have been born as far as he is concerned."[104] She compared his ideas to those of Bonnet and Buffon and suggested that they were physically impossible, ridiculing the course such particles would have to make throughout the body.

> Like the organic particles of Buffon, they travel undoubtedly in the vital fluids throughout the whole of the organized being, from cell to cell, from fiber to fiber, across solids and liquids, cell walls, and vacuoles. They are so small that nothing stops them on their way. They are less than atoms, perhaps like geometric points, and nothing in the physical world can give us an idea of them. Our imagination, plunging into the infinitely small, must imagine them. Moreover, they are so intelligent, these little germs, that—instead of allowing themselves to be swept outside the organism with all the detritus of vital combustion that it constantly eliminates—they remain forever, heaped up, multiplied infinitely, and yet latent and elusive. They give no sign of life except to produce periodically either buds or normal ovules in the living being that they inhabit in order to fertilize it or, if needed, to reconstruct the cut foot of a salamander or a crayfish or ultimately to reproduce that little piece of skin that, just now, we supposed was lifted up in order to understand the work of reproduction, cell by cell.[105]

There was no possibility, she declared, that one spermatozoid could contain the numerous "germs" that Darwin's theory required. Some of the numbers she cited paralleled Delpino's criticism of pangenesis, which, he had suggested, only a nonmaterialist interpretation could resolve.[106] While Delpino had suggested a vitalistic theory, Royer similarly offered a new theory on behalf of a dynamic materialism. She claimed that she would soon propose a rival theory of "dynamogenesis" that would solve Darwin's dilemma by integrating force (energy) into the theory.[107]

In late September 1869, the Russian translator of Darwin's *Variation of Animals and Plants under Domestication,* the scientist V. O. Kovalevsky, came from Paris to Darwin's house in Down, Kent, to meet Darwin and to discuss his Russian translation, which had just appeared.[108] Uncertain whether a copy of his Russian version would reach Paris in time for him to take to Darwin, it is probable that he brought with him a preprint of Royer's new French edition, which debated Darwin's new theory outlined not in the *Origin* but in *Variation.* Darwin, reading this preface, may have talked to Kovalevsky about it. No matter how accepting Darwin may have been of Royer's earlier commentaries as long as they did not criticize his ideas directly, her frontal attack on himself as a thinker infuriated him. Did he also hear from Kovalevsky, who had recently been living in Naples, the rumors about Royer's irregular union with Duprat and the birth of their child?

Darwin acted quickly. Already convinced that Royer's translation had damaged acceptance of his theory in France, he realized that Royer had made the gross error of not including the corrections and notes added to his last two editions. He began to rethink what Armand de Quatrefages had recently written about Royer's discussion of abiogenesis in his articles on Darwinism,[109] as well as the angry remarks of Claparède six years before. The *Origin* deserved to be translated into French by a naturalist; Darwin wanted a new translator for the *Origin* in France, and now he was given an excuse to obtain one. Reinwald had already published one of his books in France and would surely be willing to produce a new edition of the *Origin of Species* that would eliminate Royer's embarassing prefaces and notes. Perhaps J. J. Moulinié in Geneva, who had translated *Variation* and who had promised to translate his "book on man," could take on this new translation of the latest edition of *Origin* as well.

Seizing his opportunity, Darwin wrote first to the French copublisher, Masson (rather than to Guillaumin and Company, now run by Félicité Guillaumin), expressing his deep annoyance that Royer had overlooked his most recent edition, and hinted that he would take away his authorization. Masson was amazed and annoyed. He responded immediately. The publisher reminded Darwin that this was the first letter he had ever sent directly to the publishing firm. Previously he had always written through an agent. No information about Darwin's latest editions had been provided to them, nor had Royer had any recent communication from Darwin. The publisher hoped that Darwin would do nothing to diminish the value of the edition. Masson assured Darwin that the interests of both the publishing house and Royer were identical with those of Darwin. Mentioning that "Mme Royer" was still in Italy, he added that she had purchased all the new Darwin books she could find to consult them before she produced her new edition. Certainly she would have used the latest English edition had she (or Masson) known it existed. Masson tried to placate Darwin with an offer to publish an appendix at his expense that would include a discussion of points introduced in the later editions that had been ignored. The publisher ended with some sense of his own ruffled feathers, assuring Darwin of the respectability of the publishing house and its high regard within the scientific world.[110]

Darwin had no interest in resolving his differences with Masson or Royer. This was his opportunity to jump, and he took it. He wrote to Moulinié in Geneva, to his English publisher Murray, and to the French publisher Reinwald, inquiring what were the legal ramifications of a new edition published in competition with that of Royer and expressing his desire to have one produced as rapidly as possible.[111] Both Moulinié and Reinwald expressed full willingness to proceed, and Murray wished him the best success in putting down the "Parisian blasphemers."[112]

Darwin was delighted with himself. He triumphantly crowed to Hooker:

> I must enjoy myself and tell you about Madame C. Royer who translated the *Origin* into French and for which 2d edition I took infinite trouble. She has now just brought out a 3d edition without informing me so that all the corrections to the 4th and 5th editions are lost. Be-

> sides her enormously long and blasphemous preface to lst edition she has added a 2d preface abusing me like a pick-pocket for pangenesis which of course has no relation to *Origin.* Her motive being, I believe, because I did not employ her to translate "Domestic animals" [*Variation*]. So I wrote to Paris; & Reinwald agrees to bring out at once a new translation for the 5th English Edition in Competition with her 3e edition—So shall I not serve her well? By the way this fact shows that "evolution of species" must at last be spreading in France.[113]

Hooker responded with a comment that indicates Darwin's resentment against Royer was motivated perhaps as much by the fact that he was attacked by a woman—and a Frenchwoman at that—as by annoyance at the "blasphemous preface" of the first edition, about which he had made little public complaint before. "What a sell for Mlle Royer, serve her right—How nasty women are when spiteful, & French women perhaps the worst in the world."[114]

There was no clear sailing with the new French edition. The Franco-Prussian war interfered, and Moulinié, who was translating both *Descent* and *Origin,* became ill and then died before he could finish his corrections. Reinwald was forced to add an appendix of additions to the sixth English edition that had subsequently appeared. The Reinwald edition finally came out in competition with Royer's translation only in 1873 and sold well, although some scientists in France, such as Paul Broca, still preferred the language of the Royer translation.[115] Darwin, even in the heated period of his negotiation for a new translation of *Origin,* had recommended that Moulinié purchase a copy of the second or third French edition to study Royer's "vigorous style" and French terminology to make his own language consistent with hers.[116] Even Reinwald recognized that Moulinié's translation left something to be desired and had Lubbock's translator, Barbier, rework all of Moulinié's translations, that is, *Variation,* his incomplete *Descent of Man,* and the *Origin of Species.*[117]

Although Darwin cited Royer's *L'Origine de l'homme et des sociétés* only to acknowledge her suggestion that human males may have also suckled children in prehistoric times, he did add terse comments in the margin of his own copy.[118] However, he was interested enough in her comments to head a list of possible sources for a discussion of moral and social evolution with her name and the title of her book in preparation for his own study of human evolution.[119]

Royer was unlucky with her book. Although it was first advertised in late 1869, the uncertainty of the situation in France seems to have delayed the publication of some copies until early 1870, only months before the beginning of the Franco-Prussian war.[120] The outbreak of war was followed by the siege of Paris and the Commune, which severely limited both public attention and sales. As she later noted in her autobiography, "After the war, the work had become antediluvian. Moreover, it was taken for a translation from Darwin's *Descent of Man,* which had since appeared, undoubtedly due to the prejudice of a public for whom the translator of a first work never does more than translations."[121] There were reviews, but these were either unfavorable or printed too late to influence sales.

Possibly with the intention of securing her mother's help with her young child and her household, Royer returned with little René to Paris and set up a household for Duprat, keeping the rental of the apartment always in her own name to avoid challenges from Duprat's wife.[122] Returning by railroad through Italy and France, weighted down with baggage and a young child, she may have felt doubly her changed role, which was not unlike that of the primitive women described in her book.[123] Although, during the liberalized Second Empire, Duprat no longer had to fear persecution, it was not long before he was under attack from some of his old republican allies. Royer was to find her social life difficult as the unmarried mother of a young child and the companion of a married man, but she faced her situation with courage and dignity.

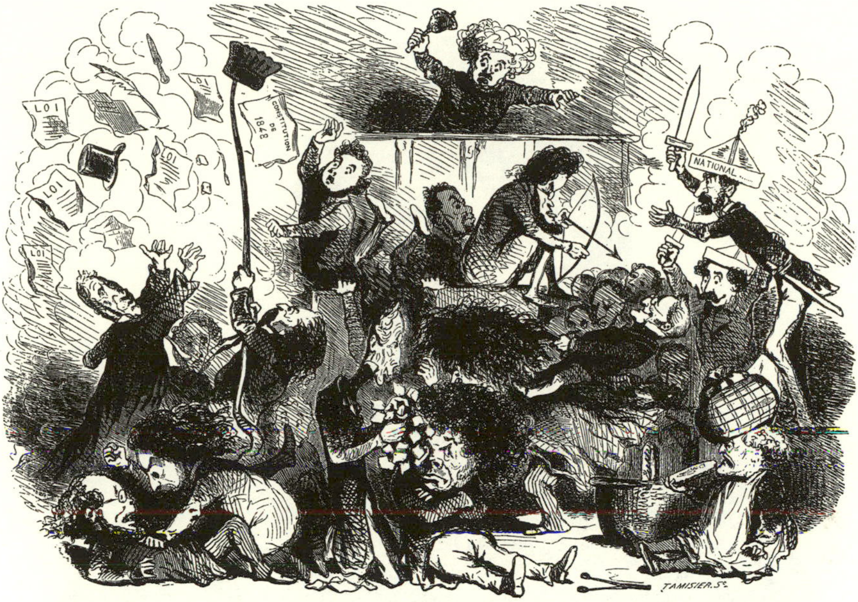

FIGURE 1. Caricature by Cham of the chaotic events at the Second Republic Legislative Assembly in February 1849. Auguste Thiers is the small man on the right leaning backwards at whom the arrow is aimed. Henri de Rochefort is the tall man with the newspaper hat labeled NATIONAL. The other man with the newspaper hat, with curling moustache, may well be Pascal Duprat. (From *L'Illustration,* February 1849.)

Seminary for Young Ladies,

CASTLE TERRACE, HAVERFORDWEST.

CONDUCTED BY MRS. LEWIS.

TERMS:—

BOARDERS—20 to 25 Guineas per annum.
DAY BOARDERS—14 to 16 Guineas per annum.
DAY PUPILS—6 to 8 Guineas per annum.

Extras.

French, German, Italian, Music, Drawing, and Painting, in various styles.

THE course of English studies embraces English Grammar and Composition; Writing; Arithmetic, including Mental Calculation; Geography, Natural and Physical; the Globes; the construction of Maps; Chronology; History, Ancient and Modern; Plain and Ornamental Needlework.

A Foreign Lady resides in the House.

Whilst Mrs. L. aims assiduously to cultivate the moral and intellectual powers of her Pupils, and to impart instruction in an attractive form, their spiritual interests will not be neglected, and the comforts and advantages of a well regulated Home are enjoyed.

Prospectuses will be forwarded on application. Respectable references given.

FIGURE 2. Advertisement for Mrs. Lewis's School for Girls, Haverfordwest. (From the *Haverfordwest and Milford Haven Telegraph,* 15 February 1854.)

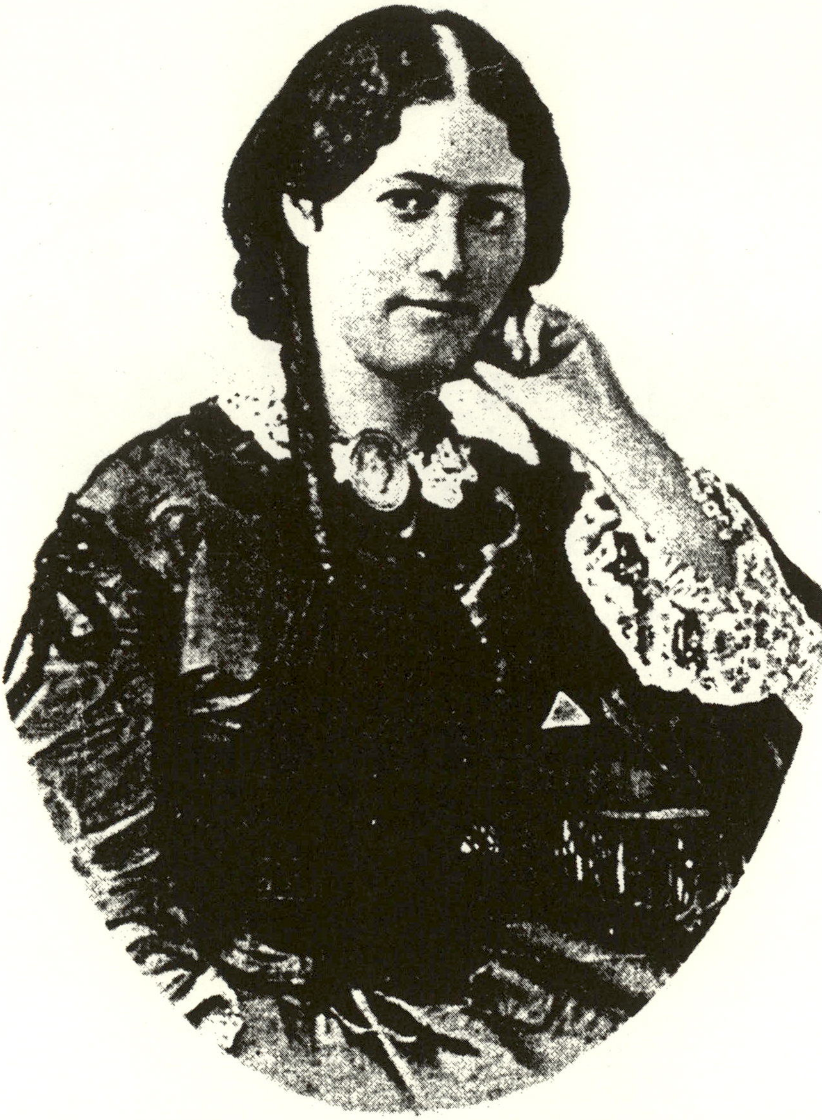

FIGURE 3. Photograph by Félix Nadar of Clémence Royer in 1865. It first appeared in print in 1895 in an article in the *Revue Encyclopédie.* (Reproduced by permission of the Bibliothèque Nationale, from the Félix Nadar Collection, n.a.f. 24285.)

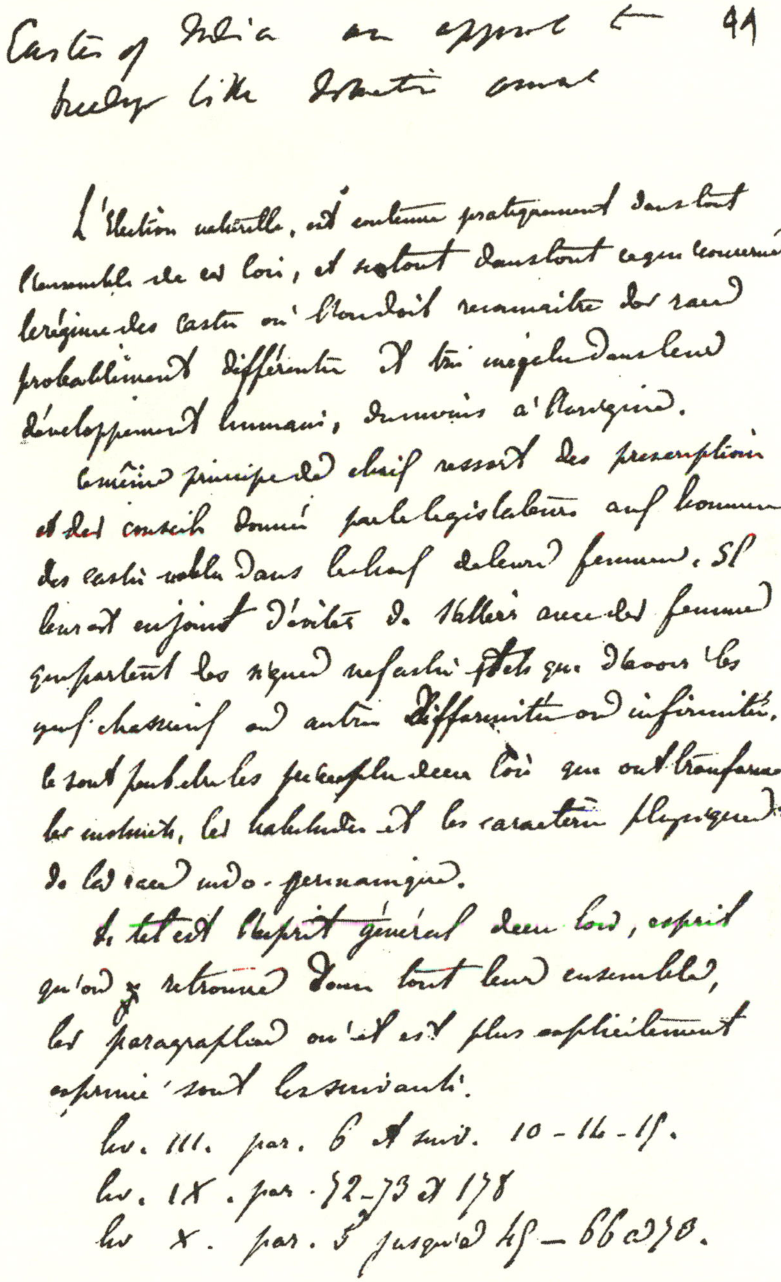
Castes of India as appert to breeding like domestic animal 44

L'élection naturelle, est entendue pratiquement dans tout l'ensemble de ces lois, et surtout dans tout ce qui concerne l'origine des castes où l'on doit reconnaître des races probablement différentes et très inégales dans leur développement humain, diverses à l'origine.

Le même principe est le chef ressort des prescriptions et des conseils donnés par le législateur aux hommes des castes nobles dans le choix de leurs femmes. Il leur est enjoint d'éviter de s'allier avec les femmes qui portent les signes néfastes tels que d'avoir les yeux chassieux ou autres difformités ou infirmités. Ce sont peut-être les préceptes de ces lois qui ont transformé les instincts, les habitudes et les caractères physiques de la race indo-germanique.

Et tel est l'esprit général de ces lois, esprit qu'on y retrouve dans tout leur ensemble, les paragraphes où il est plus explicitement exprimé sont les suivants:

liv. III. par. 6 et suiv. 10-14-15.
liv. IX. par. 72-73 et 178
liv X. par. 5 jusqu'à 45 — 66 à 70.

FIGURE 4. Appended note in the hand of Clémence Royer, intended for but apparently removed by Charles Darwin from the second French edition of *Origin of Species*. A note by Darwin reads, "Castes of India as appert to breeding like domestic animals." The references are to the Hindu "laws of Manu." (Reproduced by permission of the Syndics of Cambridge University Library from the Darwin Archive, DAR 80:44.)

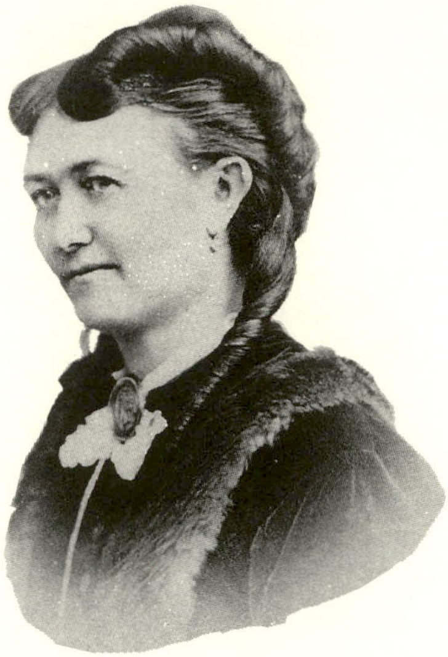

FIGURE 5. Photograph from the Archives of the Société d'Anthropologie de Paris of Clémence Royer around the time she entered the society in 1870. (Reproduced by permission of the Société d'Anthropologie de Paris. Published in *Bulletin et Mémoirs de la Société d'Anthropoloaie de Paris,* n.s. 3 [1991]:117.)

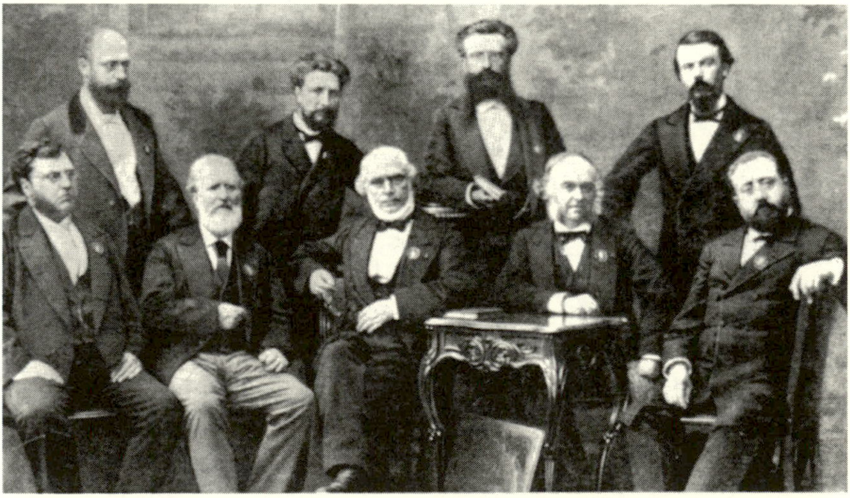

FIGURE 6. Only known group portrait of the officers and significant members of the Société d'Anthropologie de Paris attending the Moscow Anthropological Exhibition, 1879. From left to right: Standing—R. Ujfally, E. Chantre, Gustave Le Bon, Ernest Hamy. Sitting—Paul Topinard, Gabriel de Mortillet, Armand de Quatrefages, Paul Broca, Magitot.

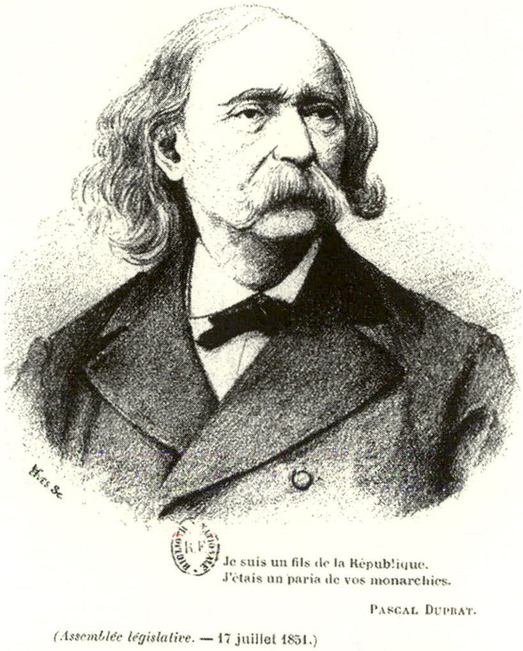

Je suis un fils de la République.
J'étais un paria de vos monarchies.

(Assemblée législative. — 17 juillet 1851.)

FIGURE 7. Pascal Duprat in old age (ca. 1880). (Frontispiece to Toussaint Nigoul, *Pascal Duprat, sa vie, son oeuvre* [Paris: E. Dentu, Librairie, 1887.])

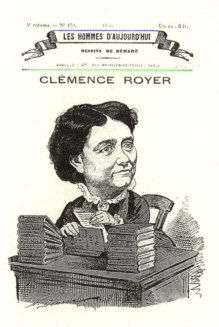

4e volume. — No 170.
Un an : 6 fr.
LES HOMMES D'AUJOURD'HUI
DESSINS DE DEMARE

FIGURE 8. Caricature of Clémence Royer dated 1881 from *Les Hommes d'audourd'hui* 4, no 170. She is reading from a copy of her new book, *Le Bien et la loi morale*. The other books include one on "Darwinisme." (Reproduced by permission of Houghton Library, Harvard University.)

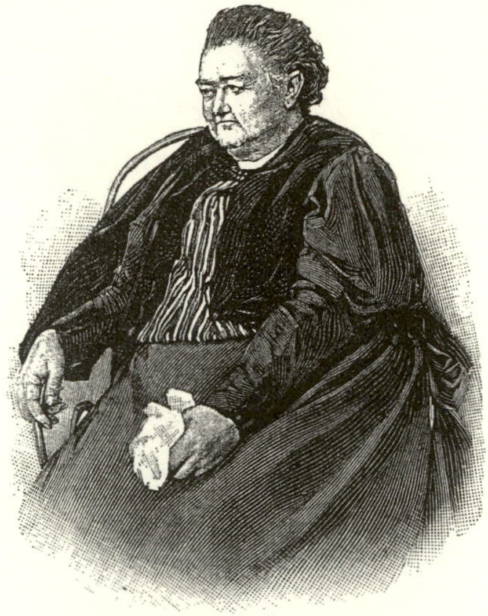

FIGURE 9. Clémence Royer about the time of her banquet of 1897. Engraving accompanied an article by Georges Clemenceau in *L'Illustration* (1897).

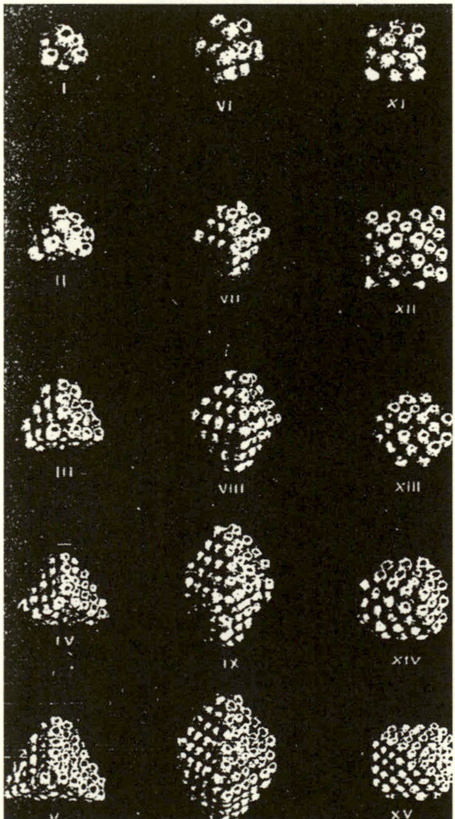

FIGURE 10. Careful constructions in various geometric shapes made from beads put together by Royer to illustrate her theories of atomic structure in her book *La Constitution du monde* (1900).

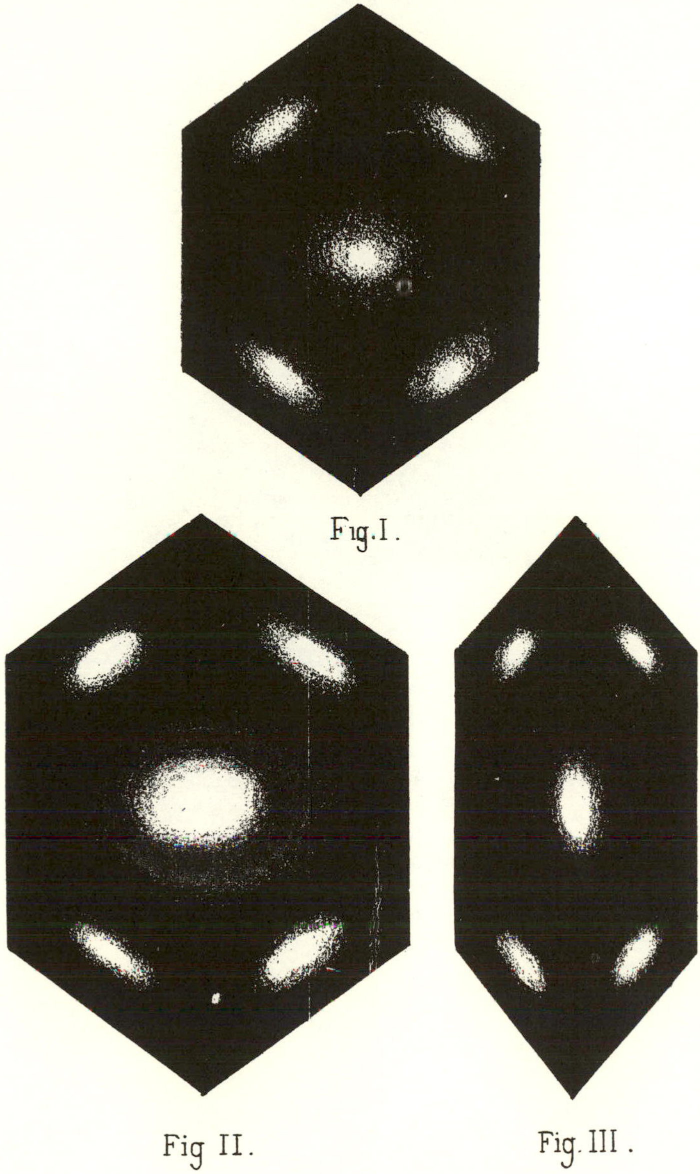

Figure 11. "The Luminous Atom," an illustration in color from the frontispiece of *La Constitution du monde* (1900)

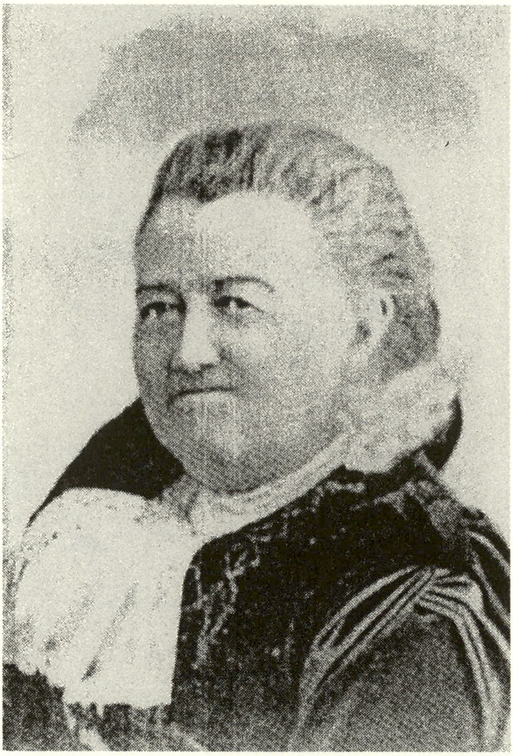

FIGURE 12. Photograph of Clémence Royer at seventy, used by Schleicher Frères to advertise her book *La Constitution du monde* (1900).

Chapter 6

"A Little Scientific Church": Royer Returns to Paris

Before Clémence Royer returned to France at the end of the sixties, she had accomplished two tasks. One was the completion of her book on a problem on which Darwin appeared unwilling to engage: the origin of the human being and human societies. The second was the production of a new edition of her translation of Darwin's *Origin of Species*. As we have seen, her mistake was to do the second of these tasks too quickly, without consulting Darwin.

On her return Royer observed something that must have struck her about Paris: the sounds of birds outside her window in the early morning. "One has to be very distracted or very preoccupied in Paris not to hear the incessant babble from sparrows hidden in the holes of our houses or from the swallows who suspend their nests from our windows."[1] Just before she returned, she had written about the advantages of city living for working people, which were not only the convenience in shopping, but the sense of not being tied to one place and dependent on a factory or other large institution, but her nostalgia may have made her overstate the advantages.[2] Royer and Duprat lived on the rue Pontoise close to the Seine on the left bank, in the heart of the intellectual life of Paris and within walking distance of the boulevard Saint-Michel and the Sorbonne. Not far away was the Société d'Anthropologie, located in the old Cordeliers building that faced the School of Medicine. As convenient as this was for her intellectual life, it may not have been completely suitable for her young child.

Life cannot have been easy for Royer and Duprat during the late sixties, although the salon they offered as a meeting place for rising young journalists and intellectuals was later remembered fondly. But Duprat had made himself unpopular by writing a series of satirical portraits of his old colleagues, those former republicans who had remained in France and participated in the government and the journalism of the Second Empire. They greeted him "like a dog, with a shower of arrows" when he reappeared upon the Parisian scene, as Royer later put it.[3] As a result, the couple was short of funds. When Duprat returned to Paris in 1869, he hoped to return as a deputy in the new, reformulated Empire, which had radically liberalized just before the Franco-Prussian war. His name had even been put up for election before he left Spain. During those heady days of the Spanish revolt, he wrote a letter to his supporters in Agen in 1868, sending enthusiastic greetings. He was unsuccessful in the elections.[4]

Duprat again turned to journalism, publishing a daily paper, *Le Peuple Souverain,* on which Clémence Royer also collaborated according to later police reports.[5] This paper stood in opposition to Henri de Rochefort, who edited the paper *La Lanterne* during the Empire and then *Mot d'Ordre* during the early republic, although the latter paper was periodically suppressed by the French government. Royer began another novel, *Jeunesse d'une révolte,* which reflected some of Duprat's youthful experiences during the 1848 revolution. The first sections of this novel appeared in print, but when Duprat's newspaper, in which this effort had begun to appear, collapsed, she abandoned it half-written, and no copies were preserved.[6]

Royer reacted to the daily reports and debates in the Parisian journals about the frightful health conditions among wet nurses, a topic that troubled her as the mother of a young child. "In the suburbs of Paris, there are entire villages peopled with women who make their living from raising babies. But alas, the cemeteries of the same villages are paved with those same creatures, who have certainly experienced the country air but also the difficult living conditions and privations that Rousseau considered so healthy and fortifying." She praised the growing number of crèches, *écoles maternelles* (nursery schools), and asylums that had opened in Paris and allowed women "condemned to work" to keep their children with them.[7] She must surely have taken advantage of these *écoles maternelles* for little René.

After 1869 Charles Darwin seems to have been unaware that Royer continued to serve as an active proselytizer for Darwinism in France. When she returned to Paris, she gave lectures on the topic of evolution at a hall on the Boulevard des Capuchines. At the very moment that Darwin had withdrawn his authorization of her translation, Royer had become a major force for the popularization of his ideas in France. A physician, Madeleine Brès, the first French woman admitted to the Paris School of Medicine, remembered the impact that Royer's appearance had upon herself and her fellow students at the medical school. One day, she reported, her much admired professor, Jules Gavarret, respectfully ushered in a woman scientist. She later recalled:

> Gavarret had a profound admiration for you, your character, and your remarkable work, as I am certain you have not forgotten. When [he] pronounced your name, everyone in the room stood up to cheer you. It is true that young people of great and generous aspirations and healthy,

> accurate judgements render homage to all that is good, beautiful, and true, even when it concerns a woman. That meeting I have never forgotten. It raised in my mind the same breath of enthusiasm. The next day I read the *Origin of Species* and learned of the immortal work of Darwin.[8]

Royer again attempted to enter the Société d'Anthropologie de Paris, this time meeting with success. This scientific society included a core of free-thinking republican physicians and scientists. Although significant moderate and even conservative scientists like Armand de Quatrefages were important figures, the central committee of the society included a large number of scientific positivists and scientific materialists who had made common cause in their interest in human origins.[9]

The circle around Paul Broca, which was interested in having evolution and Darwinism debated, was quite keen to have Darwin's translator enter the society. Charles Letourneau was a member of the central committee of the society, as was Gabriel de Mortillet, who had advertised her lectures in Italy in his journal. However, two more conservative members sponsored her admission to the society, one of whom was Darwin's French correspondent, Armand de Quatrefages. Quatrefages had met Royer at the home of their mutual friend Edouard Lartet, whose work on prehistoric archeology had helped establish that study in France, and who had recently served as president of the Anthropological Society. The other sponsor was the prestigious physician Jules Gavarret, who had introduced Royer to his class with such warm acclaim. A good friend of Broca, he was a professor of medical physics at the Paris School of Medicine and had written a book on blood with the great clinician Andral in his youth. Broca characteristically encouraged sponsorship of individuals with left-leaning credentials by centrist figures.

Many years later, Charles Letourneau described Royer's admission to the society. "The struggle was lively," he remembered. When her name was proposed, it "rang like a revolutionary alarm [tocsin], doubly revolutionary as a woman and as Darwin's translator."[10] After some debate she was admitted as a gesture towards the growing social change in France at the end of the Empire, as well as from a desire to include a woman who had contributed to the topic of human evolution. Some of the members had been deeply interested in improving women's higher education. Paul Broca, for example, had already agreed to sit on the examination committee that would award Elizabeth Garrett (later, Anderson) the first medical degree awarded to a woman by the Faculté de Médecine in 1870.[11]

When Royer entered the Société d'Anthropologie, it was with extensive experience in public debate, which she had honed in her discussions before the Congresses of Social Science in Switzerland and in her lectures. She became an active member, eventually participating in over 130 discussions of the society on a wide range of topics. She remained the only woman member of the society for the next fifteen years and, with the exception of Dr. Blanche Edwards (later Pilliet), admitted in the late 1880s, she remained the only notable woman member until the beginning of the next century (fig. 5).

Royer was later to speak of the Anthropological Society as "a little scientific church," by which she apparently meant that the participants were a dedicated group of believers in science.[12] Her first role in the society was as a spokesperson and interpreter of Darwin's concept of natural selection and the struggle for survival. For Royer, this scientific society also served as the first place in which she could regularly interact with scientists and physicians rather than social scientists and economists.

In spite of the negative reaction of many French scientists to Darwin, some important members of the Société d'Anthropologie had discussed and to some extent supported Darwinian ideas as early as 1863.[13] Among those who had spoken on Darwin and Huxley was a young physician, Eugène Dally, one of the young secretaries of the scientific society. He attempted to make Darwinism acceptable to the French thinkers by addressing their concerns in a long preface to his French translation of T. H. Huxley's book on human evolution, *Man's Place in Nature.*[14] The paleontologist Albert Gaudry applied some Darwinian ideas to sequences of vertebrate fossils found in Greece, but backed away from any applications to the human species that might "injure the dignity of man."[15] Royer's materialist friend Charles Letourneau wrote on species and variation for Littré's scientific positivist journal.[16]

Eugène Dally had touched off the evolutionary debate in the Société d'Anthropologie with a review of his Huxley translation.[17] Like Royer, he felt that it was necessary to place Darwin in a French context. His long preface to Huxley, in which he had tried to make Darwinian evolution compatible with French scientific positivism, reiterated his indebtedness to Émile Littré and Charles Robin, the foremost promoters of that philosophical school. Dally reinterpreted natural selection not as a mechanism for change but as a "form of heredity" and suggested that the term "spontaneous" selection might be more appropriate than "natural," since both artifical and natural selection were natural.[18] He proposed experiments on heredity to test some of Darwin's ideas, some of which Broca later attempted. He saw Darwinism as a form of "progressivism" and challenged some of Darwin's ideas on natural selection as increasing variation. He believed that progress in the case of humans "consists precisely in the (natural) extinction of beings that cannot support any degree of superior vitality."[19] This view of a progressivist evolution with natural selection playing a negative but never a creative role and weeding out only the weak or the maladapted was one that Conry has shown to run through much of nineteenth-century French Darwinism.[20]

Dally endorsed the polygenism of both his mentor Paul Broca and Carl Vogt. Vogt had just published a foreword to the French translation of Darwin's

Variation of Animals and Plants under Domestication. The polygenists thought that the multiplication of forms of life through time would necessitate multiple human forms as well, rather like a "forest of evolutionary trees," as Quatrefages would later express it.[21] Only by the end of the 1870s would Broca and some of his colleagues back away from their adherence to this view of human origins.

The Anthropological Society divided the debates into two parts; the first on a comparison between the primate and human anatomy began at the end of 1868 and ran throughout 1869. Royer had cited both Dally's comments and Paul Broca's lengthy analysis of the vertebrate column of man and ape in her book. The second round of debates was to be on evolution itself. The new president of the society, Gustave Lagneau, introduced the discussion with a reminder that evolution was only a hypothesis. Many of the major speakers rose to express their support of some kind of evolutionism, while the opposition was limited to a few positivists like Lagneau or museum naturalists like Quatrefages, who felt the evidence was not sufficient to support Darwinism.[22]

The first debate in which Clémence Royer participated fully in the Anthropological Society was the evolutionary debate in April 1870, a few months after she had entered the society. Although she began by answering objections raised by Eugène Dally, much of her discussion was focussed on Quatrefages's criticism of Darwinism that he directed also at her errors of interpretation in his just-published book *Darwin et ses précurseurs françaises,* originally published as a series of articles in the *Revue des Deux Mondes.*[23] She began with an attack rather than a defense. It was an error, she insisted, to regard Darwinism as a hypothesis, as Quatrefages had suggested. It was a valuable theory. The difference was that a hypothesis simply postulated a priori what might occur, while a theory brought together a posteriori many facts that were linked together in a great design. She turned to the example of Copernicus for a well-known analogy. His hypothesis of a sun-centered planetary system was later verified by Galileo's use of the telescope. Although astronomy never measured the sun and the planets directly, the theory of gravitation was not the less secure. Evolution—she used the more common French term "transformism"—she stated, was a theory based on inductions from inductions, "deriving from known observed facts but legitimately passing beyond them into space and time, as the theory of universal gravitation passes beyond the observations of astronomers and reveals to us what was and what will be. . . ."[24] She alluded to the wave theory of Descartes, which had sparked modern scientific theories of light waves. In contrast, the existence of the ether and "attraction" were hypotheses. She was well aware, she added that there were those who preferred to think of the wave theory as a commodious hypothesis only, but, she implied, this was due to a certain scientific philosophy of skepticism, which in turn had become very dogmatic.

Continuing her illustrations from astronomy, Royer suggested that if one refused to admit that living beings had successively—and progressively—evolved, one would also be unable to say that planets and stars had passed from an incandescent stage to a gaseous to a liquid and then to a solid state, on which living forms could arise. Aware of the arguments of many naturalists, such as Armand de Quatrefages, that varieties could not produce new species, she added, "You no more have the right to say to us that variability has never passed the limits that we see acting before our eyes on our domestic animals than to affirm that gravitation is stopped at the limit of our planetary world."[25]

Royer insisted that Darwin, accused of having no factual evidence, was on the contrary "full of facts." The *Origin of Species* was so much a catalogue of facts that he had left to the reader the problem of deducing his laws and his theory. "A great many people have complained of reading Darwin without finding Darwinism in it."[26] The premises were there, she insisted, but it required sufficient logic to deduce the consequences.

After Lamarck, Royer remarked, evolutionary ideas took on a new life in Darwin's hands, since Darwin's simple claims were "completely verifiable by observation." Discussing general evolutionary laws—which, she believed, were not specifically Darwinian—she argued that evolutionism required four facts. First of all, organic beings varied from one generation to another within limits. Variation was the norm, not the exception, and no two living beings were identical. Secondly, this faculty of variability had nothing absolute about it, being very unequal in different individuals, races, species, and genera. This second "fact" she discussed at great length. Plants varied more than animals, and among the animals, hermaphrodites varied more than species with two sexes (dioecious species). This was rather curious, since Darwin considered two sexes important for species variation.

Royer discussed at some length the example of domesticated animals, about which there were raging debates concerning variability. Domestication, she believed, did not lead of necessity to variation. The domestic goose and the ass had surprisingly fixed heredity, whereas pigeons, dogs, and sheep varied "to excess," she noted, taking her cue from Darwin's book *Variation*. Third, there was a general tendency for descendents to reproduce the type of their immediate ancestors: "This is the atavistic force or heredity." Fourth, every organism oscillated constantly between atavism (a return to an earlier form) and hereditary fixity (a preservation of its own type) due to a conflict between two forces, one of which was the influence of the environment and the other intrinsic or extrinsic effects. These principles, she felt, all could agree upon.

In her opinion, arguments used against Darwin—for example, that reversions of domestic animals to wild forms did not produce the same ancestral types—could be easily answered by arguing that the environment in each case had a different influence. To make this point she used not Darwinian adaptative arguments but a Lamarckian description. "If their forms are more spindly and their legs thinner and more agile, it is because their nourishment is less abundant, less regular, and because they must often cover vast expanses to procure it, as well as escape the attacks of their enemies."[27] She argued that if a monstrous variety was nonviable, it would disappear without posterity. If on the other hand the variation was not too extreme, it might create a new race like the famous Scottish short-legged sheep. Quatrefages, she added, was right in reproaching Darwin for not giving enough weight to those useful variations that appeared suddenly. In a brief response, Quatrefages commented only that Royer's acceptance of abrupt variation placed her outside Darwinian theory. As he had earlier remarked, so did her notes on spontaneous generation.[28]

Geographical distribution, Royer continued, was well explained by evolution and only by evolution, since it demonstrated the manner in which a species, triumphing over its rivals, might expand over an area until it was blocked by natural barriers. Certain organisms were found only in America, Australia, or Africa, whereas throughout Asia and Europe, where no efficacious barriers existed, one had almost the same zoological population.

Praising the final chapters of the *Origin* including Darwin's discussion of classification, embryology, and a recapitulation of his theory—"the most beautiful and the least known"—she brought up Darwin's "central law" of struggle for survival—which she called "vital competition" (*concurrence vitale*)—and what she termed his "corollary law" of natural selection. Following Darwin's use of Malthusian population laws, she reiterated that every organized being had an exuberant power of multiplication, but there was limited room for its offspring. Ignoring the primacy for Darwin of individual selection, she gave her illustration in terms of races or groups of individuals "fatally condemned to disappear from hunger, if they do not succumb to other causes of destruction." Clarifying the meaning of the struggle for survival, she insisted that this did not mean that only the weakest or inferior disappeared. Rather, it was the "least well adapted to their local conditions of life, the least able to procure substance most proper for them or to triumph over enemies of their race and multiple hazards of daily life." The best adapted alone survived, and they alone left a posterity that inherited their advantages.[29] Except for her insistence on the usefulness of "abrupt" change, much of this section of Royer's discussion of Darwinian evolution used Darwin's own examples.

Royer also took up another issue, that of infertility between human groups, upon which the French anthropologists had built their polygenist view of race. First of all, she insisted that closely related forms were not necessarily fertile with each other, but were often infertile for unclear reasons. (Darwin had emphasized this point in his discussion of hybrids of flowering plants.) She also claimed, with some justification, that other groups were interfertile only because of the interference of human agency not found in the wild. For Royer, sexual generation was only a contingent circumstance in evolution.

Natural selection accounted for the appearance and development of sexuality as well as sterility. "It explains by a simple relation of specific utility the very contingent fact of hybrid sterility."[30] Sexual reproduction was superior in localization and produced a more perfect specialization than could develop from simple budding.

Extending her discussion of sexual and asexual reproduction, she made a confusing case for hermaphroditic species, suggesting that "sexual affinities of individuals have only a rather relative taxonomic value." She went on to argue that grafts did not take between certain forms because of a lack of affinity. Successful fertility of any two individuals depended "not on an essential difference of nature or on an identity of origin, but on internal rapport, on hidden physiological suitabilities that our science has not yet penetrated."[31]

Taking up the monogenist argument, Royer proposed that Darwin's monogenism did not require a single individual from which all others developed, but only a single kind comprising a large number of individuals. A single individual would have had to reproduce asexually, but since Darwin believed in advantages accruing from sexual crosses, she concluded that he must believe that whatever the original form was, it would need to cross with others to remain vigorous. Failing to recognize Darwin's concept of sexuality as something that itself might have evolved, and perhaps misled by Darwin's heavy emphasis on sexual selection, she expressed her doubts that sexuality was a "fundamental law of the organism." "Darwin was wrong," she said, "to fall into the cult of sexuality . . . which conflicts with the order of all nature."[32] A single egg or rudimentary form, she thought, could not have been produced only once on the surface of the globe, since among billions of organisms produced at the present time only a much smaller number had any chance of developing. She believed that nowadays there might be a development of simple organisms from the debris of complex organisms—as Felix Pouchet had argued in his discussion of "heterogeneity," or spontaneous generation—but this could not explain the original appearance of life. Instead, special conditions must have been present at a determined epoch when the earth was cooling and covered with vapor. Billions of this prototype must have occurred all over the globe, even before vegetative reproduction occurred. The fact that life could only have occurred at one point in the evolution of the planet prompted her to entreat her colleagues: "Let us guard the flame of light so that beings can be transmitted from one to the other like the runners in the ancient circus. Once extinguished, the desert and the silence alone will rule over our devastated globe."[33] Her arguments echoed those she had made in her book, and she may have been prompted in her appeal for the preservation of life by the impending war with Germany.

Shortly Gabriel de Mortillet was to pick up on her last point and to question her argument limiting spontaneous generation to special geological periods when life could develop, as she had done in her book *Origine de l'homme.* This was a slippery slope, he warned, towards creationism.[34] Another colleague, Louis-Adolphe Bertillon, took issue with Royer's denigration of sexual selection. To Bertillon, Darwin's explanation was the only satisfactory one he had yet encountered. It was the only one that could explain the development of beauty in the animal and plant world.[35]

By arguing for a multiplicity of original forms, which she considered to have been almost identical, Royer could allow for a kind of polygenism resulting from parallel lines of evolution. Most of these original sources or prototypical germs would have become extinct, she thought, before the appearance of the first fossils. In response to Quatrefages, who had questioned the concept of multiple prototypical germs, she proposed the answer she had given in a note to her translation of the *Origin,* in which she speaks of "the parallelism of destiny." Through this parallel development it was possible to have a plural number of primitive forms but only a single heredity. She believed that in this way she had united supporters of Lamarck with believers in spontaneous generation and even with adversaries of evolution. Her arguments became at this point so highly involved that she moved from the simplicity of Darwinian evolution at the level of individual selection to the assumption that orders or families could evolve as units in a form of group selection.

Nevertheless, when returning to the specifics of Darwin's theory, she insisted again on its real value and its validity as scientific truth. Darwinian evolution had a capacity to explain "all biological phenomena with the most marvelous flexibility." The law of life was "the law of probabilities and results," and although one could never indicate absolutely its direction and intensity because of unknown factors, one could apply "the law of the parallelogram of forces, formulated in algebraic terms."[36] Perhaps it was this image, this kind of geometric formulation that led her to make an attempt three years later to illustrate the action of atavism through diagrams in order to show how hereditary abnormalities such as the "hairy-faced man" could have survived.[37]

In response to the often heard claim that there were no fossils illustrating transitional forms, she suggested that no museum could include all the fossils of the evolutionary organic series with all the "retrogressive or progressive transformations" or all their migrations or changes of habitat. She spoke of the difficulty of understanding even a poorly represented "species" (she evidently meant "family") like the cephalopods, whose existence was menaced in the more recent epoch after having been very important in an earlier period. Biological change could mean that they also could at some later point suddenly begin to increase and "cover vast countries with new kinds of species." Evolution was an inductive theory, she added, as much dialectical as experimental. "Transformism is not a belief, it is a series of reasonings and arguments based on observed realities that easily triumphs over the weakness of arguments that have been opposed to it. All its affirmations are positive, all the objections that have been made against it are negative. They are drawn without exception from lacunas of science, never from its recognized laws." She ended with a challenge to her colleagues. If they couldn't accept evolution, it was not because of any lack of intelligence or reason. Their sentiments, instincts, and hereditary and acquired habits struggled against the theory. Perhaps, as Quatrefages had said the other day, it was a racial influence "from which only a small number of individuals had succeeded in escaping."[38]

Quatrefages, who had remained quiet through much of the evolutionary debate, believing that his book on the history of evolutionary theory had detailed most of what he had to say on the subject, rose to the challenge that Royer held out. He apologized to his colleagues for holding them past the usual hour, but he wanted to remind them that evolution comprised a number of theories and was far from being a single theory. Darwinism relied entirely on the struggle for existence and the selection that resulted from it. All rapid transmutation outside these laws was outside Darwinism. There were no facts, as even Royer had admitted, that clearly demonstrated slow transformation. He mentioned a conversation between himself and Royer at the home of the archaeologist Edouard Lartet, then president of the Anthropological Society. He had made, Quatrefages recalled, some joking attempt to invent an alternative theory that was neither Darwinist nor creationist but could account for all the known facts. "I think it is useless to recall this pleasantry here. Certainly it is not the only one that could be invented by mixing the most precise facts with some of the great principles that have been developed seriously by many philosophers more courageous than curious about reality."[39] Quatrefages reiterated in this apparently friendly manner his censure of pure speculation about evolutionary change that had kept him from becoming an evolutionist.

The debates continued in the Société d'Anthropologie, however, and a group of individuals close to Paul Broca—Louis-Adolphe Bertillon, Charles Letourneau, Gabriel de Mortillet, and Abel Hovelacque—spoke in favor of evolutionary theories. Broca himself clearly explained what he could and could not accept in Darwinian evolution and argued on behalf of a polygenist transformism based on the evolution of multiple parallel forms. He called Malthusian selection "Darwin's law" and praised nine different points that until the present time had remained obscure and that Darwin had clarified. Nevertheless, while making heavy concessions to evolutionary theory, he added that he did not think natural selection alone could explain all of the phenomena. In his view, the importance of the environment must be taken into account.[40]

One of the most committed scientific positivists in the society and Broca's good friend, the statistician Louis-Adolphe Bertillon, rose to expand upon one of Royer's points by showing the usefulness of hypotheses. Those that Darwin had suggested were useful in the same manner that Laplace's cosmology was useful: not because it lent itself to experimental proof, but because it coordinated a large series of facts.[41] Bertillon pointed to the importance of Darwin's theory in explaining embryological facts. Although he endorsed Broca's emphasis on the active role of environment in evolution, he did not agree that natural selection failed to explain the preservation of nonuseful traits, as Broca had asserted. Darwin had answered this objection in his description of correlated characters, giving as an example deafness in blue-eyed cats.

It is important to emphasize that Darwin, taking note of Broca's emphasis on environmental influences, went some distance in his later editions of both the *Origin of Species* and *Descent of Man* to address those objections. He quoted Broca's objections to the action of natural selection as an exclusive mechanism of evolution and thereby weakened his own earlier belief in the power of natural selection.[42]

One member of the Anthropological Society, Hector George, after listening to the debates on evolution, described the wide varieties of Darwinism and transformism he detected. Royer had produced "the first transformation of Darwinism, but not the only one." Other scientists "have come as rivals or disciples of Darwin to modify his doctrine, which is already very elastic."[43] He proceeded to enumerate the varieties of transformism that he had found: "Some of them admit transformism only within certain limits. They want at least one primordial type for each class of animals, and they admit four to five successive creations. Others are monogenists: they want only one primitive type, but they admit a creative God at the beginning. Others, equally monogenist, don't want a God. They admit spontaneous generation, ascending and successive evolution, and man's development from an ancient germ. . . . Others finally admit God, admit the soul, admit successive creation, even admit the fixity of species; but since they admit also the creation of varieties and races from a single species, they call themselves transformists."[44] George detected political and social opinions "embroidering" these ideas, forming so many combinations that "even a mathematician could scarcely calculate them."[45]

Soon the evolutionary debates of 1870 were interrupted by the beginning of the Franco-Prussian war. This "terrible year," as Hugo designated the period from June 1870 to July 1871, began with some hopes. Duprat and Royer, like many of their friends, hailed the Third Republic on 4 September, following the collapse of the Empire and the flight of Napoleon III, with enthusiasm. Duprat seems to have had some role in the Défense Nationale when the government moved to Bordeaux. They both remained cautiously observant of later events, as Paris lay under siege, and the population found itself on the verge of starvation. Following the armistice with Prussia, the demand that the national guard lay down their arms and allow Prussian troops to occupy the city led to the confusing events surrounding the Paris Commune and the subsequent bloody repression by the French troops of the government, which had retreated to Versailles. Other friends took more extreme positions. Charles Letourneau, Royer's associate at both the Société d'Anthropologie and *La Pensée Nouvelle,* worked as a physician on the side of the Commune and had to flee to Florence, where he remained for six years. During that time he became a close friend of Alexander Herzen Jr. and worked on concepts of physiological psychology with Paulo Mantegazza.[46]

In 1871, during the siege of Paris and the Commune, Paul Broca had trouble preparing the *Bulletin de la Société d'Anthropologie* without his assistant Ernest Hamy, to whom he wrote regularly during the war and the Commune.[47] Royer's mother and little René may have retired to her native Brittany. Many families went to their native village as times became difficult in Paris. Paul Broca's wife, who stayed with him for most of the period, sent her children off to Broca's village near Bordeaux, Sainte-Foy-la Grande. Two childhood companions of Paul Broca, Élie and Élisée Reclus—whose youngest brother, Paul, was one of Broca's interns—were involved in the Commune as dedicated anarchists. Élie Reclus's wife, Noémie, who had participated in a group to rethink women's education with the Brocas, went into hiding with her two little boys after the defeat of the Commune.

One political letter from the early days of the Third Republic written by Royer was picked out of the papers of a member of the Commune. Undated, but probably written in September 1870, soon after the Republic was declared, she wrote from rue Pontoise in Paris. Addressing herself to the men of the Défense Nationale, she asked them to support new elections throughout France "as soon as possible"—if not by 2 October, then by 16 October—in order to gain support from the entire country rather than leave it in the hands of "two old men" whose "nebulous connections do not give one confidence in their republican faith and, worst of all, who do not know how to communicate this to the nation."[48] She thought that if elections were held and groups of supporters for the republic could be formed along the coast at Bordeaux and Nantes, this method of linking France would produce a sense of national unity that would allow "the West and South to defend the East and North." Her greatest fear was of a social revolution that would result in a reaction that could restore either the monarchy or a new Bonapartist empire. She expressed her fear that Paris would be betrayed from within by those who "urge the belly against the head," the "party of violent individuals, incorrigibles, who have twice lost the liberty of the republic by making it slip in the blood of scaffolds and barricades."[49]

Like Duprat, Royer placed the survival of a republic above all other considerations and supported revolutions only when these were political but never social, very much in the spirit of the early phase of the 1848 revolution. Many years later, a journalist remembered the exciting meetings with Duprat to discuss republican ideas at his home on the rue Pontoise.[50] Royer also presided at these discussions, which she recalled with pleasure in spite of the unhappy events that followed. Here, Paul Lafargue came to see her to try to persuade her to translate Karl Marx's book *Das Kapital* into French. He suceeded neither in this nor in persuading her to adopt socialist beliefs.[51]

Although Royer had objected to the "two old men"—Thiers was one of them—who were running the Paris government in France during the Franco–Prussian war, Duprat supported Thiers against Léon Gambetta, who was both minister of the interior and minister of defense when he sought the presidency in February 1871. Gambetta had tried to block Thiers's move to place the government in Versailles rather than in Bordeaux or Paris during that shaky period at the conclusion of the war, just before the Commune. Thiers had sent Jules Simon and Jules Favre to Gambetta at Bordeaux to persuade him not to take power. The result was Gambetta's resignation. Duprat had seconded Thiers's action in his newspaper *Le Peuple Souverain* against one-man executive power, which he believed would lead inevitably to dictatorship.[52]

Royer later explained Duprat's opposition to Gambetta as having been performed "in the interest of the republic without calculating the outcome."[53] Duprat had written in *L'Esprit des revolutions* that there was only a single step from demagoguery to despotism.[54] He insisted that individuals at the head of political movements had to know how to moderate the forces that they directed. The success of a just cause could be compromised by the behavior of its followers "and the violence of its defenders." Revolutions therefore had to "push away utopias and chimeras even when they please the crowd."[55] The reference to crowd pleasers points directly to Henri de Rochefort, the quixotic journalist and publisher of *La Lanterne,* a supporter of Gambetta during this period. Many years later, Royer believed that Duprat's assistance in blocking "Gambetta's move towards dictatorship at Bordeaux" placed Duprat in direct opposition to Rochefort, from which Duprat would later suffer politically.[56] Royer added rather wryly that although Rochefort readily injured others—he was noted as a famous duelist—he never pardoned an injury to himself. Rochefort played a rather curious role in the Commune; he supported its formation but left France before the Commune actually took power. When Rochefort was finally arrested, he was held in prison but not deported like so many others. Thiers may have hesitated, perhaps from some sense of his journalistic power or in recognition of his strong support of Gambetta. Later deported when the duc de Broglie became minister of state, he escaped to Belgium and England, returning only after complete amnesty was granted to supporters of the Commune. Rochefort, still angry with Duprat, seems to have been one of the sources of the vehement political attacks on Duprat in the late 1870s and early 1880s.

Rochefort and other socialists had another reason for their antagonism. Duprat, as a member of the Chamber of Deputies during the Second Republic, had the dubious honor of proposing the law that declared Paris to be in a state of siege in 1849. The law granted executive powers to General Cavaignac and was used to suppress by violent measures the riots by angry workingmen. Later arguing that his law had produced a dictatorship that lasted only three days, Duprat added that he had always opposed long-term unbridled executive power. However it was intended, this same law was used to enforce the bloody repression of the Commune. Duprat's role in proposing the original law to deport and summarily execute supporters of the Commune was not forgotten by his enemies and helped to drive him out of active politics at the end of his life.

Whatever Duprat's responsibility for the original law intended simply to suppress social upheaval, he was appalled at the summary executions carried out wholesale by the army of the Versailles government of men and women suspected of being Communards. One journalist, Edmond Lepelletier, a young republican friend of Duprat from 1869 and later involved in the Commune, recalled that Duprat had risked his own life to save him from death. Lepelletier had been denounced by some enemy and had written in haste to Duprat as well as to other friends to assist him. Only Duprat arrived on the scene. He insisted that the Versailles officer release Lepelletier immediately. Because of Duprat's appearance, with his long moustaches and his old overcoat, he rather resembled "a dealer in contraband disguised as a professor." The officer was tempted to execute him as well, thinking perhaps he had discovered the real Communard and novelist Jules Vallès after having executed "many a false Vallès" throughout the day. Duprat vouched for his friend, identifying himself as an old republican deputy of 1848, a claim that seemed suspiciously revolutionary to the officer. When this did not sway him, Duprat announced to the officer that he was dealing with the future ambassador to Greece. This second claim finally induced the Versailles officer to "let go of his prey," much to the relief of the grateful journalist.[57]

Although Duprat never became an ambassador to Greece, the government under Thiers had offered Duprat this post in recognition of Duprat's support and various quiet errands he ran for the government. According to Nigoul, he refused the offer because he did not wish to abandon his country during a difficult period. In fact, the offer may have been withdrawn following complaints in the press that Thiers was appointing his ambassadors in an arbitary manner or because Duprat's articles about Greek-French disputes lacked diplomatic objectivity.

After his failure to become a European diplomat, Duprat was elected by his old home district of Landes as a radical republican in the first election following the suppression of the Commune and sat on the extreme Left of that highly conservative government. Duprat's usefulness to Thiers in the 1870s seems to have been partially based on his friendship with men on the radical Left as well as in the Center, and at least once he undertook a sensitive errand for him to sound out the public sentiments of men holding widely different political positions.[58]

In June 1872 Royer began to write a political column for the Russian newspaper *Goloss,* reporting on events at the National Assembly, supporting major centrist republican figures, and commenting that the political Right "had played a sad role" in France. Following this publication, the police began to collect a dossier on Royer (they had long kept one on Duprat). The police reports seemed singularly concerned that she was writing for a foreign journal, especially a Russian one, perhaps because of their concern over Russian nihilism. Their caution may have seemed justified by her description of an attack on Gambetta and his supporters in Marseilles by a group of Bonapartists and members of the Right in which she explicitly questioned the arbitrary action of the police during the incident and recalled similar police behavior at the beginning of the Second Empire. Her dossier began to reflect concerns by the police that she regularly received letters from foreign countries. They accurately described her as "very intelligent" and the "collaborator and then the mistress" of Pascal Duprat and noted the presence of their child in the household.[59]

Clémence Royer participated at the same time in a somewhat different kind of revolutionary project, the preparation of a questionnaire about sexual and reproductive differences in various human societies. This was a project proposed by the Société d'Ethnographie headed by Léon de Rosny, a rival society of the Société d'Anthropologie. Royer had joined the society in 1860, although she does not appear to have actively participated before this committee was set up on 10 May 1870. The questionnaire was presented at the annual meeting on 28 July 1871, almost immediately after the suppression of the Commune, but published only in 1873. Royer is listed last but may have been the reporting member of the otherwise all-male committee for this questionnaire. While this type of questionnaire was not unusual in itself—late-nineteenth-century ethnologists commonly inquired into sexual habits of "native races"—the presence of a woman among the members of the committee must have seemed surprising and even shocking at the time. Royer believed in honesty about certain matters, and the questions about female menstrual periods, conception, childbirth, breast feeding, and menarche demonstrated once again Royer's interest in female reproduction and sexuality. Questions that were included about penis size and male reproductive behavior may have taken more courage to propose or to report upon.[60] The same issue of the *Actes de la Société d'Ethnographie* demonstrated an equally courageous willingness to publicly memorialize one of its members, Gustave Flourens, who was summarily executed by the Versailles government, as a heroic military leader first of the National Defense and then of the Commune.[61]

As life began to return to normal in Paris, Duprat and Royer moved to the seventeenth arrondissement in Paris after Duprat's election to the National Assembly as a delegate from Landes in November 1871. This move placed Duprat in an area close to a Paris railway station and allowed him to make frequent visits to his supporters in the provinces. Duprat and Royer established themselves in an apartment at 3, rue Brochant on the edge of the square des Batignolles. Their windows looked out over this very attractive park designed by Baron Haussmann in 1867. Its numerous trees and winding walks included a small, man-made stream with a circular basin.[62] Here a young child could run and play, as Royer remembered playing in the Tuileries. Sitting in this attractive setting must have provided Royer with an opportunity to relax from the bustling intellectual and political life she had embarked upon. Some of Royer's happiest letters date from this period. The presence of her mother nearby, if not in her own household, may have helped to give her the freedom to write and attend late afternoon meetings at the Société d'Anthropologie. This was her most prolific period within that society, and she regularly submitted articles and participated in active discussions. Later the central committee of the society took action to suppress her discussion of women's roles in society and of the consequently lowered French birthrate, which caused her to markedly reduce her contributions for a period of time.

The friends of the couple continued to be drawn from a wide range of the republican political spectrum. Royer, in spite of her ambiguous social position, was able to maintain some pleasant social relationships with her colleagues. Some indication of this is given by her friendship with François Lenoir and his wife. Lenoir, an amateur collector of anthropological items and later a railroad archivist, had first written to her in the spring of 1872 on the strength of their joint friendship for the recently deceased president of the Société d'Anthropologie, Edouard Lartet. Commenting that he had gone a number of times to meetings at the Société d'Anthropologie, Lenoir expressed his wish to become better acquainted with her, adding: "Like you, Madame, I am occupied with the origins of man. You are the master, it is true, and not a humble student like myself."[63] He invited her to see his collections. Their friendship appears to have been cemented by his offer to allow her to use his archaeological collections to illustrate her public lectures.

The families of Lenoir and Royer-Duprat were soon meeting on a regular basis, and greetings between "Mme Lenoir" and "M. Duprat" were exchanged in their letters. Royer, inviting Madame Lenoir to her home near the Batignolles, hoped that she would not hesitate to make the long trip from one end of Paris to the other. "She is of the race that couldn't be dismayed by a trip to the Indies, and I don't live in the Indies." She sent warm greetings to "your Big Baby [*sic*]" and added that "le Petit Baby [*sic*]" [her six-year-old René] embraces you."[64]

Royer discovered that Lenoir was intrigued by mathematical puzzles, and she asked him to help her solve problems that derived from her revived interest in the basic structure of matter. She set a problem for Lenoir to solve, asking him what shape spheres would take if submitted to enough pressure to eliminate any spaces between them. The result that Lenoir came up with—hexagons—delighted her, and she used this result many years later in her book

La Constitution du monde. She expressed pleasure and surprise at the trouble he had taken on her behalf.

Royer's interest in physical theories may have been reawakened by one of the comments made by Quatrefages on the value of hypotheses during a discussion at the Société d'Anthropologie. During a debate he had quoted Newton: "Everything occurs as if the bodies are attracted as a direct relation of their mass and the inverse of the square of their distances, but nothing proves to us that they are so attracted." This was a "ray of light to her," she would later comment.

She also served, in a minor way, as a patron for Lenoir, arranging for him to meet Paul Broca to exchange scientific specimens (including a gorilla skull). She asked him for feedback on her reviews, for example, of the Bordeaux meeting of the French Association for the Advancement of Science (Association Française pour l'Avancement des Sciences), that appeared in the newspapers *L'Opinion* and in *La République Française.*

In a charming letter in early 1874 Lenoir described with some humor his difficulties in deciphering both her handwriting and that of Broca, as every biographer of these two must heartily agree. "Yesterday among the letters I believed I recognized your writing, and I said to my wife, 'At last a letter from Mme Royer.' I opened it immediately, and the hieroglyphics of the contents confirmed me in the notion that I had under my eyes a sacred text of which you were the author. Only after having played Champollion for some moments, did I see my error. I had just deciphered a letter, charming for all that, of M. Broca, who thanked me for some collections I had given for his museum at the Medical School. Your pretty little flyspecks came only much later. A new task was imposed upon me. I commenced to decode it, and believe me, dear Madame, that the said task was accomplished not only with courage but with the greatest pleasure by your very devoted Lenoir."[65] The friendship between the two families seems to have lasted for many years, although letters after 1877 do not convey quite the same warmth or record a regular exchange of visits. The two families, however, shared an interest in pacifism, feminism, and social theory. Madame Lenoir, as well as Royer, attended the international congresses on the rights of women. In the 1880s, when Royer started her own scientific and philosophical society, the Société d'Études Philosophiques et Morales, Madame Lenoir was among the members.

With the publication in 1873 of the newly authorized translation by Moulinié and Barbier of the *Origin of Species* in the Reinwald edition, Royer had to defend her Darwin translation once again. Charles Lévêque, the vice-president of the Académie des Sciences Morales et Politiques, announced she had "betrayed Darwin," a comment also "insinuated" by two other scientists, Nourisson and Valroger.[66] She argued in her defense that Darwin had never indicated to her any unwillingness to accept either her preface or her notes. Although Darwin asked her to make some changes in 1865 for her second edition, he also had written to her to say that she had understood his thinking better than anyone else! "If the idea of authorizing another [translator] came to him, it was too late not to have been suggested to him for reasons extrinsic to my translation."[67]

Royer insisted that the sole reason for Darwin's withdrawal of authorization was because he found her too independent a translator. She admitted that she had been in a hurry to finish the edition for financial and other personal reasons, and this prevented her from taking more care over the changes Darwin had introduced in his later editions. Nevertheless, she remained convinced, as the evidence showed even more clearly than she knew, that Darwin's greatest complaint was directed at her rebellion against him as an authority. Royer's sense of herself as a rebel was so powerful that she could not bow even to the greatest scientific authority, as we shall see again in her response to Newton when she began to study and reinterpret physical theories.

The resulting debate within the academy was decided in her favor. The reporter for the Académie des Sciences Morales et Politiques, Arthur Mangin, declared in the *Journal des Débats* that "Lévêque recognizes today that the case of the first translator is a great deal less grave than he had believed. The protest of M. Darwin is reduced to [a] passage in a letter found at the head of the fifth edition of the *Origin of Species,* translated at his invitation by M. J. J. Moulinié." This letter contained Darwin's public explanation that he had sought a new translator because Royer's new French edition did not follow the changes made in his latest editions. Mangin added that Royer was in her right in limiting her task as a translator. He added that it was also within her right to explain and develop his thought, since she had clearly explained in her translator's notes and prefaces that she alone was responsible for this extension of Darwin's ideas. Lévêque had "implicitly recognized the justice of these claims in his corrective note." Royer added in her own appended reply that she still would have preferred a public retraction before the Académie rather than an indirect recognition of the justice of her claims. She appears to have tried to remedy this with a separate publication of her two letters of explanation to the Académie and the extract from the *Journal Officiel.*[68]

How was Royer regarded by her colleagues among the scientists in the 1870s? Some found her suggestions full of ideas and welcomed her remarks, others, like Mortillet, found her too ready to speculate and criticized her when she wandered too far onto the hypothetical field. Some of the same reasons that make her controversial in the present day made her a challenging, not always easy, colleague. An early biographer claimed that Royer tolerated contradiction poorly and found it difficult to admit her errors, which made her discussions in learned societies "painful."[69] Certainly, her willingness to construct elaborate theories in a scientific society dedicated to "positive science" had annoyed some of her colleagues. One of the young scientists, Louis Lartet, for example, complained to his friend Ernest Hamy, a young assistant secretary of the Société d'Anthropologie, "What inexcusable theories Mlle [*sic*] Royer permits herself. Fortunately, there were no geologists present."[70] A year later he made a more general complaint: "I am sick to death of our Société d'Anthropologie with its scientific claims, its encyclopedic pretensions, its sterile and impertinent verbiage. I am not so flattered as you might believe to see my prose in the company of Pictet, Garrigou, Clémence Royer, and *tutti quanti* so that something can act as a counterweight."[71] One cannot exclude the likelihood that the sharp exchanges, so common among men in scientific societies, may have sounded different to the ear when they were advanced by a strong-minded woman.

Royer had long been a colleague of many of the individuals involved in the Académie des Sciences Morales et Politiques through the *Journal des Économistes* and the Congress of Social Science. She continued to strengthen her tie to this part of the Institut de France. At times, she was to win monetary prizes for essays submitted in competition, although not always with full credit, as we shall see. The Institut, however, neither could nor would ever admit her as a member.[72]

Royer always thought that an understanding of science had a direct connection to political life. Like many of the republican figures of the time, she emphasized that science was especially important following the "unhappy disasters that we experienced from Germany."[73] As she declared in one of her public lectures at the close of 1874, the "deplorable events" of the recent past had shown the "too great ignorance which all the French had of their own country." There were no longer great men in the country because colleges and *lycées* no longer taught the philosophy of science but only specialized science with narrow practical aims. In her eyes, she added, to applause, "a man who lacked science was an empty vessel."[74]

Chapter 7

"Woman Is Not Made Like This"

Royer had been writing about the role of women in society ever since she had become articulate. Soon after she was elected as a member of the Société d'Anthropologie, she made a point of declaring that she was making a special study of the role of women in antiquity.[1] As noted in chapter 6, the differences of sexuality and reproduction in various racial groups were also of concern to her, so much so that she had worked actively on a questionnaire on this topic for travelers.

She had introduced the issue of sexuality into the discussions of evolution in the Société as she had earlier into her book on social origin, but she had insisted that different forms of reproduction could be identified: "In one [organism], it is sexuality, the relationship of two individuals, that is necessary for the manifestation of the generative force; in the other, a single being suffices to reproduce its race."[2]

In these evolutionary debates, Royer had raised the question of an overemphasis on sexual reproduction in evolutionary thinking. "Our scientists," she said, "have a disposition to find sexes everywhere," creating them before they looked for them, finding them in mosses, lichens, mushrooms, infusoria. Everywhere where scientists had found "two organs or only two tissues, two liquids, two different organic elements with different textures or properties, they have made two sexes of them."[3] This was not a new tendency, Royer asserted. People had always tried to make male and female entities out of the strangest objects. Originally occurring in mythology, it had become transferred to philosophy.

Royer gave some examples:

> One sees everywhere sexual polarization: first the gods and then ideas could only march in conjugally united couples. The atom itself had its poles. Of course the positive pole of an electromagnet or a battery has

> been called male by our scientists because—the feminine being always inferior in something—the feminine pole must be the negative. An Italian philosopher among my friends, always following the tenuous thread of analogy, that false seducer, has made oxygen the universal female, the alma mater, the Cybale and Vesta of nature. All other bodies are males, and gold is the most noble of all because it resists more than any other the attractions of the great seducer.[4]

In Royer's opinion, the sexualizing of matter was related to the relegation of females to an inferior, passive situation both in biology and society.

By 1873, she had become an extremely active member of the Société d'Anthropologie, devoting much time to papers and discussions before the anthropologists. She constantly participated in debates about Aryan origins, on atavism in evolution, on case studies of curious humans like the hairy-faced "man-dog" who passed through Paris. Yet, in the midst of this activity, she must have soon realized that membership in this scientific society had a rather different function for her as a woman than it had for the ambitious young men and the older professionals who surrounded her. Whereas for them the scientific society provided professional visibility and publication that would enhance a medical or scientific career, for her it was an end in itself. Unlike her equally active colleagues, she was not elected to a position in the central bureau of the society, she could not expect to function as an officer of the society, nor did she sit on committees. As a woman she was excluded from all that. None of her colleagues expected to be paid for their work for the Société d'Anthropologie or for the other scientific societies to which they belonged, but Royer could not anticipate even the professional payoff that the others could expect. For her male colleagues, activity in one society often preceded an invitation to belong to more prestigious societies and academies where they would form friendships destined to advance their careers.

Royer cannot have been unaware of the growing desire on the part of Paul Broca and his friends to create a school of anthropology that would provide teaching positions in that field. As I have shown elsewhere, those individuals who had spoken in support of a polygenist evolution would form the core of this school proposed in 1875 and established the following year: Eugène Dally, Broca, Louis-Adolphe Bertillon, Gabriel de Mortillet. One notable exception would be Clémence Royer.[5] Eighteen years later, requesting Quatrefages's support on behalf of a prize offered by the Académie des Sciences, she emphasized the fact that, as a woman, she had been excluded from any university or higher education teaching positions.[6]

In 1873, a long series of discussions and debates began in the Société d'Anthropologie on the falling birthrate in France. Louis-Adolphe Bertillon, demographer for the city of Paris and a close friend of Paul Broca, had just published his figures demonstrating the population decline.[7] The existence of such a fall in population raised questions about the validity of Malthusian concepts of population pressure and resulted in violent controversies. The views of the French on population were consequently very different from those of the English or the Germans who were experiencing at the same time enormous population growth. Paul Broca, in the course of the debates on evolution before the Société d'Anthropologie in 1870, discussed Darwin's interpretation of Malthusian population growth as a fundamental tenet of his theory. Broca reminded his colleagues that the laws of reproduction meant that animal and plant reproduction were potentially unlimited. But given the reality of limited food supply and space, the result was a

> fatal law of struggle of living beings, struggle between species that dispute place and nourishment, struggle between individuals (of the same species) that claim a part of the common lot of their species, the universal and eternal struggle to which the weakest must succumb. This great law, long recognized by philosophers and naturalists and unpityingly constituted in human societies by the economist Malthus, Charles Darwin has used in his turn. No one before him has formulated it with so much precision. No eye but his has seized it in its entirety. No mind has understood all its implications. Justly this should be called *Darwin's law*.[8]

Natural selection, a consequence of this Malthusian concept, led to important debates among French physicians, who formed the largest group of the Société d'Anthropologie and who did not want these arguments used to justify preventable human deaths. Broca made this point very clear when he opposed Royer's eugenic suggestions in his article "Les Sélections" (natural, sexual, and social) for his new journal *Revue d'Anthropologie.*[9]

Population was not increasing with the rapidity that was noted in Germany and England. Some individuals in the Société d'Anthropologie dismissed this as an indication of the high level of French civilization, since some thinkers linked civilization to increasing infertility. As France became more and more interested in colonial expansion in the 1870s, it also became vitally concerned with the need to populate potential colonies and develop industries. Bertillon had suggested that the encouragement of emigration to the colonies might help stimulate population growth in areas from which the colonists came, as it seemed to have done in other parts of Europe. He also sought economic and social reasons for the differences between provinces in population decline.[10] To committed evolutionists like Royer, population drop was an additional worry, since she believed that population pressure was the evolutionary motor for change and social progress.

There were a number of attempts within the Société d'Anthropologie to explain the drop in the French birthrate, but the arguments spilled over into other scientific societies as well. In Lyon during a meeting of the Association Française pour l'Avancement des Sciences in 1873, Royer had become involved in an argument with Bertillon and others over an explanation based on economic factors and differing inheritance laws in various departments of France. In her opinion, the active role of women was being left out of the equation.

In July 1874, the issue was revived within the Société d'Anthropologie with a long report by Delasiauve about the relationship between social class and birthrate in the Department of Eure. At this point, Royer's frustration came to a boil, and she spoke with heat and emotion about the extent that women were being left out of the discussion. "Up until now," she declared, "science and law, exclusively made by men, have too often considered woman as an absolutely passive being."[11] Woman was thought to have no passions, no instincts, no interests of her own. She was viewed as purely plastic material that could take any form given to it. She was thought to be a creature without any personal conscience, without will, without the inner resources to react against her education or the customary discipline she received. "No," she said, "woman is not made like this."[12] Women had played an active role in the rate of multiplication of the species.

But Royer did not end with this statement. Instead, she launched into a long discussion about women, which seemed to spring from her heart like a *cri de coeur.* "When man speaks of woman," she said, "it is to grant her those qualities that please him or those faults from which he personally suffers. Never does he see her as she is, because she always had some motive to dissimulate before him. . . . Woman . . . is the one animal in all creation about which man knows the least."[13]

Royer argued that men saw only women's actions, without realizing what they thought. Woman was a foreign species for man with whom he never really communicated. Up until now, no woman had been either able or willing to explain in general terms what she thought about the important questions that concerned her, without some personal interest being involved. Even when a woman discussed a problem with a man, she was rarely completely sincere. Neither her education nor her instincts prepared her to discuss the multiple motives for her actions with objectivity. If you wanted to know what a woman was thinking about, the first requirement was not to be a man![14]

In a section that sounds like the advice given to latter-day field ethnologists, Royer went on to say that women had to be observed and analyzed. They must be studied without being interrogated, made to betray themselves during the long conversations that took place during ordinary family life or in school. "This is what, as a woman, I have been able to do."[15]

Through her observations, Royer had come to the conclusion that there had been a real weakening of the basic maternal and sexual instincts in women, especially in the most cultivated women, as a result of their training. Extending the claim she had made in her first Darwin preface, she added that there had been a rigorous selection of women for calmness and submissiveness.

Women as a result had become much freer than men of sexual impulses, except for a pathological minority. This assertion, however, seemed somewhat contradicted by another claim in the same article that sexual instincts alone had saved the human race from extinction.

If women were so intent upon marrying, Royer asserted, it was because marriage had become their profession, often the only profession open to them. Society, by giving them no other place, had forced them to deal in "the commerce of love, legal or illegal."[16]

> Her first child is generally welcome because at the birth a weakened residue of maternal love is awakened in her. In general, her life, until then absolutely chaste, has disposed the young girl to become a mother. A mute but real need, in default of passion, pushes her to satisfy that somewhat vegetative law of the organism that woman can only achieve through maternity. But the second pregnancy is generally greeted sorrowfully or uneasily, and the third is dreaded. The fourth is almost always avoided, whatever the financial situation of the family might be.[17]

She considered that in many cases economic considerations served only as a pretext for both husband and wife. A woman, she commented rather sarcastically, tended to fill her professional role as a wife in the same way that other professional roles were filled, namely, as something to be done through necessity not through any real calling.[18] In a rather startling passage, she suggested that many wives tolerated their husbands' infidelities after one or two pregancies as long as this did not result in diminishing the life style of the family, especially once the first illusions of love had been shattered following some marital betrayal. The result was that marriage had become an association of interests, and the husband a kind of "legal fiction."[19] The wife might try to seduce her husband again through fear that he might love someone else too much. "This is the psychological moment for infertile self-indulgence. The wife becomes a mistress because she no long wishes to be a mother."[20]

Royer introduced the delicate subject of abortion by referring to the decline in birthrate among the so-called Yankee race in the United States, recently discussed by Hepworth Dixon.[21] The population in the United States had risen only because of the level of immigration and a high birth rate among recent German and Irish immigrants. She had verified this information with a woman doctor who had spent some years in the United States, both on the coast and in the interior, and who had close ties to the American medical world; she had confirmed Dixon's suggestion that middle-class Yankee women in the major cities commonly resorted to abortion.[22] Both male and female doctors performed the abortions, making considerable fortunes from their ability to gently "kill the fruit without endangering the tree" in the earliest stages of pregnancy.[23] The clientele was not needy. The women were elegant, rich women who did not want to miss a "pleasant social season or spoil their figures." Preferring to be wives rather than mothers, they often put off the first child for several years in order to "prolong the honeymoon."[24]

In the United States, economic conditions could not be the primary consideration for this limitation on the birth rate, Royer added. Education for children was free, and there were many opportunities for a career for boys and plenty of potential husbands for the girls through immigration. Royer recalled the situation of Rome during its decay, wondering aloud if the refusal of men to be soldiers was linked to the refusal of women to have babies,[25] a curious comment from a woman who later became an avowed pacifist.

Infanticide, she continued, whether practiced among "savage" peoples of Australia and Polynesia or the long civilized country of China, was often directed against female children. Whereas in China the father made the decision, in Australia it was the mother. With some sympathy, she wondered whether this decision by a woman who had submitted to a brutal and tyrannical life was motivated by the desire to keep another girl child from suffering as she had.[26] Even among the French, she believed, too many girls were rarely welcome, and many children were never born because of the fear that they would be girls.[27]

Women had the additional problem of finding their prospects limited by the number of men available as husbands. "All of those who exceed that number will be in the situation of unemployed workers, of merchants without customers, especially women of the middle classes, for whom all other work is considered degrading."[28]

If a woman had some financial resources, she would survive, but without a real social life of her own, otherwise she might augment the number of those "who, unable to buy with their dowry either a husband or social situation suitable to their education, might possibly become willing to sell themselves . . . to potential husbands of rich wives of the next generation and so increase the number of bachelors."[29] She claimed that an increase in single men meant an increase in prostitution and a consequent rise in the number of unmarried women becoming prostitutes or nuns. Thanks to war and emigration and the large number of men choosing to live alone, there were too many women. "This surplus of women, which might seem favorable to an increase in population, actually prevents its rise, since the value of a woman diminishes for a man by virtue of the great competition; the market is less in her favor."[30]

France had suffered more than most countries, partly because of wars throughout the century, partly because women did not emigrate as easily as men, and partly because the old French civilization had made Frenchwomen "the least female," by which she meant they were freer from sexual determinants without the healthy education needed to utlize that freedom.[31]

Admitting that she had used "brutal formulas in their stark reality," Royer brought up the role of the Catholic Church, which, she believed, had affected the attitude of women towards sexuality. Far from being too favorable to birth increase, she mistrusted the church's endorsement of celibacy, which suggested sexual restraint even within marriage.[32] Primitive Christianity had opposed marriage, and she insisted that the Catholic Church permitted its members to "perpetuate themselves" in order to assure its domination. But even then they had to turn to the Jewish texts in the Bible for use in the marriage ceremony to encourage people to go forth and multiply.[33]

Protestants in England, especially those in the ruling classes, she went on, were obsessed with the birthrate of the poor. Some of the same publishers in England who put out the Bible also publicized methods to decrease the birthrate of the poor and provided cheap and popular propaganda to this end. In the United States, women willing to "use the most radical procedures to suppress the population" were often "learned women theologians strongly versed in the study of biblical texts."[34] Royer asked rhetorically whether the policy of convents and priestly celibacy supported by the Catholic Church had not suppressed the number of children born as thoroughly as abortion had in the United States. There was no difference in the two procedures, she declared, at least judging by the results.[35]

While the education of middle-class boys had made them skeptical and unwilling to consider marriage a "sacred ritual equally binding for both parties," young girls on the other hand were never prepared to be mothers. "Marriage in their eyes is freedom, liberty, the right to be the mistress of a house, to have servants to command, to say 'my home,' to buy a dress that pleases them, to go to the theater, to which their mother refused to take them, to waltz at the ball with men previously forbidden to them, to have a seat in the church with their own name on it, and of course a coach with their mark or coat of arms upon it."[36] Motherhood on the other hand was generally depicted as painful, "shameful in itself, shall we say, unless preceded by a sort of anticipatory pardon by the church and by legal authorization."[37] With a personal sense of reference that few of her colleagues could have missed, she added that, although bearing a child outside marriage was no longer a crime, it could still be punished by disinheriting the child in spite of the change in modern economic conditions.

Women as a rule knew nothing about childbirth until they married. "How could they desire it? They think of it only with fright."[38] She deplored the fact that young women were never taken to watch a woman in labor or taught by their families or in school about even the minimal care they would have to give a newborn child. "Marriage, for the most part, is only a sad surprise, a terrible deception, a fall into reality from the high ideals that her imagination has painted for her until then."[39] These comments by Royer contrast with the description she gave of the wiser preparation for the facts of life given to her heroine Lucie by her mother. But she suggested the unhappy possibilities of sexual seduction or rape, again echoing Lucie's story. "When [young girls] have learned the law that presides over the renewing of generations, it is neither through their mothers nor their teachers but by chance and often the most unhappy chance."[40] If women from the countryside were better and more fertile mothers, it was because they learned about reproduction from the cowshed and the stable; they learned "from nature itself about these mysteries that are hidden with such care from young girls in the city."[41]

Again echoing the observation she made many years earlier in her novel that both young men and young women needed instruction about sexual consequences, she added that the bad effects of this lack of education about the facts of life on a young girl were aggravated by the far worse education of young men. Was it any wonder that the maternal instinct was attenuated in young girls? Having become mothers unexpectedly the first time, they refused to nurse the baby themselves and took care to avoid another pregnancy.[42]

She declared that it was surprising that the human species succeeded in perpetuating itself in spite of everything. What had saved the species, she believed, were primitive instincts accumulating "across the entire animal genealogy" that managed to resist the attempts of legislators or religions to "subdue, weaken, or make them disappear."[43] She made her point even more forcefully by showing the weight and importance she gave to instinct. "These ancient physical instincts of the brute, still latent in the species and always ready to reawaken, cause all forms of revolt. This is something that has already saved the species countless times and will save it yet again from everything that has been invented by the makers of dogmas and codes until the day when reason, enlightened by science, readily submits to the only laws that result from the interests of the species itself, once these have been studied and recognized."[44] It is important to note that here brute animal instincts are seen as the salvation of the species by promoting rebellion as well as ensuring reproduction.

If Royer had paused here, she might have carried her colleagues along with her, dedicated as they were to the same image of triumphant science linked to social progress. However, she continued with an description of the dangers that France would run if it should fail to create new social and economic principles to regulate the relations between the two sexes. She urged the need to change society to give women a new social and economic power. More importantly, she indicted the ill-advised social codes set up by men in the past, which needed to be revised by women.[45]

Humanity, she stated, would destroy itself if it had the misfortune to live "in accord with the dogmas, principles, and precepts that it has made up until now," and she suggested that egoism and economics would lead both men and women "to close off life to the child," leading to the future extinction of "all our superior races." Fortunately, human beings were contradictory and profoundly ignorant of the "real laws of nature," and this very ignorance and failure of logic would save humanity.[46]

In a brief, but alarming, note of racism almost as extreme as Theodore Roosevelt's later admonitions about the "yellow peril," Royer went on to reveal her own prejudices. There was not only the peril for France of becoming a second-rate power in Europe but a peril to the whole white race, which still counted only about 300 million. They had "opened the doors to the teeming yellow race so capable of adapting to every climate."[47]

Harping again on the need to regularize illegitimate births, she suggested that custom and law must begin to recognize the right of women to become mothers outside legal marriage. This would improve the "attenuated instinct for maternity" in woman and arouse the even weaker paternal instinct in man. Unmarried mothers must fulfill all their duties to their children and "force the law to treat these children as the equals of their brothers." In order for a woman to use such a right, she had to have a way to earn her living so that she would not be constrained "against her nature, her tastes, or her preferences to sell herself either to a husband or a lover, whom she can see only as her keeper, legal or otherwise, if she submits through interest or necessity."[48] Woman had to stop seeing love and marriage as a kind of "more or less agreeable or lucrative commerce." She had to begin to understand that marriage was not just an opportunity to "appear in a white veil covered with flowers, or surpass her friends with her clothing the next day, or even promenade with her doll baby in the arms of a nurse decked out in ribbons."[49]

Like the Italian republican mothers, she argued that a woman needed "to give the state citizens to defend it and to raise them seriously, using her reason as well as her heart."[50] Woman needed to free herself from religious prejudices, "not to inculcate them." She needed to teach herself so she could teach her children. Repeating what she had said in her book on income tax reform, she added that "motherhood is the equivalent of military service and she has to support its dangers and privations with courage," a sentiment endorsed by many men as well as women of the time.[51] She owed it to her race to provide "intelligent and robust, healthy, and audacious representatives." They would then be able to go out to "dispute" the land held by other, "inferior races."[52]

Royer did not think that it was sufficient to speak of women's duties without recognizing their rights. She began to spell out a mutual contract between equals that could be broken if all the conditions were not fulfilled on both sides. Women had to have the same education as men so that man and woman could be united in "the same beliefs, the same respect, the same sympathies, the same hatreds." They had to learn to understand and to appreciate each other.[53]

Again emphasizing the importance of reformation of male sexual behavior that she had proposed in her novel, she commented that young men, like young women, had to have the same restraints placed on them—without those "sad debaucheries"—so that when they were married they would not have learned to divorce their heart from their sensations. Thinking perhaps of Duprat's wife and their daughter, she spoke with some feeling about "badly matched" liaisons, which have "such sad results" and which "throw into the world social hybrids" who never find a proper place for themselves.[54]

With a desire to accommodate economic freedom for both husband and wife, Royer suggested that husband and wife should not be required to live under the same roof. "While young couples wait to make for themselves a place in the sun," the husband could stay with his parents, and the wife with hers. In this way, the first children could be born under the "expert eyes of a grandmother." The custom of having a family composed only of a couple and their children—what in our day we call the "nuclear family"—she believed, would result in "the death of society through egoistic individualism."[55]

The need to form a new household could also result in depopulation, since it led to late marriages. The result was a demoralization and elimination of family life that increasingly created difficulties because each couple spent more and produced less as the woman became involved in the care of her household and her children. She recommended that the young couple center their life around those of the previous generation—"under the domestic direction of the grandmother"—so that both the young man and the young woman could practice a profession "and each contribute their part to the well-being of the family," until in turn they could repeat the same pattern for their own children.[56] Royer, again, seems to have taken her own life as a model. Her mother lived very close to Duprat and Royer and probably played an important part in helping to rear René, although she was to die only two years after Royer had written this memoir.

Doubtless recalling the unpleasant relationship that had continued between Duprat and his legal wife, she warned that unless these necessary reforms were carried out, "we will see war declared between the two halves of humanity, who will be occupied in deceiving, in exploiting one another."[57] Instead there should be a "reasonable and thought-out law of selection" that would have as its principal aim, if not its only aim, "the multiplication everywhere of the most noble types of the species, both physically and morally."[58]

She again suggested human eugenical laws similar to those that she had proposed in her Darwin prefaces, but she no longer proposed the harsh elimination of those born malformed, possibly taking to heart not only Naville's criticisms but those of Broca, who had commented that no physician, trained to save life, could adopt such harsh measures.[59] Instead she suggested that social severity should be limited to those who "through venal calculation propagate unhealthy germs or badly endowed races." For those who could not expect "a posterity that is healthy in mind and body" celibacy should be not only permitted but imposed. She suggested some social compensation for this group of unfortunates, who would be permitted "every license among themselves" on condition that once they entered this state, they could not leave it or permit "any germ [offspring] to be born." If abortion or infanticide be authorized, it would be in such cases only.[60] Love could be free on condition that "it is not, as it is today, an appetite, a distraction, a blind fatality for man and for woman, a necessity, a profession, a calculation."[61]

How would this kind of social reform come about? Royer asked. Through women themselves, after they had learned both their duty and their rights. While leaving man to "write and efface his ephemeral constitutions and codes ten times in one century that are always recopied from ancient codified errors," woman would "engrave new customs upon the solid rock of hereditary instinct by giving to the world sons [*sic*] instructed by her who would transcribe these customs into laws."[62]

The publication committee headed by Bertillon had some difficulty with three parts of Royer's contribution: she had challenged the church (both Protestant and Catholic), she had challenged the Napoleonic Code, which specified a woman's legal relationship to her husband, and she had advocated some marked changes in social regulation of sexuality and reproduction. The galley proofs of Royer's manuscript were marked with blue and red editorial pencils to indicate changes that the publication committee felt Royer should make. Royer at first attempted to comply but then objected, believing that Bertillon was using his position to suppress a point of view with which he did not agree.[63]

After the election of 1873 and the rise of the monarchist party led by Marshall MacMahon to power, Gambetta, the editor of *La République Française,* cautioned his readers, "We have discovered the politic method and the method of patience and solitude."[64] The political setback for the liberal republicans had also resulted in the suppression of feminist lectures and journals. In this context the failure to print Clémence Royer's contributions on women becomes more understandable, although she took the editors' cautious attitude very unkindly and personally. The "method of patience" did not come easily to Royer.

Royer's statement on women embodied many recurring themes in her writings: the importance of human instincts as a source of correction for social errors, the capability of women to create a biologically based society, and the belief that an alliance between mothers and their sons might accomplish this.

References to matriarchy as a preferred form of society were present in her earlier writings, although more cautiously. In the *Origin of Man and Societies* she had commented—with some disclaimers—about the usefulness of such a society with a reversal of sex roles.[65] Such a society might result in economic gains because a more "fertile" [*sic*] use of time would result from a lowered capital outlay. Earlier, she had hoped for the blossoming of a "female science" that would correct masculine errors.[66] Now it was society itself that should be corrected.

Given such strong recommendations about the future of human society as well as her emphasis on the "uneasy bargains" that men and women had struck with each other, it is not surprising that her male colleagues hesitated to print her memoir. Although her anticlerical comments would not have disturbed them, since many of them shared her attitude, her attack on all forms of

Christianity may have seemed excessive for a group with a heavy Protestant membership. Her eugenic comments posed special difficulties. Paul Broca had specifically attacked this aspect of her Darwin preface, commenting that "society must grant protection to all its members or return to the savage state."[67]

Even more significantly, by 1875, when the 1874 *Bulletin* went to press, the central committee of the Société d'Anthropologie was in the process of rather delicate negotiations with the Faculty of Medicine, the municipal council, and a few important bankers to create the new School of Anthropology, the high point of Broca's long-desired Institute of Anthropology, intended to unite the anthropological facilities of the society, the laboratory, and the museum. (See fig. 6 for a photograph of significant members of the Société d'Anthropologie in the late 1870s.) This projected School of Anthropology had already come under attack by the Catholic press as an attempt to develop a "school of free thought."[68] To publish Clémence Royer's controversial remarks at such a time may have presented an unnecessary risk.

Royer, possibly unaware of the multitude of factors involved, turned to Paul Broca as a court of last resort to plead for the retention of her memoir unchanged. "Have you read my communication? she wrote with annoyance. "I do not believe it, or you would have seen that nowhere have I attacked the civil code."[69] Yes, she added, perhaps some of her statements were strongly stated, but "it is not my fault that this is the way things are." Referring to Bertillon sarcastically as "our Cato of Demography"—demography was a term he had helped define—she characterized him, perhaps unwisely, as "more scrupulous in words than in deeds" and went on to comment that she had observed this in Lyon, asking Broca to keep this comment "between ourselves". She claimed to detect behind Bertillon's prudence "a trace of that ambiguous and equivocal morality that rules so strongly today."[70]

Royer told Broca that she had shown her article to Duprat, "whom I have never known to be mistaken about the measures to be taken on behalf of courageous speech." Duprat had suggested that she make the requested changes and cuts in order to have the piece published. Unfortunately, Royer balked at this suggestion, although she had at first attempted to make the changes. In rereading it, she felt that she was accurate in everything she had said. She was not willing to make major changes, only to add a series of notes of justification and explanation. Her appeal to Broca ended with the plea that he allow these questions to be discussed "at least once by a woman who believes herself as capable as any man to pretend to the title philosopher. . . . Just because she is a woman, she is free from certain prejudices characteristic of men on these delicate questions."[71]

The publication committee headed by Bertillon must have seen this letter along with Clémence Royer's lengthy additions. The manuscript was set as final page proofs, testifying to the society's original intention to publish it, but in July 1875 it was eliminated from the volume and placed in the archives along with the galleys and page proofs and a laconic note that the author had agreed to its suppression, since she had not wished to make the necessary changes.[72] No indication of her discussion about women exists in the published bulletin. Bertillon's brief remarks in reply to Royer during the same meeting were also suppressed.

It is a pity that this manuscript was not published in even modified form, since Royer never published comments on women's social roles in quite this form anywhere else. She indicated in her note to Broca that she intended to write an extensive monograph on this subject and asked for her supplementary notes to be returned for this purpose, but the monograph never appeared. Her comments on these issues in later years never carried the same passionate originality of this censored article.

Royer must have been both hurt and insulted by the suppression of her paper, as indicated by the fact that she ceased to be an active member of the society for some time following this controversy. Although she contributed both papers and comments in discussions on a regular basis until mid-1875, after the final decision not to print her paper was made, her communications ceased for the rest of the year. The following year she offered only a single paper on a very different topic.

Royer's publications on population before this suppression in 1875 dealt only with economic and evolutionary aspects of the issue.[73] When she took up the related topics of reproduction, heredity, and sexuality in a paper for Paul Broca's journal, *Revue d'Anthropologie,* in 1877, she approached them in broader terms, no longer discussing woman's role in French society. In her paper entitled "Two Hypotheses on Heredity" she elaborated her earlier attack on Darwin's hereditary theory of pangenesis, as promised in her preface to the third French edition.[74] She insisted that Darwin's new theory "contradicted natural selection" and proposed to replace it by a "dynamogenesis" that incorporated energy into the system of material inheritance. Royer expanded her ideas of sexuality in her analysis. She also included the first detailed description of the connection between material nonliving atoms and living cells, which would obsess her from this point on.[75]

A comment in her paper on heredity hints at one source of her growing interest in the energetic and mechanical basis for living organisms. Her first encounter with the death of a family member in the home had made her realize that the living organism was a "powerful and delicate machine in movement." Death itself "from the experimental point of view" appeared to be no more than the last phenomenon of life. "[It is] a successive and not instantaneous phenomenon just like that of birth, but in general more rapid in the succession of its phases."[76] We will see how her concern with fundamental structures, both atoms and cells, would underlie all her discussions of physics, evolution, and morality over the next ten years.

One of the most interesting aspects of her discussion of heredity was an insistence on the identity between cellular, asexual, and sexual reproduction. Once more she objected to scientists who sought "two fluids, two poles" everywhere, finding two sexes "even in the stars themselves."[77] Beginning with the phenomenon of parthenogenesis, something that had intrigued her as early as her first reading of Darwin, she pointed out that, at least in some insects, females could "produce offspring for long periods of time without the action of the male." She believed that an identity had been recognized between the ovule and the bud of a plant, which "furnishes us a decisive proof, moreover, that the vital cycle can be opened up and commence without fertilization." Budding was a kind of normal parthenogenesis. "This is in sum the most general mode of generation. It is primitive, natural. It is the rule. Everything else is an exception."[78]

The fertilized female and the sterile female differed only to the degree that "organic movement" in each of the ovules was kept in a latent state. The spermatozoa of the male therefore only gave a "vital impulse" to the ovule, an impulse possibly required as the world cooled. As she put it, "Fertilization is, in sum, only an organizing snap."[79]

She stated even more clearly her conclusion that sexuality was only a contingent factor in evolution.[80] Organisms did not have to evolve separate sexes. She recognized that Darwin had pointed out the advantages of sexual generation in increasing more varied and vigorous products, while self-fertilized or asexual forms would be "incapable of sustaining the struggle against more favored relatives."[81] She connected these developments to the development of specialized cells into "cellular hierarchies" resulting in the formation of specialized organs, first in a hermaphroditic form, then as two sexes, as the advantages of "greater vigor" of separate individuals were played out. "But," she insisted, "in no way does this prove sexual separation to be primordial and necessary as [Darwin] has a tendency to claim."[82] Nor, she added, did cross-fertilization prevent self-fertilization.

Her interpretation of the retention of some forms of asexual generation coupled with natural selection acting over generations to "order the primitive disorder," accounted, she believed, for such phenomena as sexual dimorphism, the extreme variety of some species, and the wide differences within insect castes. Darwin had already accounted for the problem of neuter insects and insect castes to his satisfaction as a form of group selection. But to Royer, natural selection was an ordering mechanism producing peculiar "abnormalities" such as the radical size difference in some species between male and female.[83]

Starting with the observation that asexual or "hermaphroditic" reproduction produced less variety, while sexual reproduction resulted in both more individuality and "more monstrosity," she reintroduced her theory of "dynamogenesis" as an explanatory mechanism. Energy impulses were transmitted in a "straight line" in the hermaphrodite, whereas two impulses were provided in sexual crosses. Only in sexual reproduction was "each newly produced machine organized and prompted by two machines."[84] Like never exactly reproduced like. Accidental circumstances and "external physicochemical forces" always came to modify the initial "atavistic" direction. The result was force at "an angle of some sort" that pushed aside the straight or parallel lines of reproduction.[85] This image of heredity as a dynamic "angle" derived from an earlier argument in the paper, where she compared "organic molecules" to a large group of marbles falling on an equally resistant marble surface, scattering in all directions. By adding chemical properties to this it was possible, she believed, to get some sort of "perpetual motion."[86]

One cannot avoid the question why Royer was concerned to show that sexual reproduction had only a contingent nature. The answer appears to derive from Royer's view of woman's role in society and contemporary claims that the female role was fatally determined by nature. If, indeed, there were two sexes in nonliving as well as living things, and if the female was relegated to a passive, nourishing role and never a creative one, then, she feared, woman also could be assigned a perpetually inferior position in society. She had attacked Rousseau and Proudhon for depicting woman only as a procreative complement to man.[87] Royer, a creative, active woman insistent about her own originality, could not tolerate this kind of sexual determinism. If the option was to privilege asexual or parthenogenetic reproduction and to deny the role of sexuality as a motivating factor in nature, so be it.

In 1876, Duprat lost the election for a seat in the National Assembly from Landes, and soon after the little family moved, first to the rue Jaquemont and shortly after to the rue de Rome, providing a more middle-class setting for Duprat's successful electoral campaign as a deputy from the seventeenth arrondissement of Paris in 1877. However, at the end of 1876, gossip among individuals in the Batignolles district was reported to the police, suggesting that Royer and Duprat had quarreled publicly and "scandalously," and that Duprat had moved on his own to the rue de Rome and was about to move again because "his concubine" had followed him there.[88] Since this report is not repeated in Royer's dossier, one wonders if the "scandalous quarrels" were not with Royer but with his legal wife, that "jetting tempest," whose demands for support were always a burden in Royer's eyes.

Royer was soon holding regular soirées at the rue de Rome for Duprat, to which a variety of like-minded political and intellectual friends were invited. These friends included the Belgian writer Céline Renooz Muro, who was also exploring the world of science. She had written to Royer about her enjoyment of some of Duprat's lectures and requested further information about them. Renooz herself had begun to organize a lecture series at the rue de Bac, and she invited Royer to participate.[89] With this dogmatic and eccentric woman, also a member of the Société d'Ethnographie, Royer would have at first a pleasant, later an abrasive, relationship.

Given that nothing that Royer wrote in 1876 indicates a rupture between her and Duprat, a more likely explanation for the move was the death of Royer's mother. Again demonstrating the manner in which she always objectified her most powerful emotions, Royer wrote an article for Broca's journal *Revue d'Anthropologie* on burial rites in 1876, the year of her mother's death and the year of these moves.[90] In some detail, Royer imagined the abandonment of a corpse within one of the prehistoric caves, the closing of the cave with a stone, and the later reopening of the cave by other families. She suggested a variety of interesting interpretations of objects found at prehistoric grave sites, primitive burial rituals, and linguistic origins of words for tombs and sepulchers. Her vivid description of fear of the corpse as well as of the distaste for a place of death gives a powerful personal motive for her relocation from the rue Brochant to the rue de Rome.[91]

Royer went on to describe someone torn between curiosity and fear of looking at the dead. "In the night his sleep is haunted by the vision of the dead one, who reappears to him as living. He runs to assure himself the corpse is in the same place and accuses it of coming to trouble his repose." Cave dwellers, she said were "constrained to abandon for a time the grotto where they lived in safety because one of them has died and has been buried there, in order to look for another habitation."[92] Possibly, she added, they would be forced to move again because of a second death. She suggested that modern men and women have retained the instinctive dislike of primitive people towards places where relatives have died. "This primitive instinct of fear of the dead dominates all others in our modern populations in the countryside and even in the cities. It is never without a sort of fright, of instinctive repugnance for touching a dead person, which even very cultivated men cannot overcome. Among women and children especially this feeling has the irrational and blind power of hereditary instincts."[93] She described in detail the appearance of the dead, and the role that women played in preparing the corpse, a task left for them to attend to, "as are all other vile tasks."[94] Royer's comments reflect her concern about the role of women in society, of which her own ambiguous position had made her doubly aware.

Royer had viewed the woman question with passion and feeling in the 1870s, as a woman with a young child born out of wedlock, living publicly with a married man. Her position as wife and mother gave her a privately but not publicly recognized role. A letter she wrote in 1877 indicates that she was also aware that much of what she had said about women in society was viewed by her colleagues with some embarrassment. When asked to speak in a lecture series by Céline Renooz (then Madame Muro) at the rue de Bac, she at first replied that she was in enough physical discomfort so that she could not promise in advance to speak too long. She agreed to apply for permission to speak on "social customs and moral law" only with the understanding that she was not firmly committed. But, she added, in a revealing comment, her lack of the usual repugnance for certain topics that were considered too delicate for a woman "in the current state of opinion" meant that she was "always afraid of saying too much about them and letting escape from me the torrent of indignation that each of us carries in her as the heritage of the whole race."[95] That comment may also reflect her perception of how her memoir on women and the birthrate had been received by the members of the Société d'Anthropologie three years earlier. The death of her mother the year before may have further aggravated her sense of indignation about women's social roles, and she may have been worried about her own increased health problems.

What Royer would have said in Renooz's lecture series we cannot know, since she was prevented from speaking on this question by the police. Neither they nor the minister of public education wanted her to discuss social customs in a public forum. In the police reports, two issues weighed against her. First she was known to be living with Duprat "as a married woman," and she was known to be the mother of his son, who also lived with them. Secondly, she had been contributing political articles to a Russian newspaper. Both these factors made her potentially dangerous, although she was regularly authorized by the police to speak on scientific topics, and she participated in scientific meetings, which were not under police scrutiny. In this case, as the ministerial report to the police read, it would be "seriously inconvenient to allow public criticism of the current regulations of the police on customs, since such criticisms would provide only objections without useful results for the services of your prefecture."[96]

Royer, discovering that she had been forbidden to speak because of a ministerial decision, naturally was upset. Only two ministers (one of them being Jules Simon) had ever prevented her from speaking in public, she explained to Renooz. "You know that I was in no hurry to confront the public again, but this refusal invites me to defend a right, and at least I want to know their motives."[97]

The action by the prefecture and the ministry provides an answer to the otherwise puzzling question as to why Royer failed to speak at the first Congress on the Rights of Women held in 1878 in Paris, although she did attend the conference.[98] Having been prevented from speaking in 1877 on less dramatic issues, she may have tried to avoid the same kind of refusal only one year later. Her public silence kept her from gaining the kind of international recognition for her ideas on women she might have received from the English-speaking contingent.

Some of the prejudices against Royer's outspoken remarks in public and scientific forums may have been due to contemporary male fears of the "man-woman," as caricatured by such writers as Alexandre Dumas *fils*.[99] A political reaction to the growing demands for women's rights sought justification among the scientists. Gustave Le Bon, a colleague of Royer's in the Société d'Anthropologie, had worked in Broca's laboratory in 1877 and 1878 on the relative differences in brain and skull size between men and women. Having shown that the differences existed from culture to culture but were more exaggerated among civilized people, he concluded that his study proved the natural inferiority of women's brains, which had limited women's social roles in the past and should continue to do so in the future. Although there were women of superior intelligence, they were abnormalities, monstrosities of nature. The large percentage of women should be kept in their traditional roles, since the pressure to compete with men would result in perversion and decadence.[100] The Société d'Anthropologie awarded Le Bon the Godard Prize for this contribution on women's brains, but distanced itself from his social conclusions. Paul Broca, in the central committee meeting insisted that the report, read by Charles Letourneau, should include a clear disclaimer.[101]

Royer chose not to challenge Le Bon directly on the issue of women's brains, but she lost no opportunity to challenge him on other issues, since he often spoke slightingly of women as "inferior beings." She even entered the Laboratory of Anthropology to study craniology with Léonce Manouvrier. After Royer's death, Manouvrier, who confronted Le Bon on both his measurements and his conclusions, commented that Royer herself had mistakenly adopted the "myth of male science" by accepting that her brain must be larger than that of most women.[102] If this was so, it appears to be in conflict with her general view, which she shared with Paul Broca, that women's education, not brain size, was the key to social change.

CHAPTER 8

Years of Trial: A Search for Universal Laws

As the 1880s approached, Royer found her personal situation ambiguous. On the one hand, she was living a gracious life as Duprat's hostess in a pleasant bourgeois area of Paris. On the other, she began to realize that Duprat's political problems and her public association with him were a handicap for her own ambition to make her scientific and philosophical ideas more widely known. The family moved from the sterile area of the rue de Rome to the avenue des Ternes, a vast boulevard in a bourgeois neighborhood where they rented an apartment at a far higher yearly rental of Fr 1,500. Here, at number 82, in an apartment in an attractive new building with sculpted faces decorating the cornices, Royer would initiate her own society to study moral and philosophical sciences.[1]

Not only did Duprat have a gift for backing the wrong political and financial horses as he aged, but he made additional enemies through his rather cruel, satirical word portraits of his old comrades, fellow republicans, and fellow deputies in his rewritten book on revolution, *L'Esprit des révolutions,* published in 1879. Here, under thinly disguised Roman names, he lampooned political and literary men of all shades of the political spectrum: monarchist conservative ministers like the duc de Broglie and General MacMahon, the liberal republican Léon Gambetta, the radical Henri de Rochefort, the positivist republican senator Emile Littré, and many others.[2]

At this point Duprat had expanded his role as the rebel in the assembly, challenging the increasingly "occult power" of Gambetta, who had reached the height of his personal influence. In this fight against Gambetta, during February 1881, Duprat was supported by radical republicans like Clemenceau, without that party ever totally trusting him or giving him its support.[3]

He continued to serve republicanism by speaking regularly in the provinces on a variety of topics from income tax reform to the history of the French Revolution. He went on working in journalism as well. He took over the newspaper *Le Nouveau Journal* as editor in chief, only to leave as arguments developed between him and his colleagues and the money to support the paper evaporated. He tried his hand at a number of capital projects and sat on the board of banking ventures, but these lost rather than made money. In a period of rapid increase of capital and the spectacular expansion of the railroads, Duprat contracted only debts.[4]

Already in the late 1870s he had been under attack in his district of Paris and had won his seat only narrowly. By 1881, when the new elections were held in the seventeenth arrondissement of Paris, Duprat was pictured by his opponents as a republican of the past, not the future. The increasingly strong radicals in the area had never forgiven him for his support of Thiers during the Commune. Lockroy, a future minister of the republic who had supported him in 1877, had become his avowed enemy and lent increasingly important support to his opponent, Henri Maret, insisting upon unproved rumors of Duprat's financial duplicity.[5]

Duprat did not seem to be able to convey his own program adequately enough, although on the face of it seemed strong and liberal: separation of church and state, divorce, revision of the constitution, extension of municipal liberties, abolition of the death penalty, the reform of magistrates, the extension of arbitration between bosses and workers, equitable divisions of income tax, liberty of association, meetings, and the press. He opposed armed interference of France in Greece, yet advocated obligatory military service. Duprat insisted that he had been independent in every ministry, and he pointed out the enormous number of talks, at least a hundred, that he had given on the subject of republicanism throughout the provinces, but this did not produce support for him in Paris. The radical Left and socialist journals described him as a "shady product of politics and finance" who "hated the people, for whom he has a horror."[6] One might add that one of the regular police informers supported his opponent, Maret, even going so far as to libel Duprat in public meetings.[7] The result of all these attacks against him was the loss of his seat in the assembly.[8]

The new president of the Republic, Jules Grévy, urged the minister of foreign affairs to appoint Duprat to an ambassadorship. For a number of reasons he was not acceptable to most European governments. He had, after all, publicly supported revolution in Spain, and his position on the Greek-French disputes had not won him friends in Athens, although one might imagine that his old European ties might have made him an excellent Swiss or Italian minister.

Duprat was offered an ambassadorship in Chile; he accepted in spite of the long sea journey this entailed, perhaps to ensure a good income to his family after the loss of his seat in the assembly and the failure of his financial projects. His supporters in Landes, where he retreated in the early 1880s as his health began to fail, were concerned about his taking up the appointment. His brother's family nursed him back to health, while he spoke eagerly to his young associates about great opportunities in the New World (fig. 7).[9]

Duprat was visibly aging. His old-fashioned hairstyle and his ancient hat made him a figure of fun to his enemies, who ridiculed his appearance. One particularly cruel attack in the comic journal *Petit Caporal* described him a "rheumy old man" who could not "be tailored to take some serious role in the comedies or tragedies of Marianne," that attractive female symbol of the republic. His hat and hair would be clean enough for an uncivilized nation, the squib continued, although he would never be expected to represent France "at a hat shop or a bath house."[10] Possibly this was simply a retaliation by this right-wing paper for his nasty word picture of the duc de Broglie published in 1879.

"All these proscriptions [against Duprat]," Royer complained, "have weighed upon me, have isolated me, have closed all the reviews to me. Reduced to powerlessness, I could not ask for or receive publicity from a journal that the same morning has insulted the father of my son, still less from those who were opposed to his convictions and to mine."[11] The financial burden weighed especially heavily upon Royer, as Duprat planned to spend some years in Chile, and she sought new monetary sources of support during the early 1880s. She was no longer writing for *Goloss,* which had been suppressed in Russia since 1876. She tried for a series of prizes offered by the Académie des Sciences and the Académie des Sciences Morales et Politiques on a variety of questions. Only two of these would earn her a monetary prize, although no laurels. As she put it, quoting from an Italian proverb, "First try to live by philosophy."[12]

Royer continued her regular contributions to the Société d'Anthropologie and the *Journal des Économistes,* but these scholarly ventures, of course, brought in no income. Resigned to never earning money from lecturing in France, she also had to give up profitable foreign lecturing, since winter lectures in badly heated rooms had adversely affected her health.[13]

Royer began a number of projects to increase her visibility and her income in the early 1880s. One of the financially more successful was a new version of her Darwin edition, which was originally envisioned as a shorter and more popular edition of *Origin.* Royer wrote to Charles Darwin in 1881 to obtain his permission.[14] He gave his consent on condition that she follow his latest text. She seems to have interpreted this as a request not to write a popular edition but to produce a corrected version of her older text. The result was a reissuing of her old translation of Darwin in a new form, which came out the next year shortly after his death.[15]

Although she made few changes in the translation itself, Darwin's requirement that she observe all his changes in the last edition of the *Origin* meant that she footnoted these, along with his extensive notes at the end of the volume, as an appendix. Not only did she give Darwin's notes but commented on them and on his changes to *Origin* in this first appendix. She also added a second appendix that contained her own notes from all three previous editions, accompanied by additional notes signaling her more recent evolutionary insights described in articles she had published since the 1870 edition.[16]

While she retained her original preface in its modified form, she removed her two other prefaces, replacing them with a short note to the readers of the fourth edition, beginning with the words: "Twenty years have passed since I made the principal work of Charles Darwin known in France." The new edition had already gone to press when "the news of the death of the author came to revive and rejuvenate his now uncontested glory." The French press was experiencing an "explosion of posthumous enthusiasm" and rendering him a "tardy justice." Royer congratulated herself on having long before adopted an evolutionary doctrine, "following Lamarck," even before reading Darwin.[17] The enthusiasm for Darwin, she continued, had not been without its critics, who too often produced ill-founded criticisms. Royer saw herself as a self-appointed defender of Darwin's ideas, in spite of the corrections and additions to Darwin she permitted herself.

What Royer created in her appendices was a kind of concordance to Darwin, although few French readers can have followed the intricacies of the changing shades of Darwin's thought. Royer's own notes can be read today as her fullest commentary on Darwinism including those ideas that she considered to be her own contributions to evolutionary theory, both Darwinian and non-Darwinian, and the connection of both to her hereditary theories.

Outside of her Darwin edition, two scientific issues concerned her at this time. One was to put the "moral" or "social" sciences on a good scientific basis; the other was to develop a good hypothetical model of the molecular structure of matter. For Royer, the two were closely related, as she had explained in her contribution to *La Philosophie Positive* on "the nature of beauty."[18]

Influenced, undoubtedly, by reediting and summarizing the prefaces she had written to her translations—in which she had insisted on the application of natural selection to moral law—she began to extend this theory in a new book, which, she claimed, she had tried to publish for twenty years. She had tentatively announced these ideas in her first lectures for women in Lausanne. At the Congrès des Sciences Sociales in Gand, Switzerland, in 1863, she developed them still further. Blocked by the prefecture of police when she tried to lecture on the relationship between moral and natural law in 1877, she finally decided to publish the work she had begun twenty years earlier.

The result was her book *Le Bien et la loi morale,* which she published herself "under conditions that mean that even if the entire edition is sold, I will be left with a loss."[19] There had been objections, she noted, to the publication of her study of morality in a large review, because one group thought her too heterodox—as she certainly was in the eyes of the positivists—while another thought her proposals were too far-reaching, too sprawling.[20] She expressed a sense of pressure on her to publish for fear of the loss of priority. Already her ideas were being anticipated in England and Germany, she added. Haeckel was publishing on "animated atoms and cellular souls," and Spencer had just published *Data of Ethics,* "in which he arrived at conclusions very close to those I expose here on morality, only less extensive."[21] Again, as in many earlier situations, Royer used the work of another thinker to spark her own related ideas, which she then developed in opposition. While she acknowledged Spencer's recognition of morality within the animal kingdom, which could only be "disregarded at its peril," he granted only a passive and unconscious existence to the vegetable kingdom and drew a line "at the threshold of organic life." She invoked a "new" concept of "specific egoism" that would go far beyond Spencer's "competitive egoism."[22] This adoption of a related, but often distinct, term—as she had done in proposing "dynamogenesis" in opposition to Darwin's "pangenesis"—illustrates the degree to which her terminology as well as her concepts developed in reaction to what she read.

In the beginning of her new book she reiterated many of the points she had made in her first Darwin preface. There she had defined moral law as "that which tends towards the conservation, multiplication, and progress of every species, relative to place and time."[23] For Royer in 1862, placing what she saw as the origin of good and evil on a natural, scientific base had been an exciting project. She believed she had found a replacement for religious explanation in this description of human origin "*toute brutale.*" Animal and instinctual aspects of humanity in the process of evolution could explain the penchant for evil and the aspiration towards the good or, at least, the "better."[24]

Royer had argued before the Social Science Congress in 1863 that one should not judge people's private life during their lifetime. Although this may have served as a public defense of both Duprat and herself, she placed it in a much wider context. "Each individual tends to call good what one permits oneself and bad what one avoids, condemning or absolving according to the license allowed, and that is an evil. We know that moral law is vital for humanity, and once this is weakened, our species is condemned to degenerate. Above all, these questions call for calm."[25] She reminded her listeners that Jeanne d' Arc was condemned in the name of morality, as was John Huss and many others.

Morality changed, she said, but it did not progress. Morality was a relationship between an act and its agent; it wasn't just a human fact, but a universal fact. In animals morality was "an instinctive law," while in humans it was subjected to other considerations. Nevertheless, morality still retained its instinctual basis. Two kinds of morality existed: one was an inherited conscience, "a revelation of instinct and feeling, conserved by authority and based on the principle of submission." All fanatics employed this kind of morality, which "retained something of the beast or the domestic animal." But this morality needed to be subjected to the rational and intelligent conscience of free thought (*libre raison*). The moral law of the past, which reflected the inheritance of the entire species, had to be developed, reformulated, "enlightened" by the rational conscience, which itself must be developed.[26]

Royer argued that once moral law was perfected, there would be no need for laws or justice or rulers. "We would be like gods. . . . We have, therefore, insisted on the necessity for a serious and scientific revision of morality; we have said that this was a pressing necessity for children and the young, for whom doubt is deadly."[27]

Beyond that, Royer went on, one had to know what was good for the species. The formula for that "good" changed constantly, although she felt it could be discovered through "induction, observation, and experience" and by studying "nature and history through our sentiments and our instincts." The fundamental principle of moral law, as she defined it in 1863, was "its usefulness to the species that it directs." Moral law for humanity had to include a provision to allow it to "multiply its individuals, its varieties, and its forms" in order to increase its "faculties, its powers, and its progress" on the evolutionary ladder. Any moral law that prevented this progress was "a false, cruel, condemnable law."[28]

Her adversaries proposed ideas, she said, that were "chaotic and contradictory" by defining an absolute morality that had existed from ancient times. No one, she noted, could agree on what this morality was, except that it had progressed over time, but Royer denied that morality itself progressed in spite of her commitment to evolution.

When Royer returned to the topic of scientific morality in her book in 1881—almost twenty years later—she declared that she had discovered the basis of all moral law in the law of biological utility and progress towards happiness. In dramatic language, she insisted that moral law be based upon a biological understanding of the human being "and his true place in the organic series."[29] Extending her remarks about the effect of doubt upon the young, she added in a vivid metaphor that when religious dogmas are overturned, "the statue falls and breaks and humanity rests without rule or law." Most present-day morality, she added, consisted either of a "rewarmed stew of old adages . . . religious reminiscences and various laws" or invoked common usage or common-sense decisions. Science, said Royer, would have to provide a replacement for this unsatisfactory legal basis.

One of the more unusual features of her book was her attempt to make this "universal law" apply to the inorganic world as well. She presented her ideas as the final conclusion to the philosophy she first proposed in her 1859 lectures for women. She took as her point of departure the belief in the existence of one "main, eternal, and universal fact": a substantially fluid atom that was "infinitely active, expansive, and repulsive." While she conceded that this physical unit was hypothetical, her commitment to the existence of some sort of fundamental physical atom was total.[30]

She invoked atoms, she declared, precisely because she wanted to close the abyss between the living and the nonliving, between animal and plant, between matter and mind.[31] Still preoccupied with her old arguments concerning Darwin's theory of pangenesis, she explained that she had rejected that hereditary theory because it appeared to deny this unity and to open a gap that Darwin had previously closed. She wanted a theory that would end the Cartesian dualism of mind and matter, of physical phenomena and psychic phenomena.

This unique substance, Royer declared, was fundamentally identical with an almost infinite number of "elemental and primordial unities, which could combine in many different ways." Referring to her studies on physics and heredity—and indirectly her criticism of male-female differences—she again expressed the desire to find active rather than passive principles. She insisted on the rigor of her logic in drawing connections between heat and light and heredity and thought. Promising to write further on the connection between mind and matter, she explained that she had not drawn all the consequences of the physics because "I had the hope that a little volume on morality would find readers more easily than would arid speculations on general physics."[32]

She began with deceptive simplicity: "Good is likable, evil is hateful . . . so one must like good and hate evil . . . and from that one assumes that for most beings it is not only existence that is good, but the consciousness of existence." From this she drew the conclusion that "everything that augments consciousness is good, and what diminishes it is bad."[33] All morality could be derived from these statements. She insisted on her priority in signaling the moral law implicit in evolution, demonstrated in her Darwin prefaces. She quoted her conclusion from her first Darwin preface that depicted the law of reproduction and the conservation of the species as good by definition.[34] This and this alone, she insisted, provided an absolute criterion for good and evil. While, admittedly, upholding this moral law for one particular species might place that species in conflict with what was "good" for another species, she denied any real contradiction.

A number of problems stood in the way of creating a scientific morality. The scientists themselves had become narrow-minded, shunning large theoretical ideas as a form of metaphysics. The general public, on the other hand, considered anything scientific without immediate social or industrial applications as something to be avoided.[35]

Using a culinary image, she insisted that science was incorrectly admired for its "batterie de cuisine" (kitchen apparatus), its "instruments, machines, tools, electric light projectors, telegraphs, phonographs, telephones." Quite aside from facts that could be measured and counted by precision instruments, there were other scientific facts "no less important, no less real, that result from theory and rational induction."[36]

Evil at times could be done in the name of good, as had happened in France during the French Revolution. Moreover, the judgment of good and evil could differ "not only for men of different races and different times but for men of the same race and the same time; these judgments change in each individual according to sex, age, temperament, habit, mental culture, education of the will, state of health or sickness, personal influences, affections, and social milieu." The judgment of what was good could also vary "among that part of the population that participates more in scientific progress and has the critical spirit that results from this."[37]

In the past, she added, as she had argued in her suppressed memoir, "Sur la natalité," social customs had produced moral codes that were harmful to society. For her, the burning example would always be the rights of unmarried mothers and their children, whom she considered to be unfairly consigned to an "inferior caste of pariahs without rights and protection."[38] Prejudicial social attitudes embodied in a moral code had no place in a morality based on nature. She did not, however, apply the same arguments to social prejudices about race or class.

In spite or perhaps because of her realization that society in the past had produced harmful judgments that were later corrected, Royer wished to propose a morality not subject to changing ethical judgments. She suggested that this might reconcile "individual egoism," a particular good, with a good that would be universal, "the best possible for the ideal order of the world." This morality would apply to the organic and inorganic world as well, she added in a rather Leibnizian manner. She wanted a morality imbedded in nothing less than nature itself.

Setting out to perform this task, she tried to develop a series of mathematical formulae for designating differences between the desired good and personal egoistic pleasure. She included room for both individual enjoyment and an indefinite number of beings along a hierarchical scale, which provided her with "a pyramid of infinite dimensions." The purpose of the world, she maintained, was "absolute good, that is to say, the greatest sum of good possible. The truth is that everything that augments the sum of happiness is *good,* all that diminishes it is *evil.*"[39]

Evolutionary development was a basic element in her expansion of these ideas of morality. She identified evolutionary progress with morality, since the increase both of varietal forms and their consciousness was by definition a moral good. Absolute moral good was "the indefinite multiplication of the existence of diverse forms and their individual enjoyment in all its varieties and intensities, subtracted by their part of suffering."[40] She applied this rule not only to individuals but to "secondary collectivities," whether planetary worlds or species, nations, or families, inorganic or organic. "In sum, this is the interest of the greatest number or the greatest result of interest, which makes up law." Here and elsewhere she seems Utilitarian in her conclusions.

Admitting that the general good for a collectivity must of necessity include limited, relative, and contradictory elements, she concluded that good for humanity as a species occurred only in connection with the world as a whole. As a species, she declared, human beings must limit their ambitions for happiness and not try to subject all other things to their own desires, a statement that has a modern, ecological ring.[41]

But good and evil within the inorganic world could only exist if that world was conscious of it. In order to eliminate the barrier between mind and matter, conscious and nonconscious matter, she breached it by disallowing any true difference. This became the basic principle of the monism that she later developed in her physical theories. Her insistence on the consciousness of matter, originally invoked in order to establish a universal morality, distracts from her evolutionary arguments, which posited a link between the level of evolution and the increasing level of consciousness.

Royer presented "good" at the atomic level as an atom in equilibrium and repose and "evil" as the factor that disturbs the equilibrium that the atom tries continually to reestablish. In this interpretation, evil is the "elementary motor" for the world. Good and evil are equated with power and resistance in the universe. Her later equation of activity of mind and matter as good is hard to bring into accord with her concept of an evil disruption of equilibrium, especially since this disruption is the source of her eventual good, while her own history of rebellion taught her the virtue of a forceful response.

Perhaps Royer's political advocacy of governmental stability over anarchy led her to superimpose this preference upon her universe. The close link between her science and her political ideas was brought out more clearly as she argued for the necessity for pain and unhappiness to continue to exist in human society. "Pain [*la douleur*] is the true motor of the world, and a happy humanity would cease to be humanity. If this is its unhappiness, it is also its grandeur and its glory."[42] The day when every being could reach absolute equilibrium between its needs and desires, between its instincts and its life situation, between will and power, would result in the "realization of absolute good."[43] All social organisms tried to attain this goal, but it would be long in coming. Although needs increased as rapidly as the means to satisfy them, this would be resolved eventually with a kind of equilibrium that produced specific happiness. Her book ends with a hope for universal happiness, which seems in contradiction with the required "motor" to drive evolution.

Never free from a fundamental conviction about the competition between "races" and societies, she reiterated, as she had proposed in *Origin of Man and Societies,* that the major potential rival to the "white European race" was the "yellow race," because its enormous increase posed "a serious menace to superior human types."[44] Her attack on Asian peoples reflects a justification of the move of the French government into Indochina and its repressive colonial policy at that very moment, a position characteristic of many members of the Société d'Anthropologie and the republican politicians with whom they were linked. Royer's son, only fifteen years old when she wrote her book, would at the end of his life first serve as an instrument and then become a victim of this repressive colonial policy.

The publication of her new moral theory gained her brief attention but little income. She was the subject of a friendly caricature in the lively and famous series of popular biographies *Men of Today* (*Les Hommes d'aujourd'hui*), which depicted her as a small, energetic woman with a piercing, but pleasant, expression, lecturing from her book *Le Bien et la loi morale,* surrounded by a pile of books including one on Darwinism (fig. 8).[45] The Académie des Sciences Morales et Politiques reviewed the book, although not in an entirely favorable manner.

Although Royer needed to continue to earn her own income by her pen, she recognized that only by writing novels could she realize enough money to live on. Urged by the philosopher and literary critic Ernest Havet to pursue this kind of writing, she doubted her ability to appeal to a mass market or produce a popular novel to be serialized in the daily press. Mainly, she realized that her thinking was "absolutely discordant with the little prejudices of my time." Nor could she appeal to the "vulgar" taste of the great majority. In her one novel she had felt it necessary to draw moral conclusions and was incapable of "painting without judging as Zola and Flaubert have done."[46]

She believed that her "old reputation for audacity" since her Darwin preface also blocked her from winning the prizes for which she constantly competed before the Académie des Sciences Morales et Politiques. This body included many of her and Duprat's old colleagues and rivals in economics and political science, and she contemplated the public recognition of Jules Simon, by now a leading member of the Académie des Sciences Morales et Politiques, with some bitterness.[47] She was convinced that her relationship with Duprat was held against her in the academy, and she expressed this conviction rather bitterly to Havet, a member of that body.[48] "You see that I have been right to be discouraged and to have repented for having sacrificed my life to independent research on the true and the good. To this fault I have joined another. I have put my life in accord with my convictions."[49] French society was willing to pardon a man who had many mistresses or a married woman who had discreet love affairs, but "it banishes from its ranks a woman who has had only one lover but who avows it as a right and who practices divorce before it has been written into law. Only that would explain why a commission presided over by Monsieur J[ules] S[imon] has never made me a laureate of the academy."[50]

Her suspicions seem to have been confirmed by the reaction of the academy to her monograph "Philosophy of Evolution," proposed by the academy as a subject for the Crouzet Prize in 1883. Although contributions were submitted anonymously, her identity cannot have been in much doubt. She was awarded an amount of money, described in the academy journal as "something more than just an honorable mention." Nevertheless the award did not carry the laurels of the academy with it, since it was firmly described as being "not the prize, not even a prize but an award (*récompense*) in the amount of Fr 1,500."[51]

Since the report on this prize by the philosopher Paul Janet included a lengthy discussion of Royer's analysis of evolution, it is interesting to see just how her ideas struck contemporary philosophers who, like Janet, were opposed to evolution.[52] The competition that had been proposed by the philosophical section of the academy asked for "the consideration of evolutionary theory in relationship to the principles of metaphysics." According to Janet, the purpose of the competition was to examine evolution either as the result of direct interference with natural law by some creative power (miracles and the like) or as the outcome of established general and universal laws laid down at the beginning of the universe.

Janet complained that submissions to the academy had examined far more of the scientific than the philosophical part of the question. The first contribution of those considered was primarily a short survey of the topic. The second (Royer's contribution) was almost six hundred pages long and carried the Latin device *In nova fert animus mutatas dicere formas* (In the new, the mind acts to distinguish among changing forms). According to Janet, Royer had "absolutely confounded the case of evolutionism with that of naturalism."[53] She had opposed transformism to all metaphysical and theistic doctrines and "established an absolute antithesis between the doctrine of a world developing spontaneously on its own and that of an exterior and transcendent creative power." He complained that she failed to ask whether there was a necessary link between the former and evolution or whether they were contradictory. He felt that many intermediary doctrines could be found that did not assume either a confounding of pantheism and naturalism or an absolute antagonism between theology and naturalism. Her failure to consider those doctrines was interpreted as a lack of knowledge about metaphysical systems. "Philosophy is not as simple as that: the problems are more complex and require more delicate methods for their solution," Janet declared.

He seems to have bridled at her claim—revealing her positivist roots in spite of her many denials of any link to Comtean positivism—that theism was a "only a residue of mythology" and that naturalism developed later as "a progress of scientific reason." This, Janet claimed was contradicted by philosophy, "which teaches us that both systems have always co-existed." He cited Ritter on Indian philosophy and Zeller on the Greeks to make his point.[54]

The main criticism by Janet, one that has a more interesting general application to the style of Royer's argumentation, was that she had mingled the exposition of historical doctrines with those of the problem itself, which, he thought, ought to have been separated. He censured her for "a great many stylistic failings, too many obscurities, and views too rapidly or too little demonstrated or in some way unsuccessful . . . more science than philosophy, a too absolute bias in metaphysics due to an incomplete knowledge of these questions, a prolixity of style, a certain disorder of exposition." These were the failings that had kept her from winning the prize.[55]

On the other hand, Janet recognized the "serious merits" of her work. Her knowledge of the scientific issues was extensive, and she had given the "most complete history of transformist doctrines from the scientific point of view" that had yet been made. Among the personal points of view that Janet signaled as "useful and interesting" was the distinction between morphological and phenomenal evolution that permitted alternations of generation and insect metamorphosis. Janet regretted that this did not lead her towards a conclusion that would define differences between gradual and abrupt evolution.

She also had distinguished between chemical and biological evolution, believing that one had not developed from the other but that they coexisted. Life was, therefore, described as "coeternal" with matter. She described its origin in "ethereal and imponderable atoms," whereas chemical evolution acted only on material and weighty atoms. Janet applauded her comments about the differences between biological and chemical evolution, since, he added, modern chemistry, unlike biology, did not furnish evidence for any kind of transmutation.

This discussion of the lack of chemical evolution was used not as an argument for the absence of biological evolution but to presume a primitive heterogeneity of substances that could explain "the changes and differences that constitute cosmic development." She had also taken the occasion to criticize Spencer's adoption of the nebular hypothesis.[56] With delight, Janet signaled Royer's criticisms of both positivism and Spencer's doctrine of the "unknowable" in two chapters of "just reflections and serious objections." These constituted the most "serious and interesting" sections, according to Janet, and revealed that "the author has not abdicated his [*sic*] independence regarding the schools to which he [*sic*] appears closest."[57]

Royer had included in this exposition her new ideas about conscious material atoms, making thought a natural characteristic of matter. Matter contained instinctive impulses, desires, repulsion, and conflicts as a fundamental aspect of its existence. This natural consciousness could explain "a cosmic consciousness that has been labeled 'God.' " Janet commented that this last hypothesis "is not as original as the author thinks" but was derived from "Epicurean atomism blended with Leibnizean monadism combined with Hegel's theory of becoming, all of which are dominated by the Darwinian law of natural selection and the struggle for survival."[58] He concluded with an important question: "Do all these concepts marry well? Are they not somewhat heterogeneous?"[59]

Not long after the publication of her book on moral law, her new Darwin edition, the award for her study "Philosophy of Evolution," and possibly encouraged by the additional money that these and Duprat's ambassadorship provided, Royer decided to embark upon the creation of her own society of philosophy and social science. Having failed to obtain the recognition she had sought from the Académie des Sciences Morales et Politiques, she planned to create a Society for Philosophical and Moral (Social) Studies (Société d'Études Philosophiques et Morales). This society, she hoped, would bring together a group of interested men and women to study various social and philosophical problems in a serious manner. The new society would actively refuse to be associated with any particular philosophical, political, or even literary school. She, like Duprat, continued to uphold an independent position.

At one of the earliest meetings held in April 1882 she put forward her moral theories derived from physical laws. She spoke of mathematics as the basis for absolute truth, since it provided its own demonstration, but denied that one science could be used to verify the absolute truth of another. On a more practical level, she announced that a number of people from the provinces had expressed interest in the society, and she hoped to extend the society beyond Paris. She revealed her love of trees and green spaces once more, asking the members to suggest a garden they could rent in order to hold their meetings in the open air.[60]

Royer, as the secretary-general, inaugurated the new society by giving a series of six lectures on the "Unity of the Substance of the World: Force, Matter, and Mind." These talks took place every other Sunday from May to July 1882 at the Trocadéro.[61] She was laying out the structure of what would become her book on physics published only many years later.[62] Duprat demonstrated his loyalty to Royer and her interests by attending the inaugural April meeting, at which he was duly elected as a member of the society.[63]

By early May 1882 Royer had applied to the Préfecture de Police for public recognition of the society, which was duly granted.[64] Royer was soon contemplating a weekly journal, *Le Progrès Moral,* to be published by Hennuyer. She filed a notice for the journal stating that it would appear in September 1882, but there is no evidence that it was published, possibly through lack of sufficient funds, although a bulletin of the society appeared between 1884 and 1888.[65]

Royer was keenly disappointed at the response to her lectures on physics scheduled for May and June. Overcome by an unaccustomed lethargy and worried about her health, her concerns were aggravated by an injury to her son, who burned his hand while making soup. She thought retrospectively that her lectures had been poorly timed and badly attended partly because of her increasing ill health and depression.[66] This sense of malaise may have been aggravated by Duprat's continued illness as well as his imminent departure for Chile.

Her disappointment over the lectures was somewhat mitigated by the interest in her ideas shown by Victor Considérant, a famous Fourierist, who had written to her after hearing her first lecture. Her conception of a world formed by repulsive and expansive forces rather than by attraction may have astonished a man whose philosophy was built on the "law of attraction" claimed by Fourier as the basis for all social action. Considérant attended her first lecture and asked for further explanations about her basic assumptions concerning the nature of matter. Her reply, which extended over three very long letters, included diagrams of repulsive atoms.[67] They provide a early picture of her physical theories before she expanded them in the 1890s.

She explained to Considérant that

> according to my way of thinking, not only is the world full, but it is too full, since a single atom suffices to fill infinite space with its infinite expansion in eternity and time. Therefore, an indefinite number of atoms also infinitely expansive could only include numerous others in a manner in which each of them forms a spring under pressure, producing a tension that is the source of all the movement in the universe. Substance is found to be identified with force as an agent by its material and spontaneous action.[68]

This substance she described as

> infinitely compressible so that action is due to an expansion of the elastic atoms and not a reaction. Once my point of view is admitted, everything else follows with geometric rigor. The atom is an eternal universal being, a never drying fluid substance. Only under certain conditions can this expansive force be increased or decreased. The increase or weakening of elastic force of atoms produces all heterogeneity, and I have called this the "three states of the atom."[69]

In the first state, atoms lost their elasticity to some degree, she went on, and they appeared as "weighty matter." When the atom completely retained its "elastic energy," she considered it to be "imponderable ether." This constituted the second state. In the third state, when the "elastic energy" of the atom was increased, it produced a "vitaliferous state," a term that she claimed she had developed to combat Haeckel's "theory of the organic cell."[70]

Royer complained to Considérant about the manner in which her ideas were received. Although many physicists were not happy with current theories, she said, they preferred for light "to come to them from heaven or from abroad." She might have been listened to more carefully, she added, if she had come either from "Japan or the moon."[71]

Considérant tried to suggest ways to make both her dress and her hairstyle more attractive to her audience. Her reply was revealing of both her attitude towards fashion and her annoyance that women but not men were subject to such comments.

> As for your observations on my toilette, I have a choice only between that satin dress, which seemed very ordinary, and an old velvet dress that can no longer stand the light of day. Since I am my own dressmaker, I had no time to make another. As far as luxury items go, I only have my watch and the brooch that was given to me by the ladies of Milan in 1864. Nor is my hairstyle, which for twenty years has been the same, done by a hairdresser. It is more or less well styled only according to the degree to which the state of my nerves gives more or less accuracy to my reflex movements.[72]

She admitted that she never had spent much time looking at her own image, so that she could hardly recognize her face when she saw it suddenly in the mirror. She also ventured the thought that, as one's face aged, it would be a mistake to make those around one notice that fact by changing one's accessories. There came a moment, she added, when a woman must try to preserve former memories of herself by never modifying her dress or hairstyle in a manner that might make her friends change their memory "by new impressions less and less agreeable," a philosophy that might explain why both Duprat and Royer kept distinctly old-fashioned styles of hair and clothing.[73]

Considérant's remarks about her personal appearance were taken in good part, but in a subsequent letter she expressed her annoyance that women especially were required to please their audience. "For a long time our male professors have had the right to be as ugly as Littré, ancient as Chevreul, disagreeable as Dufource, or have the piercing voice of Thiers."[74] When men spoke, their clothing was disregarded, but when women lectured, "they pay more attention to the pattern or material of our dress than to the truth of what we say."[75]

In 1883 she finally published her refutation of Newton's concept of "attraction" that she had begun to write in 1872. She argued that by adopting contiguous fluid atoms it was possible to explain gravitational phenomena without the need for what she (and others) had seen as the metaphysical concept of action at a distance. The positivist editors of *La Philosophie Positive* published the article, but added a footnote distancing themselves from her conclusions, which questioned the authority of the great English scientist.[76]

The philosophical society Royer created continued to be active throughout the 1880s. In January 1884, Albert Colas, later one of her closest friends, gave a talk entitled "Le Mouvement philosophique" with a discussion on "the principle of authority: its necessity and its exercise." Was this philosophy or thinly disguised politics? Soon, the new society would study overtly political questions as well, taking up the issue of socialism in one meeting. Royer's young colleague Léonce Manouvrier, then serving as one of the major instructors at the Laboratory of Anthropology, soon took over the direction of the society.[77] By the end of the 1880s, Royer abandoned her control over her little society, although she may have continued to edit its bulletin.[78] Her later explanation for this withdrawal was her distress at finding it "weakened by utopian socialists or spiritual dreamers." As a consequence, she gave up her position as secretary-general and "renounced a degenerating project that went against her [original] intent."[79]

The event that would dramatically change her life was the death of Pascal Duprat in 1885. He had finally taken up his ambassadorship in Santiago, Chile, in the fall of 1883, after a delay occasioned by shifts in ministries as well as his own ill health, and had tried to interest young politicians in Landes in following him to South America where, he believed, both new financial and social opportunities awaited them. Arriving in Santiago, he made a welcoming gesture towards the Chilean journalists, inviting the editors in chief of all the Santiago papers to join him for dinner in his role "as an old journalist."[80] Although he was turning seventy, his health appeared to improve, and he wrote of new hopes for the future to both family and friends. Encouraged by this renewed energy, he unwisely undertook a journey to Valparaiso to investigate commercial possibilities for the French, which aggravated his old ailments. His former constituents in Landes in southern France wrote to him, asking him to place his name before the voters once again in his home province. As his ill health returned, Duprat was given a leave of absence to return to France.[81]

In June 1885 Duprat left Santiago for Valparaiso and there waited for passage to France. Because of his increasing weakness he was taken off the boat bound for Europe in Rio de Janeiro, where he was attended by doctors provided by the Brazilian government and remained for two months. On 6 August 1885, knowing he was fatally ill, he insisted on continuing towards France. Against medical advice, the Brazilians carried him sickbed and all on board ship with the pomp that his position as ambassador called for. Later reports describe Duprat in the care of a woman, his "mistress," who had accompanied him from Europe and who sat by him as he expressed his fear that he would die and be buried at sea. Was this Royer rushing to Brazil to the deathbed of the one love of her life?[82] The only hint that Royer might have made this journey to Brazil to accompany Duprat back to France is an article she published four years later on the abolition of slavery in Brazil, followed soon after by another article on recent progress in Argentina.[83]

In sight of the African shore, Duprat died on board *Le Niger* on 17 August 1885. In spite of his emphatic wish to be brought back and buried on French soil, he was buried at sea on 19 August, since the ship lacked any provisions to embalm his body.[84] The press duly noted his death and wrote short biographical articles about him. With some exceptions, his death made little stir in France, except among his former constituency of Landes, where even the Bonapartist paper admitted he had been an honest opponent and a marvelous orator.[85]

Royer must have contrasted his death notices with those accorded to Admiral Courbet, who had also died at sea within a few days of Duprat, but was returned to Paris with great pomp and circumstance, meriting lengthy illustrated notices in the Paris journals.[86] Royer was convinced that the attacks in the journals and his last "exile" had killed Duprat, a sentiment shared by her colleagues in the Société d'Anthropologie and his colleagues in Landes.[87] He had never achieved the importance in politics, journalism, or political science that so many of his fellow former exiles and "forty-eighters" obtained. The independence that Royer and Duprat claimed from all schools of thought and all ministries cost them both a great deal.

Royer's circumstances began to alter radically. She no longer shared Duprat's income, and she could not alone support the yearly rental of Fr 1,500 for the apartment on the avenue des Ternes. She applied for a state pension as the "widow"—in fact, if not in law—of Duprat, but this could not be legally accorded to her. The new minister of education, Paul Bert, had come to her aid even before Duprat's death. She had written a series of scientific articles for his science column "Revue Scientifique" in Gambetta's newspaper *Republique Française,*[88] and he was also a colleague of hers in the Société d'Anthropologie. Before he left for Tonkin in Indochina as governor general of that newly established French colony, he mentioned the existence of a list of "indemnities" for scholars and the widows of professors. "This," he told her, "is a list of honor." He saw no reason for it not to be granted on a continuing basis, mentioning the possibility of a yearly amount of about Fr 2,000. He also thought it would not require personal begging letters on her own behalf.[89] Unfortunately, in his note to the ministry he did not specify an amount or his intent to make this an annual grant. The ministry granted her an initial award of Fr 1,200 as Darwin's translator, beginning in April 1885.

After Duprat's death, as Royer found herself in increasing difficulties, she wrote to Bert in Tonkin. The grant, which was not automatically renewed, was made again for the same amount. The third year, when she had begun to depend upon this grant, she had to request a senator, Carnot, to write on her behalf. Paul Bert had died unexpectedly in Vietnam, and although the new minister apologized for his action, he nevertheless reduced the amount.[90] The indemnity continued to dwindle every year, requiring new letters both from herself and from her political and scientific friends. She tried to write for foreign journals in order to supplement this amount, but this never produced a guaranteed income.[91] Her son René was by this time nineteen years old and a student at the École Polytechnique, where his living expenses and tuition were covered by the state. She pleaded to the Ministry of Education that, since he was unable to inherit anything from his deceased father, she needed to support him while he finished his education.[92] René appears to have been a kind and loving son, very interested in her work. He copied out at least one lengthy contribution for the Académie des Sciences Morales et Politiques for submission for a prize.[93] Her "autobiography," written in the third person in an immature handwriting somewhat similar to that of Royer with corrections in her own hand may have been dictated by her to René, since it is recorded in a student's notebook. Royer envisioned a future for him as an engineer in the French colonies, but meanwhile tried to earn supplementary amounts to help him.

Two years after Duprat's death, as her real income dwindled, she moved to a tiny apartment in the fourteenth arrondissement, which she rented for Fr 500 a year, a third of the rental of Duprat's more luxurious apartment. This apartment sat in a building, now destroyed, on the corner of the boulevard Jourdan on what then was an extension of the rue Gazan.[94] Although her neighbors were unpleasant, the apartment had one outstanding virtue, which for Royer was always an important one. The windows overlooked the beautiful new Montsouris Park, which in design resembled a large-scale version of her beloved square des Batignolles, with winding walks, flowers and trees, and a stream flowing into a large artificial lake where ducks and waterfowl could gather.[95] This park, like the Batignolles, was designed by Baron Haussmann but opened only in 1878. In an article describing the difficulties of raising children in big cities in France, Royer described a distraught mother attempting to control her children during a visit to Royer's small apartment instead of sending them out to play in the open air of the parc Montsouris.[96]

With that wonderful mixture of the personal and the general so characteristic of Royer, she proposed to the Société d'Anthropologie that it build an experimental station for evolution in the park. This suggestion was enthusiastically endorsed by Mathias Duval, an embryologist and convinced Darwinist, then head of the Laboratory of Anthropology.[97] A meteorological station already existed in the park in one of the buildings put up for the Universal Exposition of 1878. The new laboratory was built with the aim of studying comparative embryology and served as the basis for a later bacteriological laboratory in the park.

After completing her book on morality, she returned to her interest in social evolution, reconsidering animal psychology. In November 1882, fascinated by the "social instincts" of animals at all levels, she accused the Société d'Anthropologie of being more concerned with organs than with their functions. She pleaded again for a study to include what we might call motivations, but which she referred to as the *passionnel* (emotive) and which she linked to both social and instinctive actions. Reiterating what she had said in her book on human evolution, she stated, "Without motives to act there is no action possible, without being moved to activity, intelligence itself remains inert."[98] Meetings of a scientific society, she added, in which members were driven by the love of science would be useless without a push from curiosity or a wish to understand.

She discussed in detail not only the studies of primate cooperation by Jean-Charles Houzeau, but also new studies on herd animals, birds, fish, reptiles, and other animals. She discussed social insects, particularly ants and bees, "those little sisters of man and his elder sisters in sociability," whose brains were so tiny but who seemed to realize "the ideal of the social instinct in its supreme power without that excess of chauvinism . . . in human groups."[99] Giving many examples, she wondered whether there was a general law that all organic types produced some kind of social behavior among their highest forms. She questioned whether in increasing collectivities in nature as well as in human societies there would be some loss of individuality.[100] Her paper led to lengthy discussions, in which she was criticized by Eugène Dally for not having introduced new facts, not even the most recent ones, but rehashed well-known examples.[101] Stung by the criticism that she had not been innovative, she challenged him and gave as her contribution the general law of social behavior at the top of every major evolutionary branch. Later she added a little experiment she had attempted in the summer to see if she could induce the ants in her garden to use a complex of tunnels constructed for their use.[102]

Her interest in animal psychology continued over the following five years as she began to follow this road opened up some years earlier by Darwin and his disciple George Romanes. She began to read further about animal behavior, especially primates, a topic that had intrigued her while writing *L'Origine de l'homme.* The popularity of this topic for the general public is demonstrated by the wide publicity given the young orangutangs at the Jardin d' Acclimatation on the edge of the Bois de Boulogne, whose charming games were illustrated in popular journals.[103] In 1886, Royer wrote a paper for the *Revue Scientifique* on primate faculties and instincts, based on many of the sources that she had indicated but not directly cited in her presentation on social instincts at the Société d'Anthropologie four years before. This was reprinted the following year in the American journal *Popular Science Monthly*[104] and followed by another article on animal psychology, in which she incorporated some of her long-term interest in mathematical concepts into her discussion of primate evolution, taking up the question about whether primates and other animals had a sense of number (translated into English as "animal arithmetic").[105]

This spurred her to produce a more general discussion of mental evolution, presented as one of the important public lectures on "transformism" annually sponsored by the Société d'Anthropologie. The society had engaged in a long and acrimonious debate on the title of this series of conferences, some members preferring the designation "Darwinian evolution" to the more general term "transformism" to describe the proposed lectures on evolution, but the more general term, which included Lamarckian as well as Darwinian evolution, won out.[106] Royer's lecture, "Mental Evolution in the Organic Series" ("L'Évolution mentale dans la série organique"), was the fifth annual lecture. Delivered in two parts on 11 and 16 July 1887, the lecture appeared in the *Revue Scientifique* the same year.[107] Charles Letourneau had already lectured on social evolution, Abel Hovelacque on language evolution, Gabriel de Mortillet on paleontology and prehistoric man, and Mathias Duval on comparative embryology and evolution, leaving Royer the task of discussing both brain and mental evolution.[108]

In many ways, these public lectures must have seemed the highlight of her connection with the Société d'Anthropologie. Finally she was treated with respect as one of the inner circle, on a par with those teaching at the School of Anthropology, entrusted with the public promotion of evolutionary thought, although, of course, the lectures were unpaid. After this point, increasing illness meant that she rarely climbed the stairs to add comments in society meetings, although she still communicated by letters read at meetings and published by the society.[109] In 1889, Royer was made an honorary member, something that allowed her in principle to sit in on meetings of the central committee, although records of the society show them consulting her on only one issue, how to recover their tables with inexpensive green cloth! Royer, an able needlewoman, did not take this amiss and, provided with measurements, made some practical suggestions.[110]

In her lectures on mental evolution, Royer put forward a number of interesting concepts. Designed as popular talks that would outline general principles, she took great care to make her points clearly and precisely. She started out with a question about the existence of a possible special substance of mind. Distinguishing between psychologists, who study the mind through its functions by internal reflections, and physiologists, who study external organs, she spoke of the hybrid school of psychophysiologists, who had studied sensory thresholds and motor reactions, citing Weber, Wundt, and others. While she considered sensations as purely passive like a mirror reflecting light, she insisted that an active response to sensation was required before that response could occur. The proper reactions of living things, "the only ones that are really subjective," were those with "sentiment, with emotion, the particular impression that makes the sensation agreeable or painful." Human beings, she argued, varied a great deal in these reactions to music or to odors, and, if they were suffering from diseases, perversions of taste were even greater. These "passionate emotivities" were the single variable that transformed sensations into emotive sentiments. The "progressive complication of the passionate scale . . . constitutes the specific instinct that poets call the 'heart.' " She was convinced that all species and all individuals had intellectual functions and sensations in common, ruled by identical laws, even permitting humans and animals to communicate to some limited degree with each other. There had to be logical laws ruling the mind and all living organisms or there could be no connection between the self and the universe. There were direct relationships between the mental organization of a living being and its physiological constitution. If an organism had no instinct to flee what was dangerous and to seek what was necessary, and if it was not sensible or intelligent enough to find the means to survive, it would "perish with all its race and leave the place for other beings better adapted psychologically to their needs."[111]

She questioned the usefulness of the idea of hereditary instincts and innate ideas applied to either animal or human intelligence. By explaining too much, she said, it explained nothing. She suggested that instincts were perhaps only a collection of predispositions resulting from certain sensations, emotions, sentiments, or needs that in turn produced acts. These might call up additonal emotions or sensations in a sequence until the whole "instinctive act" was accomplished. There was, she argued, a kind of intelligence in animals and humans that could detect methods for accomplishing particular results suggested by their needs, sensations, and so forth, along with "all their conditions of adaptation to time and place."

Although humans varied enormously in intelligence, she believed the same logical laws were at work whether one was a great thinker like Aristotle or Lamarck or a cave man making tools, but the difference lay in the need driving the intelligence and self-interests. Those "freed from the slavery of hunger" used their intelligence to satisfy their higher passions of justice and beauty and public welfare, whereas more egotistical interests drove the same intelligence among the lower ranks. Practical industrial activities and practical inventions derived from "the application of superior verities . . . by geniuses who are led forward through curiosity about the truth."[112]

A recurring theme was Royer's designation of a "passionate element" as a "motor of the will," recalling her earlier evocation of passion as the driving "point of action." She pointed out that automatic actions and functions continued even while one thought or acted and suggested that the same logical laws occurred in both higher and subordinate functions. Neuroses that "annul the will" resulted from conflicts and resulting hesitations between motives and needs in some "superior natures." But she questioned (misquoting Pascal) whether man was a "thinking brain," since the greater part of humanity never questioned whether it thought or not but only used its intelligence "to satisfy needs, fears, angers, and desires and, to do so, used marvelous aspects of intelligence such as courage, sagacity, ruse, and hard work or vices like duplicity, lying, violence, and cruelty." In this respect the human was not in advance of the animal, since both were driven to excess by the same passions, and their limits often came only from their own powerlessness. To quote Houzeau, "man has only what the animal has in germ."[113]

At the end of the first section of her lecture, she invoked Darwin in a section describing perfect, but ongoing, adaptation. "Each living form has just the acuity of sensibility and activity of intelligence measured by the complication of instinctive needs that it must satisfy under particular conditions of life. The only marvelous thing is the perfect adaptation of its mental organism to the same conditions of existence and of its sensorial organs to the physical environment in which it lives. But Darwin has shown how this adaptation can be produced and is produced incessantly."[114]

In the second half of her lecture she showed the structure of the brain, first the indication of nervous tissue in the early embryo (after Bischoff), then the cerebral hemishpheres, the midbrain, and the cerebellum of fish, frog, tortoise, and finally human, as depicted in standard texts (Müller, Gegenbaur, and others). Intelligence she assigned to the cerebral hemispheres and control of movement to the cerebellum (citing Flourens), and she discussed reflex action at the lower levels of the brain. She thanked her colleague Laborde for much of this information. Reviewing this history, she suggested that the midbrain may serve to mediate between sensation and action and be the site of attention and of voluntary action (to act as the will or the mind). Flourens had, indeed, made the medulla oblongata (part of the midbrain) the seat of both respiration and the place where motion was excited, although not the seat of mind or soul. Although Flourens had sought a unity of action of the brain, he insisted, as Royer did not, on a Cartesian dualism between brain and mind. Royer's denial of Cartesianism reflected that of many brain anatomists of the late nineteenth century in France, as Flourens's influence waned after his death.[115]

Turning to the nerve cells, Royer reiterated some of Haeckel's ideas of the "soul of the cell," an analogy that she would return to again. She suggested that the pyramidal cells with their nuclei adjacent to the cerebral layer (*écorce*) might also serve as a focal point for attention and will. She stressed that the nervous system was hierarchical and depended on functions at various levels but added that some images of sensations were stored in an organized and logical manner as though in "drawers," allowing them to be retrieved.

In her article on primate intelligence Royer had played with the possibility of domesticating primates, something proposed by the science popularizer Louis Figuier and much satirized in the literature.[116] The fantasy of having domestic help in her increasingly difficult situation may have contributed to her imaginative speculations, which she expanded in a second article.[117]

Royer also made brief comments at the Congress of Criminal Anthropology in 1889, at which Léonce Manouvrier challenged some of the studies on brain size and intelligence. For her occasional remarks on determinism built into brain structure and on mixed marriages as the cause of crime, in support of Cesare Lombroso, we have only a short résumé by the chairman of the meeting.

Poor health and an increasingly difficult financial situation may have contributed to Royer's uncharacteristically subdued communication as chair of the history session of the International Congress for the Rights of Women that same year (1889). Her friend Maria Deraismes had designated Royer as one of the honorary presidents along with Léon Richer. Finding herself before an audience of women, she did not rise to the occasion in her usual manner, nor did she discuss science, mostly ignored by this congress. Presiding over the historical section in that centennial year of the French Revolution, she urged women to study history and to teach it as the best method to exercise their civil rights. Rather than advocating women's suffrage, as many of the American and English speakers had done, she reminded her women listeners that they were a small elite. "Premature" voting rights would permit "the millions of [unenlightened] women to render useless the struggles undergone for a century and lead us back to the theocracy of the Middle Ages."[118]

Did Royer envision a change in the thinking habits of French women as part of their inevitable evolution? Certainly this position of caution was one generally held at the time by French feminists, who feared the loss of the republic if women, educated by the Catholic Church with its close ties to the monarchy, should vote. Secular education was the first requirement.[119]

The only exciting scientific presentation was made by a man, Léonce Manouvrier, her colleague in the Société d'Anthropologie, who presented his evidence at this congress that women were superior rather than inferior in brain size compared to men if their body weight was taken into account.[120] Royer's dramatic rhetorical style was evident only during the banquet, which concluded the meeting. Warmed by food and wine, she raised her glass, offering a toast to the inventiveness of women. She urged her women colleagues to drink to "the first woman who had the idea of taming a lamb instead of killing it; she who kept the first fruit seeds or wheat grains to place in the earth; she who invented the rude spindle or who thought of molding a clay vase to keep water during times of drought." Her belief in the good sense of ordinary women even during prehistoric times and her vivid use of language returned only for that brief toast.[121]

The same year in which Royer spoke before the women's congress, Céline Renooz, whom she had encouraged in the early 1880s, became quite hostile to Royer. Renooz blamed Royer for her exclusion from that congress because of anti-Darwinian statements Renooz had made. The experience that Renooz details in her journal, seeking but not receiving acceptance from scientific men, is an indication that the era had passed when a woman could educate herself in science and gain some degree of professional recognition, as Royer had done thirty years before. Renooz may have felt a particular annoyance at the recent publication of a number of articles by Royer in the *Revue Scientifique.*[122]

Renooz began to publish a short-lived journal *Revue Scientifique des Femmes* in 1888. This review had the explicit intent of serving feminist scientists and women physicians in France as a forum in direct competition with the *Revue Scientifique,* the French equivalent of *Nature* in England or *Science* in America. (Admittedly, the scientific review had never published many contributions by women.) The new journal survived only a single year in spite of its bold intent of "reconstituting society" through a new feminist interpretation of science. It failed to get the kind of support within the feminist community that Renooz envisioned. For that one year, however, it did celebrate the successes of women scientists and physicians, including the first doctorate in science awarded by the Sorbonne to a woman, Amélie Leblois. Renooz also published a scathing attack on Charcot's methods of research on hysteria.[123] She may have antagonized the potential audience for this journal, including the women physicians, by using it to promote her own science, printing long excerpts from her rather mystical book on force, *La Nouvelle Science,* which she had published at her own expense. In her book she attacked Darwinism and depicted oxygen as "the God Oxygen" incorporating a trinity within itself, opposed by nitrogen, the evil enemy.[124]

In her private journal, Renooz recorded that "all the women" were enthusiastic about her work except for Clémence Royer. Renooz was convinced that her writings, because they were "intuitive" rather than observationally based, were feminist, whereas she condemned Clémence Royer for doing "masculine science."[125] Nevertheless, she quoted Royer warmly in her books as an opponent of Newtonian views.[126]

Perhaps Royer would have expressed some interest in the feminist aims, if not the scientific views, of Renooz's journal, if her own financial situation had not become increasingly desperate. She had even tried to obtain a tobacco concession from the state in 1888 on the strength of the military service of her father and grandfather, something often resorted to by soldiers' widows or impoverished relatives of former government employees. The tobacco shop, or *bureau de tabac,* has traditionally been associated in France with a café, selling matches and other items as well as tobacco. Although her request was endorsed by the Préfecture de Police, either she had no head for business or her health made this impossible. There is no indication in the archives that she ever ran such a tobacco shop, although the request may have reflected her growing addiction to tobacco. Her situation must have been truly desperate for her to make this request, for it must have invoked bitter memories of Duprat's wife who she knew had run a *bureau de tabac* in Paris, at least since the 1870s.

With her usual pride she overestimated her income on application forms, listing the amount of her award from the Ministry of Public Education as Fr 1,200 (the initial award, which had never been matched again) and adding that she could probably earn another Fr 1,200 from writing for foreign journals.[127] This overly optimistic claim may have resulted in the very small award she was granted by the Ministry of Education in February 1889—no more than Fr 800—resulting in an abrupt diminution of her income. This amount was only Fr 300 more than her yearly rent, leaving her with very little to live on. When the amount was reduced once again in December 1890 to Fr 500, her yearly rental, Royer must have panicked.

By January 1891, her colleagues in the Société d'Anthropologie who had supported her lectures on evolution became concerned on her behalf. They wrote a letter to the Minister of Public Education, signed by Abel Hovelacque, Gabriel de Mortillet, Charles Letourneau, and Léonce Manouvrier, all members of the central committee of the Société d'Anthropologie and teachers at the School of Anthropology (École d'Anthropologie). They cited her worthiness as a scholar and her desperate financial need. "Our colleague finds herself in a deplorable situation," they wrote. "This is a question of life or death . . . it would be deplorable for our country if it arrives too late." On the following day the minister authorized a payment of an additional Fr 500 to be made to her. Hovelacque, then a deputy as well as the new head of the School of Anthropology, thanked the minister, adding that this grant would "literally permit her to live."[128]

Every subsequent year, Royer complained to the ministry, urging her claims and soliciting support from political and scientific figures. Every year, some major scientific or political figure supported her request for an increase of the grant, urging the ministry to convert it into an annual stipend—without success. Étienne-Jules Marey, the great physiologist, member of the Institut de France, wrote on her behalf. Yves Guyot, minister of public works, who had managed to change the status of the privately organized School of Anthropologie to that of a school recognized and supported by the state, had no better luck against the bureaucratic obstruction by the ministry. Only in 1900, when Royer had been awarded the Legion of Honor, the minister of public education finally raised her grant to Fr 2,000 to be paid on an annual basis. Like many such honors, this came too late to provide much comfort, coming a year and a half before her death.[129]

In the extremity of her poverty, Royer wrote an essay that won fourth prize from the Académie des Sciences Morales et Politiques for an essay supporting public assistance to the poor, quoting the biblical admonition "The poor you will always have with you."[130] While this can be read as sympathy for the poor, among whom she briefly lived, it can also be seen as another example of Royer's vision of the role of the great underclass to provide, with its greater population increase, the motor of progress driving social evolutionary change. Where social evolution was concerned, Royer continued to see natural selection as "election" favoring the few, in spite of her own sad experiences.

Royer's difficulties help to explain the letter that she wrote to her colleague Armand de Quatrefages, requesting his help in obtaining financial support from the Académie des Sciences. She argued that she had anticipated Darwin on human evolution, had discussed monism before Haeckel, and had raised many social evolutionary questions before Spencer. Although at least one historian of science has read this self-description as another example of Royer's arrogance, such an interpretation overlooks her own explanation that she had always given her scientific investigations freely without expecting payment but saw the prize as a recompense for the "many [academic] chairs, prizes, and awards not available to me as a woman."[131] Reading this in the context of her situation at the lowest point of her life, it reads like a cry for assistance rather than the trumpet of self-promotion. In a very short space of time, however, her life would change dramatically.

Chapter 9

"I See Young and Old Coming towards Me": The Final Years

In the depths of her poverty and despair Royer never forgot her love of science. She continued to contribute long monographs not only to the social science wing of the Institute of France, but also to the prestigious Académie des Sciences. Her theoretical memoirs on physical structures of atoms were taken seriously enough to be referred to the academy committees in 1889. Her name, though not the articles themselves, appeared on the lists of papers presented at the Académie des Sciences published in other journals.[1] She discovered in 1890 and 1891 that a Belgian free-thinking journal, *Société Nouvelle,* was interested in publishing her original observations on matter and life. A series of her articles began to appear in this journal, although they remained little known in France.[2]

Her discussion of an American philosopher in another Belgian journal, *La Revue Belgique,* shortly would place her name before the American public. In 1890, she discussed the philosophy of the monist Paul Carus, who had founded the Monist Society and published two monist journals, *The Open Court* and *The Monist* in Chicago. She praised his affirmation of "monism," or "the unity of the substance of the world," along with Spinoza and Haeckel, but she ceased to agree with Carus, she added, "when he attempts to reconcile the synthetic view of the world with a remnant of Christian religiosity."[3] Carus reprinted her article with his own reply that the "God-idea" had developed over time and that he was no more a Christian than he was a Buddhist, although he retained Christian ethics. His comments produced a letter, in turn, from Royer, who asked whether the idea of God was tenable. She suggested that "the modern mind ought to rid itself of obsolete words that no longer correspond to its thoughts and divest itself of the old worn-out forms of the human world." Carus published Royer's original review and their correspondence in the pages of his journal *The Open Court.*[4] Soon her views on a unified concept of matter, force, and mind began to appear regularly in discussions of that journal, reported and reviewed by the French correspondent to the journal.[5] But this interest from America produced no new income. Her attempts to rethink science, like all her scholarly work, remained unrecompensed.

Although Royer felt isolated, the community of women had not forgotten her, nor had she forgotten them. Mary Léopold Lacour, a young feminist journalist, married to the journalist Léopold Lacour, became interested in her. A mutual friend, the editor of the moderate feminist journal *Avant-Courière,* Jeanne Schmahl, knew her through other republican feminists. Schmahl introduced Lacour to her at the end of 1890. Mary Lacour subsequently visited her, first alone and then bringing her husband to those small rooms overlooking the Montsouris Park.[6]

The first action the Lacours took to improve Royer's situation was to suggest that she apply for a place in the prestigious retirement home for men and women of letters in Neuilly-sur-Seine, on the border of the seventeenth arrondissement, not too far from her earlier homes with Duprat during the 1870s and 1880s. This retirement home, the Maison Galignani, had been endowed by an American philanthropist, who had given money to the Assistance Publique specifically to found a home for retired booksellers, publishers, writers, and their relatives. It was situated on a lovely street in an area still remarkably serene, surrounded by a high wall and a beautiful garden. Paul Nadar, the photographer brother of her old friend Felix Nadar was there, suffering from some form of dementia.[7] In addition, there were always some places available at no cost for those who had no money or wealthy relatives to support them.[8]

As proud as she was, Royer saw the immediate advantages of residence in the Maison Galignani, where her food and shelter would be guaranteed. She could leave a situation in which she had found herself repeatedly ill-treated by her concierge and robbed by other inhabitants of her building on the boulevard Jourdan. She also had a firm wish not to be a financial burden to her son. She was a little nervous about living with a large group of unknown individuals after she had lived alone for so long but finally decided to enter the home in late February 1891.[9] Although she could not take her books or furniture into the home, she was able with the small grant from the Ministry of Public Education, now reduced to Fr 500 a year, to rent two small rooms on an adjoining street.[10] Here at 58, rue de Villiers, she could continue to work, and René could visit her when he was in Paris.

Beginning in 1892, the Lacours began to write a series of articles for various papers and journals to which they contributed in which they described Royer as an unusual "woman knocking at the doors of the Institute."[11] Lacour had urged her to put herself forward as a candidate at the Institut de France. When she heard that Jules Simon had expressed the opinion that a woman would not be acceptable to the Académie, Royer bitterly commented that she was not only unacceptable as a woman, but that she would not have been acceptable even if she had been a man. She added sadly, "My mistake precisely is to not have chewed only a single leaf of the tree of science. I have chewed on several, plentifully."[12]

With more flattering evaluations of her life and work in the papers and journals, Royer's name acquired new currency among Paris readers. She never lost a feeling of gratitude to both the Lacours. Eight years later, when she was awarded the Legion of Honor, she wrote to Léopold Lacour, thanking him for all his efforts on her behalf. He had been the first to lead her back from the dead "as though with a Herculean golden bough" just at the time when she felt she had "descended alive" into Hades.[13]

She remained actively involved in various societies. In May 1892, she attended a meeting of the Congress of Feminist Societies as a commentator.[14] The following year she became one of the sixteen founding members of Le Droit Humain, the first "mixed" Masonic lodge, started by Maria Deraismes, and one of the first in France to admit men and women as equals.[15] Royer had close ties to the world of freethinkers and Masons originally through Duprat and remained an interested participant in Masonic activities. Exactly eleven years earlier she had attended an anticlerical congress in the Grand-Orient Hall at which she spoke about the effects of Christianity on women, proposing a toast at the dinner "to the complete separation of woman and priest."[16] But the rules of even the liberal Grand-Orient had forbidden women as full members, after allowing Maria Deraismes to join a lodge in 1882. The new lodge founded by Maria Deraismes was under the Scottish Rite.[17] As a founding member, Royer continued to be an active member of the Masonic lodge, as she was of all communities to which she belonged.

In spite of her improved situation, she continued to have periods of ill health, which left her very depressed. She had published her physical theories in a Belgian journal, convinced that no one in France cared to listen to her ideas about the atomic structure of matter, in spite of the encouraging response from the American monists. By 1895, after her failure to obtain any further prizes from the Académie des Sciences Morales et Politiques and the rejection of her initial bid for the Legion of Honor, she began to believe that she would die with no chance of making her conclusions known to the public at large.

Royer made a will that year (1895), which reflected a very gloomy view of her lack of success in the masculine world of science. "A victim of those prejudices that still are opposed to the intellectual development of women, I have worked all my life without pay to illuminate a blind humanity that has only created obstacles to the construction of my philosophical work by closing off to me schools, academic chairs, and laboratories. Everything that I know I have acquired after a great struggle, and I was obliged to forget everything that I was taught in order to learn everything by myself. I shall carry with me to the tomb useful truths that others will have to discover anew. Because I have had the bad luck to be born a woman, I have lacked all means to express, to correct, or to defend my thought, and I have done only the smallest part of what I could have done."[18] She had made similar complaints to Havet fourteen years before, but the addition of the phrase "to correct my thought" reflects her realization of her scientific isolation and her difficulties in developing her physical ideas without a chance to test or exchange ideas with others.

In her testament she went still further, gaining in rhetorical fury: "I shall die cursing human stupidity and deploring having been born in a period of intellectual decadence into an old world overcome by senile dementia. Under the pretext of art, turning its back on reason, it is ready to move backwards once again and abandon itself to a new period of morbid mysticism that will maintain its retrogression and its social dissolution."[19]

This document, for all of its railing against the stupidity of the day, reflects one of her black moods rather than a final evaluation of her life. Two events were about to occur in Royer's life that would cause her self-image to be completely overturned and enhanced. The first event was a result of the decision by Marguerite Durand, a former actress and well known contributor to *Figaro,* to start a daily feminist newspaper *La Fronde,* aimed at middle-class women in 1897. As Mary Lacour reports, Durand wanted Clémence Royer to write a regular column on science for that paper. Royer sat down with some excitement to inform one of her new friends from the feminist community, Ghénia Avril de Sainte-Croix about the news.[20] The paper was "to be exclusively written by women (in the American manner)." Royer remembered a precedent. Thinking back on her brief connection with the *English Woman's Journal* more than thirty years before, she added, "A similar journal existed in England around 1863, but I don't know if it still exists." She felt that in a woman's journal serious discussions on a wide variety of questions were a way of demonstrating that there was "a climate of progressive adherents" among women. In addition, the production entirely by women would be an original touch, although she worried about the readership: "But where can one find women who love reading and common sense?"[21]

La Fronde succeeded as an important voice for women in France over the following twenty years. It soon put out its first issue with a regular column by Royer. Since she had asked to comment on political issues as well as on the natural sciences, her earliest column was not on science but on the Dreyfus case. She, like Émile Zola, supported Dreyfus against the howls of the Right.[22] The newspaper generally took a strong pro-Dreyfus stance, and she wondered how it could sustain its readership once the case was decided. Royer had urged that the paper adopt a wide political range of opinion and hoped there would be no personal polemics among the contributors.[23] Her new friends joined her as regular columnists on *La Fronde,* with Ghénia Avril de Sainte-Croix writing on women's social issues such as female prostitution, and Mary Lacour discussing literary issues and theater.[24]

The second event that changed her life occurred soon after Royer began her column for *La Fronde.* Her feminist friends on that journal had the happy idea to hold a banquet in Royer's honor with those women and men who had been affected by her writings and her work. They asked Royer for a list of famous scientists both in France and throughout Europe and America who might be interested in attending. Royer explained that she had never been in direct contact with the English scientists and doubted that they valued French contributions. She had never known Darwin personally and had corresponded with him only at the time of her translations. She had some correspondence with his son George when she prepared a fifth edition some years after Darwin's death.[25] "If Lyell and Huxley were still living, I would want you to write to them, but they are dead. And Romanes is dead also, the most faithful and the most intelligent of Darwin's disciples. In sum, there is no Darwinist school in England. There are some naturalists who have all more or less adopted the doctrine of evolution. There is in London a Society of Anthropology whose great majority, if not minority, is Darwinist. My name ought to be known to them, since there is an exchange of bulletins betweem them and the Société d'Anthropologie de Paris." She suggested that other anthropological societies be contacted, "notably those of Russia, Italy, and Lisbon."[26]

Of the great evolutionists still alive she suggested Herbert Spencer, "the philosopher of evolution," and Haeckel at Jena, "although it would be better to have M. Letourneau or M. Manouvrier write to them." She thought that Virchow had a "little difficulty with chauvinism," and she had already given her friends the name of Mantegazza in Italy. Looking again in her address book, she found "a crowd of connections almost forgotten in London. . . . You could ask for the support of Sir Lubbock, naturalist and anthropologist, of the Royal Society of London."[27]

When Ghénia Avril de Sainte-Croix tried to follow up on these suggestions by soliciting the help of the secretary-general of the Société d'Anthropologie, Charles Letourneau, he replied that he was unable to be of much help. He no longer had close ties to the foreign scientists. Spencer was old and sick and no longer answered letters. Virchow, who was also very old, was "the reverse of an amiable man." Haeckel, though not as old as the others, was in such a doubtful state of health that a number of journals had falsely announced his death. Perhaps it would be preferable, he suggested, to propose a subscription from both the French and foreign scientists who could not attend the banquet. Capitan, currently the president of the society and a self-professed admirer of Royer, had suggested either an album of signatures or an award of some sort.[28]

Among the responses was that of Alfred Giard, the first holder of a chair in evolution at the Sorbonne, subsidized by the municipal government. Although he regretted that two recent deaths in the family made it impossible for him to attend, he wanted to testify his admiration for Royer. His letter to the organizers of the banquet reads:

> In 1867 I entered the École Normale [Superieùre]. Darwin, undervalued by our official scientists, was made known to me only by an article published in *Le Magasin Pittoresque.* The translation of the *Origin of Species* had just appeared, and when I bought it near the Odéon it was a revelation for me. It had an enormous personal influence on the orientation of my ideas and on all my scientific life. So, without ever having met her personally, I contracted an enormous debt of recognition towards Madame Clémence Royer. But I do not forget the services of a more general order that this anthropological writer has rendered to science, to the socialist ideal, to free thought, and I regret not being able to join on the tenth of May to witness my gratitude and lively admiration.[29]

At her banquet, Royer proudly entered the hall at the Grand Hôtel on the arm of her son, René Duprat, described by a reporter from *L'Événement* as a "brilliant *capitaine de génie.*" Having obtained his degree from the École Polytechnique, René was now an engineer completing his national obligation through service as a colonial army officer. Charles Letourneau, representing the Anthropological Society of Paris and the School of Anthropology, recalled how—upon first reading her "admirable preface" to Darwin's *Origin of Species* that had so "bravely broken all the windows" and drawn out "all the consequences of evolutionary doctrines"—he thought it was written by a man who had adopted a woman's name to shield himself from the Second Empire.[30] He described Royer's Darwin translation as an "explosion of truth," "creating a new era" to which a small number of free spirits rallied but to which official science had remained "resolutely hostile."[31] He praised her for her contributions to this new era.

Royer's Darwin translation also figured as an important icon for Madeleine Brès, who had been the first French woman physician to graduate from the École de Médecine. She recalled the impact of meeting Clémence Royer when she was introduced to her class by Gavarret and her subsequent response to Royer's preface and "the immortal words of Darwin."[32] She also wanted to celebrate the woman in Royer "with all the qualities: goodness, grace, and modesty, the very beautiful halo of her intelligence." She had been told that Royer would have liked to be a doctor. "That would have been for you, with your great intelligence, a rather modest ambition, but for us, Madame, what an honor it would have been! With what brilliance [*éclat*] you would have decorated our beautiful profession so worthily exercised by the young women, my distinguished colleagues, whom I see here grouped around me. . . . We ask you to continue to consecrate your youthfulness and the vivacity of your admirable intelligence to the cause of women who, while remaining women, mothers, and wives, consecrate their intelligence to the good, to the beautiful, and to the true."[33]

Royer's good friend Léopold Lacour also spoke, praising Royer for demonstrating the aptitude of women for the highest levels of science and thought. He recalled other women of science from the eighteenth century to the present and called Clémence Royer "a hero [*sic*] in the independence of her thought," adding that he saluted in her "the thinker and the hero together."[34]

For the first time Royer had the opportunity to make contact with the younger generation of women professionals. In her speech at the banquet, her response was ecstatic and charming. She spoke of her perception of herself as isolated and abandoned, "saddened at having worked in vain, I expected nothing more of life. I believed that my thought, rendered sterile, would never reach that rare elite intelligence that alone can comprehend and judge it. I believed myself forgotten by my generation, unknown by the current generation. Suddenly I see coming towards me young and old. These remembered me, these discovered me, such a great crowd hold out their hands to me to encourage and resuscitate me." She remembered her childhood ambitions to make a name for herself. "When at fifteen I burst into tears reading *Corinne,* I was far from thinking that one day you also would give me my Capitol."[35]

She thanked the learned men and women who attended this banquet in her honor, the officials of the Masonic orders, the members of scientific societies, the journalists, but it was to the young women to whom she particularly addressed her words: "I am happy to see pressing around me all these young women, these young girls who want to thank me for having opened up new ideas to them, opposed facts to opinions, dissipated prejudices, for having taken my rights instead of asking for them. I am happy to see that they approve that I have dared to do what so scandalized those who were already old when I was young."[36]

Given the many difficulties that Clémence Royer had experienced during the previous seven years, it must have been with a sense of irony that she listened to Charles Letourneau praise her at the banquet as someone who had given her life to science without hope of monetary gain. Too many scientists had pursued science for its ephemeral benefits of fame or as a livelihood without the intention to promote science for its own sake, Letourneau noted. Royer's response was to pick up, not on the theme of unpaid labor for science, but his other comment that he had thought her remarkable translation and preface were written by a man hiding under a woman's mask. "This Roland hiding under Bradamante's armor would have been ill advised, since the Empire proscribed women as well as men. I never had the honor to be proscribed."[37]

Although she had worked energetically against the Second Empire, she went on to praise it as a period during which philosophy and science had flourished "just because one could speak less about politics." She recalled this as the "heroic era of the Société d'Anthropologie." Extending Renan's idea that science would be the new religion, she commented: "We were a little church. I love little churches; they are life and liberty. . . . In our little church we worked with fervor, we struggled valiantly, shoulder to shoulder, hoping to discover greater truths, founded on more numerous facts and more general laws."[38] Royer thanked Letourneau for having valued her anthropological work. Not only had she used his contributions and that of "all our colleagues" in her anthropological writings, but she had "only transformed into ideas the facts that they furnished me."[39]

With celebrity came negative reviews as well as pleasant ones. Intellectual and personal attacks were exemplified in an article by Eugène Tavernier, who exclaimed at the long list of sponsors for her banquet, which included the writer Émile Zola, the radical deputy and journalist Georges Clemenceau, and the physicist Berthelot, but Tavernier expressed his doubts that they would have agreed with the majority of her writings. Characterizing Royer as someone who went from one extreme to the other from her childhood, the journalist pictured her as impatient with Darwin for having hesitated to declare that man descended from the ape: "Give us that good news, hurry up." She had, he added, scolded Spencer for having refused to attribute thought to inorganic life. "But the stones live and think like us. Only God has no reality." Wanting to play Aspasia, Pericles' mistress, in politics, she found "no Pericles but only Pascal Duprat."[40] Her algebraic formula for happiness in *Le Bien et la loi morale* had not worked for her. As for her one novel, it was "a pretentious, suspect, and puerile amalgam" that combined the "declamations of George Sand with Eugène Sue," with a mixture of sentiments from Jocasta and Phedra. Instead of seeking to explain the life of the universe, he concluded, Royer ought to study something that would explain her own personal existence. She should imitate the "modest nuns who administered her asylum," who might "suggest to this learned lady some thoughts infinitely more useful and beautiful." The journalist added that even Clemenceau, one of the sponsors of the banquet, had smiled a little at Royer's pretentious formulas for happiness.[41] But at least one reporter came to jeer and stayed to appreciate the keen intelligence and modest dress of Royer surrounded by aging beauties in their finery and by old generals in uniform.[42]

Georges Clemenceau, former radical deputy and later hero of the First World War and premier of the republic, offered his own interview of Royer to counter Tavernier's negative view. He interviewed Royer at the Maison Galignani following the banquet and reported back to the popular journal *L'Illustration:*

> This woman whom I knew for so long through her writings, I saw in her modest asylum full of peace and serenity. I found her happy in the

> joy of elevated thought, which escapes the attention of the wicked world. Her features remain fine, her great blue eyes singularly lively, her manner of speaking simple and easy; her clear language testifies to her precise, firm thought, evoking in me the memory of the highest female minds, which were the honor and patrimony of our great eighteenth century.[43] (fig. 9)

At least one woman, Clemenceau added, was willing to be concerned with cosmological problems, although his remark conveyed a touch of condescension. He observed that Clémence Royer's theories "await criticism along with those that they have the pretension of supplanting," but he praised the attempt.[44]

With the increased confidence that her banquet had given to her, Royer wrote a generous comment on the work of the feminist writer Jenny d'Héricourt, whom she had met so many years before in the salon of Marie d'Agoult. Royer, in the course of praising the new book of Léopold Lacour on feminism, *L'Humanisme intégral,* described the book as "a real trap in which to catch the antifeminist wolves. . . . Only a man could have told them such blunt truths." But, she added, why had he not spoken of Jenny d'Héricourt's work *La Femme affranchie,* which also spoke bluntly on these topics? "Such an omission is an injustice. Her book was written under the Empire, soon after that of Proudhon, . . . [in] language that was superb and worth more than that of Proudhon." She added that Maria Deraismes had a copy of d'Héricourt's book, "but it appeared to me at times that she did not like to speak of it, because after those two heavy volumes so full [of matter] it was very difficult to find anything else to say."[45]

When Léopold Lacour pressed her further for information about d'Héricourt, she explained that she regretted that "our contemporary feminists have forgotten that she was the first of them to open up the road and march along it faster and straighter than anyone else. If they had cited her more often, you would have had her in mind and would not have omitted her yourself. If I had known more precisely the subject of your book, I could have prevented this lacuna. . . . Only the rarity [of d'Héricourt's book] excuses the ignorance of our contemporary feminists about this fundamental classic of feminism. This is a book worth republishing for which you could give some lovely accounts or review articles."[46]

Although Royer was concerned about feminist issues,[47] she gave priority to her full-scale elaboration of the nature of matter and mind. The process of intellectual work had always been her greatest pleasure, and she wrote with excitement to her friends about her new solutions to old problems. She told Ghénia Avril de Sainte-Croix that she had experienced a number of "eureka" moments. Her innovations would serve, not to *épater les bourgeois* (shock the bourgeois), as Voltaire had suggested his work would do, but at least to "lessen the well-known pride of the officially recognized scientists."[48]

Cosmologies of one sort or another were a common pastime of late-nineteenth-century scientists. The most famous were those of Haeckel and Spencer, but many other scientists in Europe and America were publishing general theories of matter. Royer's old rival in the Société d'Anthropologie, the sociologist Gustave Le Bon, had just begun a series on philosophy of science that would soon include his own extravagent physical theories.[49] As Royer worked on her book, she tried to unify theories of physics and chemistry from the smallest atom to the farthest extent of the universe and tie this in with all aspects of living matter from simple cells to the complexity of human mental functioning.

Royer was well aware of the difficulties of working in isolation. She spoke of her early theories and the doubts that had come into her mind. "This new theory of the fluidity of atoms, which supposed their mutual repulsion, struck against the hypothesis of mutual attraction that the great majority of my contemporaries still believed to be scientifically demonstrated. The objection appeared to me so strong that after having searched in vain for some means by which to reconcile two such contradictory facts—and too respectful of Newton's authority to dare to emit a doubt about his doctrine—I thought myself duped by a seductive illusion and I regretfully abandoned my preliminary studies."[50]

She recalled that when she for the first time had an opportunity to read a copy of Newton's *Principia* in Mme du Châtelet's translation—difficult for her to obtain in the 1870s—she "never felt a joy to equal" that experience. Her pleasure came from the statements of Newton himself that explained that "attraction" was a metaphor to explain gravitation, opening the door for her own theories of repulsion.[51]

In the introduction to her book she insisted on the necessity for science to overturn a preliminary interpretation in order to find the correct one, giving Ptolemy and Copernicus as examples. She made a valiant attempt to bring together all scientific knowledge into a unified theory. In the preface and introduction she celebrated science and its accomplishments, defending science against the antipositivist attacks of *fin de siècle* France.

> How dare they accuse science of being bankrupt at the end of a century in which it has renewed the face of the world and created a new humanity, in which it has enlarged astronomy towards the infinite, created geology, remade history, resuscitated humans who had disappeared [in prehistoric archaeology], in which it has given man those powerful and gentle slaves, steam, compressed air, and electricity, in which it has been able to transmit thought by telegraph, speech by telephone, and recorded song with the phonograph?[52]

Once again she scolded scientists for their overspecialization and their retention of outmoded belief systems. Too often, as she put it, they had held "their science in one cerebral hemisphere and their religion in another," not realizing these contradicted each other. Claparède and Darwin were her prime examples. Darwin, she remarked, didn't want to offend his friends in the House of Lords or in the Anglican Church. He wanted "to be accepted as a gentleman and a Christian and be buried in Westminster Abbey."[53] Royer saw this as a personal flaw.

Her book attempted to set down laws of logic from which she could build her atomic theory and her interpretation of chemistry, physics, astronomy, and life itself. She proceeded as Lyell's *Principles of Geology* had done, from a historical account of concepts of matter. Her emphasis centered on early ideas of the fundamental unity of force and matter, and she gave a rather detailed history of Greek theories from early mythologies through pre-Socratic philosophers like Thales and Heraclitus to Aristotle, with some discussion of the atomists as well, a study that she had developed for one of the Académie des Sciences competitions.

Emphasizing both monist and feminist ideas, she objected to dualistic theories as she had done in her Darwin prefaces. She noted that from ancient times active and passive principles of matter had been associated with male and female. Although Thales had described water as a single primary substance, this in turn required an "active" principle to move it, "lapsing back" into the more ancient male and female principles of primitive mythology. Throughout her discussion of these early theories, she expressed her preference for single active, generative principles in physics, as she had preferred vegetative, nonsexual reproduction as a fundamental aspect of life, warning her fellow supporters of evolution in the 1870s to avoid the "cult of the sexual." For Royer the division of the world into two parts was another example of this "cult."

Although she utilized algebraic equations throughout her book, she adopted no new mathematical tools. Instead, she defended Euclidean geometry against Riemann and the non-Euclidean geometers. A rigid logic had been a guide to her thought and her mathematical interpretations. In this she was not too remote from Klein, who emphasized pure logic assisted by geometrical models. Klein had denied that "pure logic can do all," pointing to the "suggestive power of geometrical construction and representation."[54]

Sitting in her small room, she tried to develop models of chemical molecular structures, using closely packed geometrical models constructed of lead shot and beads, which she had someone photograph when she was finally satisfied (fig. 10). Her models of molecules had caused her many days and nights of anxiety, as the fragile constructions of beads and shot collapsed. "Over a little more than a month I have been at this task night and day, a true task of Penelope with a far distant goal, because whenever I believe I have finished a figure, all contact collapses and I have to start all over again."[55]

She tried to illustrate the connection between different chemical elements, without the advantage of Mendeleyev's periodic table, not yet incorporated into French science. Instead she included a chart describing chemical elements along a graph, which resembled one included in Adolphe Wurtz's 1868 book on atomic theory. Ideas of protoplasm at that time were often based on different structural ideas, including those of bubbles. Royer extended this idea to visualize all matter in the universe expanding and pushing together like multiplied soap bubbles, an idea that is experiencing a recent revival.[56]

In one diagram illustrating luminescence Royer referred to this as "light" created by crystals under pressure. This physical effect, later termed piezoelectricity, had been studied originally by the physicist Antoine Becquerel in the early 1850s.[57] Clémence Royer had attended his lectures on this topic, her first introduction to physics. She may have absorbed the impression that light was always a result of pressure, and this in turn could have pushed her to adopt repulsive rather than attractive forces (fig. 11).

Her concept of matter was opposed to the new idea that there were planetary atoms because of the necessity in her system to have a plenum, although this was not an attack on Rutherford and Bohr's planetary atomic models, which would not be proposed until later in the twentieth century. She was disturbed by the possibility that radiating particles penetrated matter, as Crookes had recently suggested. Her image of the universe was one composed of ether and active (energy-containing) atoms in fluid contact with each other through the medium of ether. In this cosmos there was no action at a distance, all action was a result of pressure, which varied locally by producing movement in waves as the atoms continually expanded. At each point she related her atom directly to living cells in order to demonstrate the continuum between living and nonliving matter, and many of the oddities of her physical world seem to have originated from a need to demonstrate this continuum.[58]

Royer expanded her idea of an intrinsically conscious atom, the "egoistic atom"; she first explained this concept in a section called "The atom—monad, motor, and conscious center of the world": "The atom is essentially egoistic; it is one of the multiple centers of an infinite space."[59] Carrying Darwinian evolution to the level of the atom, she described a struggle for survival among these atoms and their forces. "The aim of atomic forces is to occupy the greatest space possible, to extend themselves to the exclusion of all other forces." It is the opposition of forces, "their struggle," that produces mutual action and reaction. It is a self-conscious struggle as well, since "each atom is a *moi* [a self] that knows itself only by encountering non-self."[60]

She believed that her expanding atoms, as she put it, "tend unceasingly to expand, to dilute themselves in space, and to form spheres of rays more and more extended."[61]

> The sensation of obstacles limits their expansion and that of the forces opposed to them. All atoms, then, are elementary minds, or souls [she

> used the word *âmes,* as Haeckel did, and as she did some years earlier in her discussion on mental evolution]. These have some knowledge of existence and will; they exist by themselves for themselves. They have a vague consciousness of their environment [*milieu*]. Any state of realized consciousness in living beings is only the result of a more complex evolution . . . becoming souls of organic cells.[62]

Eventually this atomic psychic activity could evolve to the point where living beings compared sensations and looked out on the cosmos. These developed organisms, human beings, then became the "optical centers of the world." The centers were not only human eyes but also the optical tools humans created, which produced "an always confused image of reality." Only through logical relationship could these images of reality produce knowledge of the laws of the universe. The mind and brain were, therefore, a necessary part of seeing—a comment that recalls her own myopia, which required a constant subjection of everything she saw to her logical knowledge of the world.[63]

She produced a cyclical cosmology that explained the evolution of a universe in which suns with accompanying planets were continually created out of condensing gases and then eventually exploded back into gases. Our planets were also spiraling into the sun until the sun itself, heating up and expanding from this mass, would explode into nebular gases, which she believed to be cooler than suns or stars, and the cycle that produced planets would then be repeated. She depicted the earth as liquid magma within and liquid seas without and, therefore, subject to deformation in various ways as it spun around. This deformation, she concluded, produced an alternation of magnetic poles.

When she came to write a section on gravitation, she commented to her friend Ghénia Avril de Sainte-Croix that she was advancing in her work "by force of will," in spite of trouble with her lungs—she was developing severe asthma—and the threatened loss of her last few teeth, "which want to join the others." "I have finished my 'gravitation.' It is a great task to correct Newton, and I believe I have done so."[64] As she completed the proofs on her book, her eyes began to trouble her.

In 1900 she published her cosmology *La Constitution du monde* with the materialist and scientific publisher Schleicher Frères, who had taken over from Reinwald, publisher of the rival translations of Darwin (fig. 12). Almost eight hundred pages long and filled with diagrams and photographs, this work was made possible by the financial contributions of a woman by the name of Valentine Barrier, whom she did not even know but who had been impressed by her work.[65] She sent copies of the book to many literary and scientific men, including the gentle anarchist and geographer Élisée Reclus, Lord Kelvin, Anatole France, and Émile Zola, who sent pleasant notes in return. She had a letter of congratulations about the book from Léonce Manouvrier, soon to become the new head of the Société d'Anthropologie, in a tone "warmer than his normal temperature."[66] She confided to Ghénia Avril de Sainte-Croix that the letter she received from Lord Kelvin pleased her above all others.[67] His approval of her ideas may have stemmed from his own "quasi-rigid" ether theory.[68] The book generated many reviews in scientific journals in England and the United States as well as in France, not all of them complimentary. One reviewer in *Science* deplored her "lamentable lack of scientific training and spirit."[69] A reviewer in *Nature* was kinder, remarking that "some of the ideas give one the idea that there is much to say in their favour," but concluded with the question, "But is it new?"[70]

Soon after the book was published, a second banquet was organized for Royer to celebrate her receiving the Legion of Honor, which had finally been awarded to her.[71] Royer was touched, not simply by the cross of the Legion of Honor but by the smaller cross presented to her by her coworkers on *La Fronde,* "the first diamonds I have ever possessed."[72] This banquet was organized by the Bleus de Bretagne (Blues of Brittany), the republican organization of Brittany, recognizing her Breton heritage. The famous novelist Anatole France was at this banquet, along with the Freemasons, feminists, physicians, and scientists who had honored her earlier, although some were too old or too ill to attend. The new minister of education placed the Legion of Honor cross around her neck. He had finally increased her stipend to Fr 2,000 a year, now too late to make the significant difference it might have made in her life and that of her son some years earlier.[73] René was ill in Indochina at the time of this banquet, and Royer felt his absence keenly. At least one speaker sympathized with his absence and toasted his safe return.[74]

Royer's thoughts returned to her father, who, although not from Brittany, had embraced that failed Bourbon rebellion still honored among the people of Brittany. She was in no danger of relapsing back to his monarchism, she told her hearers, but she honored his sense of duty.[75] She spoke again of her belief in the power of reason as a kind of religion. She was very sensible of the honor she was being given since no woman had yet been decorated for scientific or literary work. The award, therefore, to her "fellow sister" [*consoeur*] Daniel Lesueur—awarded the cross for literature—and herself was "a new victory for women overcoming ancient prejudices." She carefully honored as well the men who had "labored to obtain this for me." Speaking directly to the minister of education, she remarked that had she belonged

> to the sex of our fathers, I would have been a chevalier for some thirty years. . . . I would have become, like others, some kind of professor. But I would have specialized in our deplorable parceled-out education, which, by accustoming men to look at only a tiny corner of things, seen always from the same angle, destroys the judgment of the highest intelligences. . . . I would have, like so many others, become entangled

> in a series of observations of reduced proportions . . . so that I would not have known how to come to any conclusions. . . . I would have asked nature questions left without response because they would have been badly posed. . . . Finally I would have cost the state a great deal of money over the past thirty years. . . . I would have never done my synthetic work . . . to which I hope my name will remain attached.[76]

She had finally come to realize that her original views could not have come from the sort of formal education that her own son had received.

Her concerns about her son had increased since he had left the École Polytechnique. Although trained as an engineer, he remained first under military discipline, to which he never responded too well, having a rebellious streak like his mother. Then, as a civil engineer, he went to Madagascar and sent his mother information about the problems there that she incorporated into an article under a pseudonym so as not to embarrass him.[77] "He is such a big baby even with his great mustaches," she wrote fondly to Ghénia Avril de Sainte-Croix.[78] Having proposed some improvements to the great railroads being built in Indochina and other French colonies, he was to go to Tonkin and Saigon to supervise railroad construction by the end of 1899.[79] During the long ship voyage, he had regaled the sailors with Royer's theories of the ocean tides and found them interested and responsive.[80] Royer's anxieties increased when René became ill, first with smallpox and then with a continuing abscess, as his health continued to fail over the next two years. She was amazed at his continuing cheerfulness in his letters, although he was no longer the "handsome captain" of which one of the celebrants had spoken at her Legion of Honor banquet.[81]

In her old age, engaged as she was in rethinking the politics of the past as well as worrying about her son's future, she commented to Ghénia Avril de Sainte-Croix about the earlier illusions of her fellow republicans. She looked back on the Congress of Social Sciences, at which Jules Simon, the Garniers, and so many others began their political careers. "What beautiful illusions they expressed. They spoke of the abolition of ancient permanent privileges as something that could be realized the next day. They judged the great wars that were to come as impossible. They believed in the fraternity of peoples and the opening of frontiers to free exchange without customs. Never would we have been able to believe that the Republic would choose to do what it has done, even more so than the Monarchy."[82]

Her son's acquaintance with the people of Indochina gave his mother an expanded view of the world. Her fears of the threat of the rapidly growing population of the "yellow race" changed as she despaired of the direction in which Europe was going. She worried about the future and thought that "horrible and absurd things" would occur in the coming century. "My opinion is that the Chinese are less bestial than we are and that we will perhaps one day be one of their colonies." Perhaps, she added, if she could come back in a future life, she would find Peking preferable to Europe.[83]

Her continual worries about René were not unfounded. He would die in Indochina less than six months after Royer's death, from a liver abscess.[84] A friend writing back to France about his death told of his last days in the hospital and a well-attended funeral that lacked the expected glowing elegies to this young man. Perhaps it was fortunate that she was to die before him, but his ill health was of great concern to her in her last years.[85]

Although Royer's health worsened, she still continued to write her regular column for *La Fronde.* In the summer of 1900, she was too ill to attend sessions at either of the two feminist congresses held in Paris that year, although she was an honorary president of the Congress for the Rights of Women. At the Congress on Feminine Work and Institutions (Congrès des Oeuvres et Institutions Féminines) one of the rising young women physicians, Dr. Blanche Edwards-Pilliet, who had been a colleague of Royer's in the Anthropological Society and had attended both her banquets, commented on the sad absence of Royer. She proposed that a delegation be sent to Royer's bedside to express the regret of the women present that "the greatest French woman scientist" could not participate in this important feminist event. Royer was deeply touched by the gesture.[86]

Royer continued to be in very poor health through the next year and became a recluse shut in her room, not even having the strength to walk a few blocks to her little study. The publishing firm Schleicher Frères had suggested that she publish all her articles and books in a twenty-volume edition. She thought the possibility an excellent one, but the prospect of rereading everything she had written over forty years fatigued her. Her articles, she explained, had often appeared in periodicals that were not easy to find or in scientific bulletins and proceedings of congresses. The whole collection of articles would require "library rats" to find them all.[87] The collection as a result never appeared, partly because René, whom she had wanted to be her literary executor, was not there to oversee the production and because none of her friends took on the task.

Royer felt rather overwhelmed by her increasing fame, which meant that floods of manuscripts and letters arrived at her door that she had no strength to answer, and she begged her friends to explain that she was too ill to correspond with the general public. A typewriter that René had given her at the end of 1897 had made her letters finally more legible, and at first she found it delightful to write as though she were playing on a piano, but she did not always have the strength to use it as she weakened.[88] She was greatly cheered by news that her cosmological book was selling well, especially in university towns like Oxford and Cambridge, even in the United States at Harvard.[89] Her publishers spoke of a second edition of *Constitution du monde,* and she had acquired a Spanish disciple of her new theories on matter, Fernando Tarrida, then living in England, and wrote to him with pleasure during the early part of the year. Her closest women friends, often too busy themselves to visit, came less often.

Although she felt better towards the end of 1901 than she had towards the end of the previous year, she began to fail and suddenly lapsed into a coma in the spring of 1902, shortly before her seventy-second year. Mary Lacour, not finding her usual column in *La Fronde,* rushed to her bedside, to find the nurse giving her oxygen. She slowly returned to consciousness.[90] Lacour realized that Royer was extremely agitated that the religious sisters, who served as nurses in the home, would try to obtain a final deathbed conversion. She had placed in her will a specific denial of any future claims that she had returned to Catholicism. As she murmured, "No conversion, not Catholic," Mary Lacour, who had spoken to the head of the Maison Galignani about her wishes to die with her freethinking beliefs intact, relieved her mind. As Royer relaxed, she asked her, "What would you like?" and Royer said simply, "Something good." These were her last recorded words, she died peaceably but unattended at a moment when both the watching nurse and Lacour had left her alone.[91] Shortly after, one friend arrived to sketch her. Another, preparing a plaster death mask and a cast of her hand, was struck by the moistness of her body some time after she had breathed her last. In spite of her years of devotion to the Société d'Anthropologie with its customary policy of post-mortem brain analysis, Royer had forbidden any removal of parts of her body, neither brain nor skull. Perhaps she had recalled with a bit of a shudder the entire skeleton of her former colleague Louis-Adolphe Bertillon hanging in the Musée d'Anthropologie and his brain residing in a jar. In true Victorian style, she allowed friends to take only strands of her hair to remember her.

Royer had requested a simple coffin made of wood and lined with sand. She did not want her tombstone to reflect the actual place of her burial. Instead, she had suggested that her coffin be placed in some cave by the seaside, perhaps in memory of her Breton heritage, perhaps thinking of those days of quiet thought by the Welsh sands, or perhaps in the belief that in this way her molecules could mingle with the remains of her only lover, Duprat. Without her son being present to make a decision, she was buried in the old Neuilly cemetery in the seventeenth arrondissement, where she had lived for fifteen years, and her name was placed on her tomb.[92]

At her funeral, representatives of scientific, feminist, and Masonic societies spoke, as they had at the two banquets in her honor. Some were missing. Many of her old friends and colleagues had died or would die soon after. Quatrefages, Letourneau, and Mortillet had died. Albert Colas was ill. Marguerite Durand, the publisher of *La Fronde,* passed out little bouquets of violets to her friends to place on the coffin. Durand used these flowers as a metaphor to express her delight at the feminine gaiety and coquetry that Royer displayed even in her old age, which seemed to her as though "a rock was revealing unexpected flowers in its crevices."[93] Throughout the lengthy speeches at her funeral, a small bee buzzed over the carpet of flowers. It seems fitting to end the biography of Clémence Royer there, with the image of the bee that she had invoked so many years before as a representative of female genius. But it is important to remember that neither the bee nor Royer was working in isolation. Both were part of a far wider community, perhaps not visible at the moment, but present at the center of all their activities.

Perhaps this single bee is too quiet an image for a woman whose whole life was lived in rebellion. Royer's image of the real motor of the universe had never been attraction, as the bee had been attracted to the flowers by their smell, but repulsion and reaction, closer to the action of a swarm of bees rising and dividing to move far away from its original home. If she was a bee, she was not the docile neuter worker in the hive, but a rival queen rising out of the hive, intent on taking part of the members with her. She had reacted against her family, rejecting its politics and social values. She had rebelled again, against her religion. Even when adopting scientific principles, she continued throughout her life to declare her independence even from those scientists whose ideas had most stimulated her. She had found a new world for herself of thought, reason, and science that brought her a happiness that no personal event could ever equal.

Clémence Royer and Her Biographers

Clémence Royer seems to have received some attention every decade or so since her death in 1902, each response reflecting something characteristic about the era in which her writings were read. Within eight years of her death, André Moufflet, a sociologist, wrote on Royer's theories of social evolution and her monism, including brief, but intriguing, comments on her life with Duprat and recollections of her life in Italy.[1] The article was published in the *Revue Internationale de Sociologie,* a journal that emphasized "organic sociology" as promoted by the French school of René Wurms. A few years later, an analysis of Royer as one of the few real monists in France was published by J. B. Saulze with a preface by Ernst Haeckel.[2]

In 1918, Aristide Pratelle—Albert Milice, Royer's first real biographer, writing under a pseudonym, according to Geneviève Fraisse—called attention to her Darwinian terminology, especially her use of the term *concurrence vitale,* or vital competition, instead of the more militaristic "struggle for survival."[3] Writing in the period at the close of the First World War, he hails her pacifism and her belief in a nonviolent struggle between organisms, exemplified by the term *concurrence vitale.* In an era that reacted to German Darwinians like Ernst Haeckel, who had glorified life as a battle, this gentler approach seemed to him to provide a preferable view, close to but not identical with that of the gentle anarchist Peter Kropotkin.

In the first full-scale biography of Clémence Royer, published in 1926, Albert Milice glorifies her life, depending upon her early autobiographical writings, but adding details from his research at the public library in Lausanne, biographical information on Pascal Duprat and her son René Duprat, and highlighting the final years of her life, about which he had the most material. Milice, the son of a former friend of Royer, attempted to produce a coherent philosophical view of her science as "Royerian philosophy," integrating her evolutionary interpretations with her cosmology. He analyzes and praises her lengthy notes to her Darwin translation that were criticized by her contemporaries and modern scholars alike. Milice goes so far as to praise her one novel, *Jumeaux d'Hellas,* as a fine piece of literature. His hagiography even extends to a recitation of various important places along the route from Praz-Perey in Cully, where she wrote her first serious pieces, to the small writing room she rented at the end of her life. Milice reports her death scene with the reverence usually reserved for saints. He describes her scientific theories, devoting a section to each science, while insisting on the unitary nature of her science and philosophy. He also depicts her elitist social views as a significant contribution to the twentieth century.

In 1930, stimulated in part by Milice and members of the feminist community who wished to celebrate a French woman scientist, Marguerite Durand and the other editors of the feminist daily newspaper *La Fronde* and a group of scientists and feminists held a centennial observation of Royer's birth. For this celebration, a special issue of *La Fronde* was produced, with long excerpts drawn from her writings along with portraits and biographical notes. This celebration of Royer as scientist, writer, humanist, and rationalist thinker was sponsored by a committee that included Raymond Poincaré, then president of the Third Republic. Adrien de Mortillet, the son of Gabriel de Mortillet, spoke about her as a paleontologist, Milice about her work as an evolutionary thinker. The French woman physician and feminist Blanche Edwards-Pilliet, who had honored Royer in 1900, spoke of her encylopedic interests. Most surprisingly, the great physicist Paul Langevin, associate of Pierre and Marie Curie, also honored Royer at this event. He spoke not about her science, her physical theories of matter, or her cosmology, but about her strong rationalism and her faith in science. The celebration included, in true 1930s style, poetry by a well-known poet and politician, Clovis Hughes, who had also recited a poem in her praise at the 1897 banquet, songs by a folk group, and dances "in the Greek manner."

One of the organizers of this event, Harlor—nom de plume of Thérèse Hammer, a famous French feminist of the early decades of the century—recalled Royer to the intellectual public once again after the Second World War when she wrote about her in 1954 for the *Revue des Deux Mondes.*[4] She reiterates much of the material used for the centennial celebration and by Milice, giving an enlarged and flattering portrait of her as a scientific thinker. Yet by the early 1970s, Royer was forgotten, even disappearing from the biographical section of Larousse.

Yvette Conry in her magisterial work on the introduction (or, in her view, the non-introduction) of Darwinism into France, *Introduction du Darwinisme en France* (1974), brought Royer back to the attention of the intellectual community, but in contrast to Milice's inflated praise Conry lays much of the blame for that non-introduction at Royer's door. Going further than Robert

Stebbins, who saw Royer as brilliant but insufficiently trained in science for her task, and who indicated that the fundamental lines of French opposition were well drawn before the translation appeared,[5] Conry includes contemporary accusations of enemies and friends alike. She accuses Royer of mistranslating Darwin to the point of "fraud," of having introduced "intelligence" into natural selection, and of collapsing Lamarck into Darwin or rather Darwin into Lamarck, especially by misreading adaptation. Although Conry admits that the term Royer had used for natural selection, *élection naturelle,* was drawn from the term *élection artificielle* (artificial selection) used by breeders and scientists, she seems to have overlooked the point (recently raised by Miles) that the French terms were first coined by Darwin's Swiss admirer and reviewer, the scientist René-Édouard Claparède, who assisted Royer on the translation. In Conry's opinion the use of *élection* itself led to unnecessary attacks from scientists such as the perpetual secretary of the Académie des Sciences, Pierre Flourens, who opposed Darwin's anthropomorphic appeals to nature—but those are endemic in the English text.

Conry accuses Royer of scientific vanity and personal pique in post-*Origin* interpretations; she cites the first half of the letter to Quatrefages from 1891 to illustrate that vanity.[6] Conry quite correctly points out Royer's deviations from Darwin: her insistence on an innate force within the organism that drives evolution towards perfection and her various descriptions of the origin of life in multiple unicellular forms. Many of these beliefs Conry attributes to Royer's prior Lamarckism. The question remains whether Royer's translation can be charged so heavily in the face of multiple readings (and misreadings) by other, far better trained French scientists. One cannot deny that much of the argument and the incredible richness of detail surveyed by Conry demand thoughtful attention by every scholar who follows her. Some specific accusations have been more recently challenged, as noted below by Sara Joan Miles, although Miles's conclusions have been questioned in turn by Claude Blanckaert.

Linda Clark and Geneviève Fraisse both published their studies of Royer in 1985, a little over ten years after Conry. Linda Clark studied Royer within a group of other French social Darwinists, after making a study of girls' primary school in the French Third Republic.[7] This earlier study led her to the Marguerite Durand Library and to the rich materials on Royer. Her study, which focusses on Royer's writings on social evolution, also incorporates some significant biographical material. Clark's interest in French feminism and her thorough historical knowledge of Third Republic politics allow her to place Royer's social evolutionism within the politics of her time. For example, she skillfully demonstrates that Royer's reflection of a centrist republican point of view ("solidarism") in the 1880s made her ideas far more acceptable to the French establishment. She also balances Royer's social evolutionary ideas against those of her immediate contemporaries and demonstrates varying shades of evolutionism. She demonstrates that Royer supported and endorsed Spencer's social Darwinism on one hand while attacking him on the other. Clark manages to effectively define Royer's position in contrast to English and German social Darwinists. Like Fraisse, she utilizes contemporary police reports and commentaries of contemporary feminists like Juliette Adam.

The first modern biography of Royer, *Clémence Royer: philosophe et femme des sciences* (1985) by Geneviève Fraisse, manages to compress within less than a hundred pages a vital, wide-ranging examination of Royer's philosophical ideas. Going beyond the limits of an intellectual biography, she provides a number of new insights into Royer's life and describes in detail every biographical source known up to that point, including letters, archival materials, and manuscripts, all of which provide a rich base for any biographer who follows her. Fraisse, now known for the first time to a wide American audience, has placed Royer squarely within French philosophy and political economics. Like Clark, she brings insights on French feminists and women writers to her analysis.[8]

Fraisse is also the first biographer since Milice to offer a discussion of Royer's novel as an important aspect of her thought, pointing out themes of rebellion and free choice in marriage and divorce in its preface, and the importance of the proposed constitution in the conclusion of the novel. Fraisse points out that Royer questioned here, as she did in her Darwin preface, whether a "law of nature" could rule marriage when it could be so easily violated. Importantly, Fraisse discusses Royer's articles written on economics and political science for the *Journal des Économistes* and places these articles in the context of nineteenth-century political science debates. She also carefully analyzes Royer's economic and social ideas in *Théorie de l'impôt* and relates its themes to other aspects of Royer's thought. Taking up Royer's interpretation of human social development, she points out that Royer, while denying an initial matriarchy, saw a likelihood of future matriarchy.

Fraisse points out the important division—today as well as in the nineteenth century—between feminists who stress differences between men and women and those who emphasize sameness in order to argue for women's rights. She demonstrates Royer's commitment to those who emphasized difference and integrates that with Royer's belief in human inequality as a source for human development. At the end of her biography she makes available two important pieces of Royer's writings, the "Introduction to the Philosophy of Women" (1859) and her Darwin preface of 1862. Fraisse takes Royer's claims to be a philosopher very seriously, as does Miles, but finds in both Royer's Darwinism and her social Darwinism an implicit, often unacknowledged but genuine, reflection of Spencer's social theories.

Sara Joan Miles's dissertation for the University of Chicago on Royer's synthetic science (1986) places Royer within the German Romantic tradition (following the lead of Timothy Lenoir) and within the framework of Spencerian social Darwinism.[9] Like Fraisse, and to a lesser degree Conry, she finds Royer's sources in Spencer, but adds the caveat that in 1869—when she was working on *Origine de l'homme*—she could have just as easily obtained many of her ideas from French sources on social evolution. As a historian of science rather than a philosopher or historian, she emphasizes the scientific aims of Royer. Miles considers Royer's monism and syncretic philosophy to be well thought out from the beginning of her studies of science, rather than developing as she matured, as I have tried to show. She discusses Royer's astronomical and cosmological writings, her geological theories, and her interpretations of the atom, matter, and force, the first biographer since Milice to take up these topics in detail. While absorbing fully the claims of both Milice and Saulze about the development of Royer's monist philosophy, she makes little analysis of the reaction of the American monist philosopher Paul Carus to Royer's work in the late 1890s. Like Fraisse, she provides the text of the first Darwin preface (in translation) at the end of her thesis and also includes Royer's two autobiographical writings in both the original French and in translation.

Miles followed up her dissertation with a concise attempt in 1989 to refute Conry's claim that Royer had betrayed Darwin with her translation.[10] While recognizing some minor errors and omissions, she insists that significant French scientists in the early 1860s read Darwin in English, as shown by their use of the English language. She points out that some of the commentaries by Royer were made first by Darwin in his third English edition (the edition that Royer translated), for example, the parallel she drew between elective affinities and *élection naturelle.* Miles points out a number of cases in which Royer rendered Darwin's often convoluted sentences, as Royer explained, in a manner more in accord with French style. More crucially, Miles indicates that Royer changed the "probable" reasoning that Darwin uses following the English hypothetical-deductive school to the more didactic statements of French positivist science.

Miles also shows that Royer found Darwin's utilization of "one long argument" problematical. Based on English legal arguments, this was something unacceptable from a French scientific point of view, in which proven facts alone can be employed. Miles has more difficulty with other crucial elements introduced by Royer. However, she accepts Royer's adoption of the term "perfection" of organisms in place of Darwin's use of the term "advancement," since Miles believes that Darwin himself considered the perfection of organisms and progress the same. Although this is an arguable point of view that has been debated ad nauseam by scientists and historians of science alike, it is worth mentioning that Miles's thesis advisor, Robert Richards, also considers Darwin to be a believer in progress.[11]

Miles argues that a crucial text on the adaptation of the eye—in which Royer introduced the adjective "intelligent" to expand Darwin's phrase about natural selection acting as a power "intently watching each accidental alteration"—is not, as Conry argues, a "fraudulent" reading but a fair one, given the ending of Darwin's paragraph in which he mentions a "Creator." Miles, however, adopts the argument that Royer introduced a teleological reading of Darwin, making him more like Lamarck, and implicitly incorporated an internal life force driving the individual rather than chance so crucial to Darwin's natural selection.[12]

Miles demonstrates Royer's continuing attempt in her later writings to rehabilitate Lamarck by asserting that his third law (adaptation to the conditions of life) prefigured Darwin's natural selection. This, says Miles, shows that Royer did not accept natural selection, even as a passive (negative) agent. She argues that Royer saw natural selection only as a product, a result of a modifying force, not as the agent itself, thereby depriving natural selection of any real capacity for major change. This Lamarckian commentary saturated Royer's notes, Miles observes, rather than the translation. It was here that she questioned the action of natural selection. Royer was defending, says Miles, the concept of evolution as a general concept rather than an exclusive focus on the mechanism of natural selection. At the same time, she pushed Darwinism to include not only an original abiogenesis but a link between the general progression of species and the Enlightenment scale of species as well as the Leibnizian notion of the best of all possible worlds, ending her preface with a vision of "perpetual perfectablity" as a consequence of evolution.

On the topic of religion, Miles insists—in contrast to Clark's and my own reading—that Royer did not oppose religion as such but held an anti-Christian and antidogmatic position. She believes that Royer's Deistic ideas, first demonstrated in her preface to Darwin, continued in her later writings, collapsing God into Nature, in spite of Royer's claim that she abandoned all religion after 1867.

Claude Blanckaert came, as I did, upon Royer through research on the history of anthropology and specifically of the Société d'Anthropologie, although our conclusions have been rather different. In 1982, in a biographical as well as analytical article on Royer, Blanckaert examines Royer's comments on women in her published and unpublished writings, beginning with her Darwin preface. He interprets her Darwin preface as prefiguring in germ her later explanation of many of the evils of modern society, such as warfare and murder, and of the reduced position of women both intellectually and in society. Blanckaert uses Royer's writings on political economy in the 1870s as well as her articles for the Société d'Anthropologie to illustrate her belief that women's inequality had derived from a slow dispossession of their original equality with men. He hesitates at Royer's application of a rigourous progressive view to condemn other, "nonprogressive" races even to the point of extinction, and hints at the dangerous link between such ideas and the philosophy of monism leading to the Holocaust.[13]

In his 1991 article Blanckaert supports Conry's thesis against Sara Joan Miles on Royer's social Darwinism, utilizing both *Origine de l'homme,* which had recently been republished in France, and her articles for the *Journal des Économistes,* including a previously unpublished portrait of Royer in the archives of the Société d'Anthropologie.[14] Describing Royer's preface as both eugenic and racist, driven by her feminism, he cites contemporary challenges to her application of Darwinian natural selection to the human species, particularly to the elimination of the weak. While Blanckaert gives all credit to Miles's careful reading of the preface and her rethinking of the controversy over *élection naturelle,* he denies Darwin's acceptance of a Lamarckian progressivist interpretation of evolution and cites contemporary French writers who were unhappy with the Lamarckian reading that many of his fellow Frenchmen gave to Darwin, partly due to Royer's preface and notes.[15]

Blanckaert is struck by the number of contemporary commentators who found Royer's unwillingness to tolerate doubt disturbing within scientific debate. Most tellingly, he cites those put off by her theories of social evolution, which supported an anthropological basis for the human derivation from simian origins and began with an attack on Rousseau's belief in human equality. Her metaphysical and philosophical approach did not always sit well with a scientific society that prided itself on a positivist science cautious about hypotheses. He also examines the comments by those from the other end of the spectrum who rejected her ideas because they were materialistic and, even worse, because they came from a woman and a Frenchwoman at that. Blanckaert concludes that it is not sufficient to ask if Royer betrayed Darwin, but to question whether she was any more faithful to Lamarck.

Royer's suppressed communication on women, presented before the Société d'Anthropologie in 1874, (here given in the appendix) was published for the first time in French by Claude Blanckaert with Albert Ducros in the *Bulletins et Mémoires de la Société d'Anthropologie,* allowing it to finally appear in the journal for which it was first intended, although now as a historical note some 115 years later. Together with her article on the birthrate, they also published the letter from Royer to Paul Broca in 1875 reacting to the suppression of this paper, as well as a short discussion by Louis-Adolphe Bertillon referring to her suppressed remarks.[16]

Although I began in 1983 with an account of Royer as only one of the actors within the Société d'Anthropologie, my approach has been to search for the woman within the writings, to try to understand how and why a nineteenth-century woman turned to science to make her life, her society, and her world comprehensible to herself and to others. I have focussed extensively on the networks within which Royer moved and her response to her contemporaries as a child in France and later in Britain, Switzerland, Italy, and Paris. I have shown how she reacted as a member of various scientific and feminist communities, as a sensitive reader of texts, as a promoter of ideas, as a participant in scientific and political societies, as a partner in a difficult social situation, and as a mother raising an illegitimate son. At the same time, I have tried to integrate her major ideas expressed through her life as well as her writings.

Given the offense that many scientists and writers, both contemporary and in the present day, have experienced in reading Royer, I cannot resist suggesting that some of the problems that Royer experienced on all sides stem partly from her apparent violation of the implicit "gentlemanly" rules of scientific evidence that have been recently described by Stephen Shapin for the seventeenth century.[17] Was the annoyance of a Mortillet or a Louis Lartet in the Société d'Anthropologie in part due to their criticism that she accepted as "true facts" the evidence that they considered to derive from unreliable witnesses or poor scientists? Was this further aggravated by the fact that she was a woman and therefore not seen as subject to the "gentlemanly code"? Is one of the sources of even Conry's annoyance with Royer, for example, partly due to the feeling that she stepped beyond the bounds of decorum towards the author of the book she translated, especially when that author was the highly esteemed scientist Charles Darwin? This deserves further consideration.

A great deal of ink has been spilled over nineteenth-century women writers. Few of them tried to come to grips with the science of their day and tackle scientific questions head-on. Clémence Royer did attempt that task, along with a very small number of women of her era. She was conscious of the difficulties of being accepted as both a woman and a scientific thinker, and she made an attempt to bring a thoughtful understanding to defining those difficulties. One must admit that she often reacted passionately to any obstruction. She was not an easy child nor an easy woman to know, and her reaction often made her appear prideful or overbearing. Although like Blanckaert and Fraisse, I hesitate at some of Royer's comments on social class and race, I believe her to be worthy of our attention. As Darwin said with grudging admiration, "She makes some good hits." She knew how to pick up an idea, turn it over, and always find something new within it. Her writings as well as her life convey a sense of the contributions that women have made and will make to both science and philosophy.

APPENDIX
Clémence Royer on Women, Society, and the Birthrate

The following text is a suppressed communication by Clémence Royer read before the Société d'Anthropologie during a discussion on depopulation in France on 16 July 1874. It was originally scheduled to be published in the *Bulletin de la Société d'Anthropologie,* 2d ser., 9 (1875); the proof pages are numbered 598–613. This was accompanied by unnumbered galley proofs containing some editorial changes in red and blue and the following formal note from the Publication Commission of the Société d'Anthropologie dated first May, then July, 1875:

"Since the commission has refused to allow this work to appear in the proofed edition (attached) and did not judge the corrections and changes made by Mme Royer to be sufficient, she has consented to the entire suppression of her discourse."[1]

A letter from Royer to Paul Broca dated 3 May 1875 accompanied this note and the page proofs, but the extensive notes of justification she mentions in that letter have not been found, presumably because they were returned to her at her request. Both the memoir and Royer's protest against the changes they wished her to make is discussed at length in chapter 7, "Woman Is Not Made Like This."

Clémence Royer, "Sur la natalité"

In the last meeting we were in agreement, I think, that the question that concerns us is complex, that the relatively lessened fertility of the wealthy classes and, more generally, the reduction that one notices in France in the rate of population increase has multiple and diverse causes, some of an economic kind, others moral and social, rather than physiological.

As for economic causes—derived all more or less from Malthus's population principle as well as from Ricardo's theory and general laws of supply and demand—I have already remarked that the formula given by M. Lagneau summarizes in a very exact manner their resulting effects on each particular social class. If I did not fear extending myself too much here, I would very much like to prove that, in fact, there results from all economic laws a whole group of determinant motives. By acting in the same direction and with the same power on all the individuals that compose the same social class, these cause each family to limit the number of their children to conform to the opportunities offered to them in order to assure them a social situation comparable to the one the family now occupies. This demonstration, which would take me too far afield, I will reserve for a memoir in which I propose to assemble all the facts and all the observations that I have been able to collect for a long time on this grave and serious question.

Today I intend to draw attention to the fact that the formula of M. Lagneau is a new idea offered by an anthropologist to the economists, showing once more the close solidarity between the various branches of science and the help they can bring to each other, when they do not closet themselves within too narrow a specialization. The solution of a scientific problem very often can be found not in the special science to which it seems properly to belong, but among those specialties that are, so to speak, on the periphery.

However, this solution, although effective, is partial and incomplete. In fact, the economic laws that act on each family can well furnish determinant motives for more or less limiting the number of its children according to the degree to which they are strengthened, fortified, or on the other hand counterbalanced by motives of another kind, namely, by instincts or passions acting in parallel or opposite directions.

Especially from this point of view, the question that has been neglected up until now and that I think needs to be discussed is the part played by woman in this matter.

Up until now, science, like law, has been exclusively made by men and has considered woman too often an absolutely passive being, without instincts, passions, or her own interests; a purely plastic material that without resistance can take whatever form one wishes to give it; a living creature without personal conscience, without will, without inner resources to react against her instincts, her hereditary passions, or finally against the education that she receives and against the discipline to which she submits following law, customs, and public opinion.

Woman, however, is not made like this. One must recognize that, since she is always at least one half responsible for the reproduction of the species, she must play a role—and a predominant role—in its more or less rapid multiplication.

When man speaks of woman, it is in general to grant her those qualities that he is pleased to discover in her or those faults from which he suffers personally. Never does he see her as she is, because she always has some motive to hide from him. He never judges her other than in relationship to himself and is never impartial in his judgment, always more or less influenced by memories of rancor or regret stemming from personal experience. That is why, from everything that has been written about woman, one must conclude that she is the animal in all creation about which man knows the least.

What he knows are facts and actions, but how can he know the motives for these actions, the secret physiological or organic causes of these facts? Woman really constitutes for him a foreign species with a brain with which his brain does not communicate at all, since no woman has up until now had either the power or the will to discuss in general all the serious problems that concern her, without being personally interested. And when she lays out a particular problem, she has always more than one reason not to be completely sincere. Neither her education, nor her instincts have prepared her sufficiently to study herself, to know herself, and to analyze those multiple determinant motives for her actions.

If man is completely ignorant about her, she is equally ignorant about herself, dominated as she is, in general, by her prejudices, by her mental habits, by the convictions or beliefs that she has received ready-made and without criticism through her education and the tradition she has inherited. Most often, then, when asking her about the determining motives for her conduct, one does not obtain anything other than her own illusions that her mind borrows from current opinions. To understand woman, it is first necessary not to be a man, since before any man she acts and shows herself instinctively, not as she is, but as she believes she ought to appear. Moreover, it is necessary to watch her living, to live with her, to study her without interrogating her, to analyze her, to make her betray herself, without her knowing she does so, during long, casual chats about her family or school life. This is what, as a woman, I have been able to do.

As a result, I have arrived at the conclusion, which is contrary to what in general is believed, that in woman there has been a real and considerable weakening of the maternal instinct and of the sexual instinct, which is correlated with it, in the human species as well as in all other species. This weakening is evident especially among the most cultivated classes and almost a direct effect of that culture. The domesticated woman has been so profoundly modified by hereditary education that nearly nothing of the primitive, wild animal remains. What remains of it is transformed to the point that, although it may produce the same actions, these occur by virtue of completely different determining motives.

Since human societies have existed, there has been a rigorous selection of women, already very free from violent instincts, as a result of the action of law, customs, and public opinion. There has been a selection favoring the calmest feminine temperaments or the most submissive to reactions of the will. Woman today has become, in a word, freer, a great deal freer than man, from sexual fatalities, and this liberty, if education does not direct it, can be fatal for the species. If there are some exceptions to this rule, they are few; they are pathological cases due to chance reversions.

If, in general, every woman marries or desires marriage, what motives lead her to accept it, often to seek it, by every means that ruse or coquetry can provide? The reason is that marriage is for woman, above all, a profession, the only profession open to her. Society, by making no other place for her, has forced her to live by the commerce of love, a legal or illegal commerce with or without legal guaranties. Outside of legal marriage, except when first surprised in cases of precocious seduction to which her inexperience exposes her, she escapes maternity only by excessive license. If she accepts it within marriage, it is without desiring it and as one of the risks and the perils of a trade, or as a compensation offering her a social situation more or less agreeable or advantageous. Her first child is generally welcome because at his birth a residue of maternal love is awakened in her; because, in general, a life up until then absolutely chaste has disposed the young girl to become a mother. A mute but real need, in default of the absent passion, drives her to satisfy this rather vegetative law of the organism that woman can only complete through maternity. But the second pregnancy is very generally accepted with sorrow, uneasiness; the third is dreaded; the fourth is almost always avoided whatever might be the financial situation of the family. Nor do economic considerations enter except as a pretext, which the wife as well as the husband is happy to find. Woman, therefore, fills her profession as a wife in the same way in which all accepted professions are filled as a rule—through necessity rather than through a vocation. That is to say that she takes her duties as they come but foremost tries to utilize her rights and to enjoy her benefits.

The number of women who would willingly suffer their husbands' infidelities after one or two pregnancies if they were not afraid of seeing part of the family welfare and their own luxuries taken elsewhere is a great deal larger than is believed. Especially after the first discovery of inconstancy has destroyed the first illusions of love along with esteem and confidence, marriage, in their eyes, is no more than an association of interests that it is in their own interest not to break off. The husband is no more to them than a sort of legal fiction to whom they submit through fear of seeing him profit from the liberties that law and public opinion grant him. From that moment, the life of the woman is a struggle between outward behavior and spirit, in which the senses are docile instruments and in which neither heart nor love are involved. The wife still seeks to seduce her husband, even if she no longer loves him, solely because she fears that he may come to love someone else too deeply. This is the psychological moment for all infertile submissions: the wife becomes a mistress because she no longer wishes to become a mother.

Such judgments would appear quite harsh if they were not supported by a fact that is both eloquent and strange and that I expected to be brought up in the discussion.

It is quite true, as they say, that already in the large American cities the increase in population has been arrested and that families have few children, especially in the upper classes. It has been established now that the first Anglo-Saxon population is rapidly decreasing. The ranks of its generations can remain filled only thanks to German and Irish immigration. The American race, if not America, lacks children—a fact that Hepworth Dixon has established in his book on the United States. A woman who has spent long years in the United States, not only in the large cities along the coast but in the cities of the interior, and who, being a doctor, has been in contact with the American medical world, has confirmed to me what Dixon gives us to understand.[2] The true cause for the deficit in the middle-class Yankee population in these cities is abortion, tolerated by public opinion, if not permitted by law, which turns a blind eye. It is practiced almost in public on a vast scale, and a great number of specialists of both sexes have made considerable fortunes by their recognized skill in being able to kill the fruit without damaging the tree, from the moment the flower is set, by the most gentle means. Their clientele is in no way composed of needy or troubled families that have to calculate the additional expense of raising a child: free education, liberally open to all, would always permit them to provide the child with a career in this new country where there are wide open spaces and where the population can so easily expand. Rather, it is composed of worldly women, both elegant and wealthy, who calculate that another pregnancy would spoil their figures, make them lose a season of pleasures, or be disagreeable to their husbands whom they skilfully watch and understand how to hold with an admirable art. In order to be better wives they refuse to be mothers, and the first child is often delayed for several years to lengthen the honeymoon.

This fact demonstrates clearly that outside all economic laws one must take into account the causes for the diminished fertility of the upper classes, which are of a totally different order, since in America, where every human being who is born can find an open space, this decrease occurs among families who are the most capable of raising a great number of children and assuring them a fine social situation, whether they be boys or girls, because immigration provides enough husbands so that even without a dowry the girls can be assured of a free choice.

Isn't this reminiscient of what happened in Rome at the time of Juvenal, when the name Locusta became more celebrated among its citizens than that of the generals or the senators? This was a time when Rome, no longer finding soldiers among its citizens, had to entrust the empire to troops of barbarians to defend it against other barbarians. Is it not, in fact, a philosophical law that when man refuses to be a soldier, woman refuses to be a mother?

Couldn't this be related to still another factor? Among savage people in Australia, Polynesia, India, and even in China, that is to say, in states that have been civilized for a long time as well as in the most rudimentary societies, one finds the practice of infanticide. Nor did this occur because European conquerors consequently diminished their subsistance level so Australian mothers were reduced to restricting the number of their tribal defenders. Our first colonists, our first explorers found infanticide flourishing when they arrived there. Everywhere our missionaries have fought it in vain. In China, the government in order to restrain infanticide now welcomes all abandoned infants. A special public cart picks them up in the morning in front of the gates.

In Australia, as in China, one finds in particular infanticide or the abandonment of girl infants. Chinese law is precise: a girl has the right to live only if her father permits it. In Australia, the mother herself decides her life or death. Is this not because woman, who is everywhere subject to the most tyrannical laws, to the most arbitrary and brutal domination, who carries the heaviest and the most painful part in the reproduction of the species as a duty without a correlative right, soon becomes aware that to stifle a girl is to stifle a life destined for suffering?

Even among us, the birth of a girl is rarely welcome in families. The second and third birth often occur because the father and, even more, the mother desire to have at least one boy. Conversely, the fear of seeing more daughters born has often prevented boys from being born.

For a long time woman has had no other situation in society than marriage, no other possible profession than the exploitation of maternity or the commerce of love. The number of women who will be able to live with honor and security is determined by the number of men who marry them. All those who exceed this number will be in the situation of unemployed workers, of merchants without customers, especially women of the middle classes for whom all other work is considered a failure. If they have some resources, they can certainly vegetate, if not live, outside all social activity. If not, they will increase the number of women who, not being able to buy themselves a husband with their dowry or a social situation commensurate with their education and their accustomed style of life, will instead sell their love, at a discount and by the hour, to the husbands of rich women of the previous generation. The result is an increase in the number of bachelors, because they find it easier to live without the care of a family or children. This is a vicious circle that becomes larger as it turns upon itself. One might say that for every man who turns to prostitutes there is one more woman for prostitution, if not for the confessional and the convent.

In a word, thanks to war and emigration and the increasing tendency among men to live outside a family, there are too many women. This surplus of women—which ought to be favorable to increasing the population—is perhaps what stops its expansion, because the value of a woman diminishes for a man when, by virtue of great competition, the market is less in her favor.

I hope you will forgive me for using these brutal formulas in their stark reality, but they are a direct expression of the truth, from which we have no right to avert our eyes when it puts the nation and the species itself in peril and when we must seek remedies for an evil that could kill civilization.

This is the moment, I believe, to examine the influence of the Catholic religion, which I was surprised to hear M. Coudereau accuse of being too favorable to the multiplication of the species. Far from Christianity in general meriting this reproach, it should rather be reproached for the opposite. What it preaches and has always advised is celibacy, even abstinence during marriage. That is what is recommended in all the most authentic texts in the Gospels and the Apostles, as well as the complete collection of the Church Fathers. For them, all marriage is a failure; the law of generation is a shame, an affliction of the race, and the only conception that, according to them, is immaculate occurs outside natural law. Primitive Christianity being no more than a preface to the end of the world, it can not be favorable to the multiplication of a species destined to disappear soon in the midst of convulsions of nature and heavenly chastisement.

Since then, the Catholic Church, seeing that the world has obstinately continued to exist, in order to ensure its domination over a submissive people, permits people to perpetuate themselves but it does so with regret, by giving up its principles, in one of those multiple contradictions that fill its entire history. A single text in the Scriptures invites man to multiply his race, and this text, drawn from the first chapter of Genesis, is Jewish, not Christian. This is the one that Catholic liturgy adopted to consecrate marriage; the Gospels did not provide one.

Protestantism, on the contrary, returning to the evangelical texts in order to search for the rules of its laws, tends to return through the backdoor to the spirit of the doctrine's founder. England among others, annoyed by its Poor Law, which it does not dare to repeal, would like to suppress the poor man, by preventing him from being born. Under the influence of this preoccupation of the ruling classes, there is born a literature in which the most appropriate means for damming the rapidly increasing tide of a needy population is studied and discussed. This literature, made popular by design, published cheaply, often comes from the same offices as the Bible and is distributed in profusion by philanthropic or propaganda societies. The authors are often theologians, and it is quite curious to find that those American women who have been the quickest to adopt the most radical of measures to curb population growth have in general been educated theologians well versed in the study of Biblical texts, which they cite at every chance. They follow the sermons of preachers of renown very assiduously and discuss their merits with a perfect knowledge of the question. But does not the Catholic Church, for its part, have its convents, its priestly celibacy as repressive means against the multiplication of the species, which have suppressed as many infants as abortion has in America? From the moral point of view, there is no difference between one or the other procedure.

If our Bretons, more Catholic than their neighbors, the Normans, are also more prolific, it does not seem that this difference should be attributed to the influence of their religious beliefs but rather to other economic conditions, to a different division of landed estates, which in Normandy are cultivated above all by the land owners, and which in Brittany are cultivated by farmers or salaried workers. But it can also be attributed to a social situation closer to nature, to a lesser influence by civilization, that has not attenuated the instincts of the species in Brittany to the same degree as in Normandy. This is true especially for the women, who willingly fulfill their duties as mothers when the men for their part are more mindful of their duties as husbands. But the Catholic religion, when sincerely practiced, has at least one good result among our Breton country people: that the man, a believer like the woman, feels obliged to accept for himself the duties that it imposes on him.

The influence of a completely skeptic civilization which only recognizes civil law with its wide tolerance for man has acted to the contrary with all its power on our bourgeois classes, and education tends to aggravate the effects from generation to generation. The education of young people tends to alienate them more and more from family and marriage so that in their eyes it is no longer a bilateral contract equally sacred for both parties. Nothing in the life of young girls prepares them to be mothers. Marriage in their eyes is emancipation, liberty, the right to be the mistress of a house, to have servants to command, to say "my home," to buy a dress that pleases them, to go to the theater to which their mother refused to take them, to waltz at the ball with men previously forbidden to them, to have a seat in the church with their own name on it, and of course a coach with their number or arms upon it. As for maternity, religion, customs, literature, public opinion agree in presenting it to them as something hardly desirable, painful and—why not say it?—shameful in itself since it is excusable only if it is preceded by a kind of anticipatory pardon from the church and the authorization of the law. No longer daring to punish, they still stigmatize her by disinheriting the child born outside marriage, although modern economic conditions may offer a change on this point.

Maternity. Do women even know what it is before they are wives? It is hid from them like something mysterious, unacknowledged. It is for them up to the day of their delivery a terrible unknown, something fearful. All they know is that it could cause their death. How could they desire it? They think of it only with fright. Never is a young girl led to the bed of a woman in labor, never at school or in the family does she learn the first care of a newborn child. A young woman could be surprised by her delivery without even knowing that she must hurry to tie off the cord that attaches it to her entrails. No one has prepared her for the cares of maternity, unless by chance she has seen the birth of some late-born brother. Marriage, for the most part, is only a sad surprise, a terrible deception, a fall into reality from the high ideals where their imagination soared until then. If they have heard beforehand about this law that presides over the renewal of the generations, it is neither from their mother nor their teachers but by chance and often the most unhappy chance. If our country women are the best mothers and the most fertile mothers, is it not largely due to what they learned at a young age in the barn or the stable, from nature itself, about these mysteries that are hidden with such care from young girls in the city? Therefore, with such an education of our young girls—whose effects add to the even worse education of young men—it is not surprising that the maternal instinct is weakened in women. Nor is it surprising that, having become a mother the first time by surprise, she refuses to nurse the child and looks for ways to suppress any pregnancy. If anything is surprising, it is, on the contrary, that the species has perpetuated itself up to the present in spite of the convergent action of so many fatal influences. We ought to be grateful to the violent, primitive, savage instincts that have accumulated by heredity in the human race, across the whole animal genealogy, that have resisted everything that legislators and religions have undertaken to subdue them, weaken them, or cause them to disappear. These ancient physical instincts of the brute, still latent in the species and always ready to reawaken, cause all forms of revolt. This is something that has already saved the species countless times and will save it yet again from everything that has been invented by the makers of dogmas and codes until that day when reason, enlightened by science, readily submits to the only laws that result from the interests of the species itself, once these have been studied and recognized.

On the other hand, the day may come when humanity has the misfortune to live completely in accord with the dogmas, principles, precepts that until now have served and currently serve as the foundation of its beliefs and customs, dogmas that differ on every point except on the absolute domination over sexual instincts through ignorant will. Then, economic determinants will only serve to furnish each individual egoist, masculine or feminine, some motive to close off life to the child. This will happen within a few centuries to all our superior races, which will soon be extinguished through every kind of license and prostitution mixed with superstitious abstinence. What has saved man from his profound ignorance about these real laws are his contradictions and his logical errors.

We have to consider not only the danger menacing France of becoming a second-rate power in Europe but also the more general danger to the white race, which does not yet number more than 300 million people. They are faced by a yellow race that is ready to expand through all the world routes opened by its pioneers and inventors, a race that is multiplying rapidly and has already too much of an advantage through its easy acclimation to all zones.

The weakened maternal instinct of women must be reanimated by every means, and in men the paternal instinct, even more enfeebled, has to be developed. The single life must be made less easy for the man and more accessible for the woman. Customs must be put in accord with the law to recognize that women have the right to be mothers, even outside legal marriage, on condition that they fulfill their duties towards their children. The law must be forced to treat these children as equals of their brothers. However, in order for woman to make use of this right of maternity, it is necessary that she find in society some means of existence through her labor without being constrained—often against her nature, her tastes, her preferences—to sell herself either to a lover or to a husband, in whom she can see only a source of support, legal or not, if she submits to him through interest and necessity. Finally, woman must stop seeing marriage or love as something more or less agreeable or a more or less lucrative form of commerce; she must understand that marriage does not exist for the purpose of providing her an occasion to appear in a white veil crowned with flowers, to outdo her childhood companions the next day with her fine clothes, or even to walk along the promenades with a doll-child in the arms of a beribboned nurse. Marriage exists to give citizens to the state to defend it, to raise them seriously and strongly, with reason as well as with heart. Woman must free herself from clerical prejudices instead of inculcating them in her children and instruct herself in order to direct their education. It is necessary that she comprehend that maternity is the equivalent of military service for a woman and has the same perils and privations, which must be borne with courage. It is necessary that she tell herself that she owes to the race intelligent and robust individuals audacious and healthy enough to go out one day to wrench new lands from inferior races. These pioneers of civilization will have to pay tributes to harsh climates that are no heavier than those that war will continue to levy upon them until the royal dynasties, finally banned from civilized societies, will have been forced themselves to venture outside Europe to find crowns among still barbarous people.

In order for woman to comprehend and accept all these duties, her rights must be recognized. Above all the mother must find compensations in her husband so that the marriage becomes a contract between equals in which the duty of one corresponds to the duty of the other and that can be broken at the moment that all conditions are not fulfilled on both sides. Man must ask from woman only what he can and wants to give himself. The same education must reunite the two halves of humanity in the same beliefs, the same respect, the same sympathies, the same hatreds and teach them mutually to understand and to esteem each other. A young man must accept the same restraint as a young girl, so that early marriages preceded, if necessary, by long engagements, will prevent him from developing the habit of those sad debauches that succeed in forever divorcing the heart from the senses or those ill-matched liaisons, which always have such sad results and throw out into the world social hybrids who are always suspect and have no real place. But the prejudice that spouses must always live under the same roof must also be renounced. On the contrary, while the young couple is waiting to take its place in the sun, the young man could remain with his parents and the young woman with her family, where the first children would be born under the expert eyes of a grandmother. The closed-off family, narrow and composed exclusively of a couple and their children as it exists today, is the death of society within an egoistic individualism. It also results in depopulation, because it entails delayed marriages, it results in demoralization, because it puts family life to flight by rendering life conditions more difficult. Each couple spends more and produces less, and each woman becomes absorbed by the cares of her household and of her children. On the contrary, if the young couple lives with its parents under the domestic direction of the grandmother, young women and young men could both have professions and contribute their part to the well-being of the family until the time they leave and establish a family household in turn.

Until all these related reforms (rendered necessary and determined by the modern economic order) take place, there will be open war between the two halves of humanity occupied in reciprocally or alternately betraying and exploiting one another until they are finally reduced to selling what should be freely given—and never given except to the most worthy to raise their children—and then only as long as they remain worthy.

Marriage must cease to be a lottery, a game of chance in which life is the forfeit, a market that provides a profit to the most malign and wily of the partners to the detriment of the best or the most honest. Instead it must become a law of reasoned and reflective selection, having for its principal aim—if not its only one—the multiplication everywhere of the most noble types of the species, both physically and morally. Severe public criticism should be reserved for those who by venal calculation propagate unhealthy germs or badly endowed races. As for the single life, it should be permitted to and even imposed on those who could not expect a posterity that is healthy in mind or body. In compensation, they would be given full license without interference on condition that once having entered this world of outcasts, no one would be permitted to leave it, and no germ would be allowed to develop within it. If abortion and infanticide could be authorized, it would be in such cases only.

Given these conditions, domination of the will over the sexual instincts could without danger become increasingly complete. It could then become a benefit to the species, instead of, as it is today, a menace or a peril. Love can be free on condition that it be the reason itself and not, as it is today, an appetite, a distraction, a blind fatality for man and, for woman, a necessity, a profession, a calculation. Who will accomplish this reform? Woman herself when she comes to understand that it is both her duty and her right. Leaving man to continue to write and efface ten times in one century his ephemeral constitutions and codes, always recopied from ancient codified errors, she will engrave new customs on the solid rock of hereditary instinct by giving to the world sons, instructed by her, who will transcribe these customs into laws.

NOTES

Foreword

1. See Joy Harvey, "Strangers to Each Other," in *Uneasy Careers and Intimate Lives: Women in Science, 1789–1979,* ed. Pnina G. Abir-Am and Dorinda Outram (New Brunswick, NJ, and London: Rutgers University Press, 1987; 1989), 147–171.
2. For a special attention to Royer's ideas, see Geneviève Fraisse, *Clémence Royer: Philosophe et femme de sciences.* See also note 3, Abir-Am, "Afterword: Clémence Royer's Twentieth-Century Biographers Interpret a Nineteenth–Century Life," in *Women in Modern Scientific Research,* 373–381.
3. For a concise overview of the history of women and gender in science, which also includes a basic bibliography, see Pnina G. Abir-Am, "Women in Modern Scientific Research: A Historical Overview," in *World Science Report* (Paris: UNESCO Publications, 1996), 348–356.
4. See the essays on Mitchell by Sally Gregory Kohlstedt, on Kovalevskaia by Ann Hibner Koblitz, and on Hertha Ayrton by Marilyn Bailey Ogilvie, all in Abir-Am and Outram, *Uneasy Careers* (note 1).
5. For recent works on the Curies and the Joliot-Curies, including the Nobelist history of Marie and Irène Curie, see the essays by Helena Pycior and Bernadette Bensaude-Vincent, respectively, in *Creative Couples in the Sciences,* ed. Helena Pycior, Nancy Slack, and Pnina G. Abir-Am (New Brunswick, NJ, and London: Rutgers University Press, 1996).

Introduction

1. Néron, "Clémence Royer" (on occasion of the award of the Legion of Honor). She continues, "Mme Royer is simply a genius." Dossier Clémence Royer, Bibliothèque Marguerite Durand (BMD).
2. Heilbrun, *Writing a Woman's Life.*
3. Holmes, introduction to *Coleridge.*
4. Clémence Royer, *Clémence Royer par elle-même* (unpublished autobiography, hereafter cited as *Autobiography*), Dossier Clémence Royer, BMD. This is written in the third person, possibly dictated by Royer to her son, René.

5. Preface to translation of Charles Darwin, *De l'origine des espèces,* 1st ed., 1862.
6. Alfred Lord Tennyson, "The Princess" (1847).
7. This comment, often quoted in Somerville biographies, appears in a letter to Josephine Butler dated 10 May 1869 and in her unpublished memoirs. It was first published by James Stuart in his essay "The Teaching of Science," 121–151.
8. Royer, *Introduction à la philosophie des femmes,* 16. See also Fraisse, *Clémence Royer,* 106.
9. See chapter 9 for a discussion of this final judgment of herself in her speech at the Legion of Honor banquet given by the Bleus de Bretagne, as reported by Jean Brémond in *La Fronde,* 17 November 1900. Dossier Clémence Royer, Archives Nationales, F17 3216.

Chapter 1 ***A Fire of the Mind***

1. Royer, *Autobiography,* 9. BMD, Paris. This autobiography, written in the third person, is for the most part written in a childish hand, possibly that of Royer's son, most likely at dictation, since there are additions and corrections in Royer's own hand. A third handwriting ends the autobiography with a description of the banquet in her honor in 1897. One of the most interesting aspects of this document is a careful list of published materials, prizes, and submissions for competitions, including amounts she earned from these sources.
2. Adolphe Brisson, "Mme Clemence Royer," in Portraits *intimes* (Paris: Armand Colin, 1897), 121–127.
3. In her only novel she had one of her protagonists declaim: "I am a bastard and breeder of bastards," a comment that carries more than a touch of bravado mixed with anger. Royer, *Les Jumeaux d'Hellas,* vol. 1.
4. The effect of the Napoleonic Code on paternity searches will be discussed at greater length in chapter 7.
5. See Royer's speech to the Bleus de Bretagne on the occasion of her Legion of Honor award, in which she simultaneously invokes her father's dedication to the cause of the duchesse, mentions her treasuring of the document, but insists on her own republicanism. Dossier Clémence Royer, Bleus de Bretagne banquet (1900), BMD.
6. Augustin-René Royer's mother is listed as Marie Launay in his military records placed in Clémence Royer Dossier, BMD.
7. Moufflet refers to her as "a seamstress." Moufflet, "L'Oeuvre de Clémence Royer," 658–693.
8. The service record of Joseph Louis Audouard shows that he was born on 10 January 1751 at Saint-Malo as the son of André Audouard and Marie Guyonne de Saint-Verguet. This was copied out by ship captain P. Chack, head of the historical service, in July 1930 and placed in the Dossier Clémence Royer, BMD.
9. At the end of her life, Royer became a "Brétonne Bleue," one of a group of dedicated republicans who claimed Breton heritage. She considered that inheritance should be in the maternal line, a claim reiterated throughout her life.
10. Royer's speech before the Bleus de Bretagne at the banquet organized in her honor (1900). See note 3.
11. Royer, *Autobiography,* 9.

12. Ibid., 4.
13. Ibid.
14. Marie d'Agoult, *Mes souvenirs* (Paris: 1877). See also Vier, *La Comtesse d'Agoult.*
15. "So thoroughly had she amalgamated the genies of Zoroaster, the angels of Mohammed, and the Bible in a syncretism half-pagan, half-Christian, that at the age of ten she said a novena to the Virgin to obtain Aladdin's lamp. [She was] determined to use its magical virtues to give Henri V the throne. She flattered herself that in this way she would be a new Jeanne d'Arc." Royer, *Autobiography,* 23.
16. Ibid., 17.
17. Royer, "Rectifications biographiques," 2, BMD. This is a typed, unpublished autobiographical memoir by Royer, written in response to an inaccurate biography by Adolphe Brisson, who wrote a series of biographies of men and women for his newspaper in the late 1890s and collected them for publication some years later. Brisson, *Portraits intimes,* vols. 1–3. Royer's biography appears in the second part. This "rectification" was probably written for Ghénia Avril de Sainte-Croix around 1897, judging by the probable date of Brisson's interview and the year (1897) when René presented his mother with a typewriter because her handwriting was becoming impossible to read. See letter to Mary Lacour (1897). Sara Joan Miles has given a translation of this memoir into English in her dissertation, "Evolution and Natural Law." The quotations from the French given here are my translations.
18. Royer, *Autobiography,* 25.
19. Ibid., 27.
20. Ibid., 29.
21. Royer, "Rectifications," 2.
22. Royer, *Autobiography,* 33.
23. Ibid.
24. Ibid., 31.
25. Ibid., 35.
26. Royer, "Rectifications", 3.
27. Ibid. Note in connection with this idea of "monstrosity" that before the admission of women to medical schools the reference to a female "doctor" often implied a woman who performed illegal abortions. See Mary Putnam Jacobi, "Woman in Medicine."
28. Ibid. The reference is to Anne-Louise-Germaine de Staël, *Corinne, or Italy.*
29. Moers, "Performing Heroinism, 174.
30. Among the literary women so affected, Moers signals Margaret Fuller, who was called the "New England Corinne" even before she left for Italy, and both George Eliot and George Sand. It is worth noting that Dr. Mary Putnam Jacobi, another courageous woman of the nineteenth century, had been named by her mother "Mary Corinna."
31. Royer, "Rectifications," 3.
32. For details of Rachel's life as well as some interesting portraits of her at different periods, see Richardson, *Rachel.*
33. This is Royer's own description of her father's mental state.

34. Royer, *Les Jumeaux d'Hellas,* 2:195.
35. Royer, "Rectifications," 1.
36. Lamartine, *Histoire des Girondins.*
37. Royer, "Rectifications," 1.
38. Royer, "Rectifications," 1; Royer, *Autobiography,* 37.
39. Royer, "Rectifications," 6.
40. Ibid., 4.
41. Ibid.
42. Cited in Milice, *Clémence Royer,* and in Miles, "Evolution and Natural Law."
43. Royer, "Rectifications," 5.
44. Clémence Royer's metaphor. Royer, *Autobiography,* 41.
45. Ibid., 41–43.
46. Ibid., 47.
47. Ibid., 45–47.
48. Ibid. These were certificates issued by the Hôtel de Ville to teach secondary school, making her a "licentiate." No program was available to women at that time equivalent to the baccalaureate for young men. For further information on these certificates, see Daubié, "L'enseignement secondaire pour les femmes," 382–402, discussed in chapter 2. Julie-Victoire Daubié would receive the first baccalaureate awarded to a woman in France in 1861.
49. Michelet, *Histoire Romaine.*
50. These may be the lectures later published by Antoine-César Becquerel, *Des forces physico-chimiques et leur intervention dans la production des phénomènes naturels.* (Paris: Didot, 1875). Both Antoine-César Becquerel and his son Édouard Becquerel were lecturing in the late 1840s, and other lectures were published in the 1840s and early 1850s.
51. Royer, *Autobiography,* 45–47.
52. One of the first physics articles Royer wrote that had wide currency was "Attraction et gravitation d'après Newton," in which she questioned Newtonian science. Her book *La Constitution du monde,* which appeared only at the end of her life, incorporated her ideas of molecular and atomic structure.
53. The first announcements appeared in January 1854 in the *Pembrokeshire Herald.*
54. *Haverfordwest and Milford Haven Telegraph,* 15 February 1854.
55. For a contemporary description of the city, see *Black's Picturesque Guide through North and South Wales and Monmouthshire,* 8th ed. (Edinburgh: Adam and Charles Black; Chester, England: Cathedral and Prichard, 1858). At that time the population was about 6,580.
56. My description is drawn from archival material in the historical archives of Haverfordwest, now part of Pembrokeshire County Archives, located in the old dungeon and jail of the castle, from a visit to the city, and from accounts in the *Haverfordwest and Milford Haven Telegraph* for 1854–1855.
57. Royer, *Autobiography,* 49.
58. Strauss, *The Life of Jesus;* Renan, *Vie de Jésus.*
59. Colenso, *Village Sermons.* He began to write criticism of the way the church handled polygamy among the Zulu when he reached Africa, and then wrote a startling book on the Bible itself in 1862. He had begun in the 1840s writing school texts on algebra and geometry.

60. Ten years later Bessie Rayner Parkes wrote to Barbara Bodichon (18 May 1863): "I was kept away from Xtianity for years by a notion that Straus's [*sic*] *Life of Jesus* was 'incontrovertible.' it was not till I happened to read extracts of a French translation that I said to myself, 'Gracious! What stuff!' " Bessie R. Parkes Papers, Cambridge University, Girton College Archives, BRP V 117.
61. Naylor, *Time and Truth.*
62. Royer, preface to *Les Jumeaux d'Hellas.* The novel is discussed at greater length in chapter 2, although of course this insistence on moral intentions can be found among many novelists of the nineteenth century.
63. Frederick D. Maurice, *Lectures.*
64. Clémence Royer, "Rites funéraires préhistoriques," *Bulletin de la Société d'Anthropologie de Paris* (BSAP), 2d ser., 11 (1876).
65. Beale, *Reports.* The reports were issued 1868–1869.
66. *Report of Commissioners of Inquiry.* This study of boys' schools for the poor includes a number of mixed schools for boys and girls. Private schools (referred to as "private adventure") schools were considered outside this inquiry if they charged any fees above a minimum.
67. This advertisement for an English School appeared on the same page as the advertisement for Sarah Lewis's school. *Haverfordwest Telegraph,* 15 February 1854.
68. For a contemporary account of the reform efforts of Mary Carpenter, see Frances Power Cobbe, *Life.*
69. W. H. Channing, *Memoirs of Margaret Fuller Ossoli* (Boston: Phillips, Janson, 1852). See letter from Bessie Raynes Parkes to Barbara Smith (Bodichon) of 31 August 1855: "I have M. Fuller's life here: Matthews' book. Dear, what a woman; as before it affects me almost to tears. She had such a deft and thoroughness." Bessie R. Parkes Papers, Girton College Archives.
70. Impressed by Stowe's novel, a report in the newspaper mentioned a fund being organized: "The Birmingham Ladies' Anti-Slavery Society kindly consented to superintend the machinery for the English collection with very successful results from nobility, gentry, middle class, and working class to be used for the emancipation and elevation of the Negro Race in America." *Haverfordwest Telegraph,* 19 April 1854.
71. Report on Frederick D. Maurice's speech at the opening of Working Men's College, *Haverfordwest Telegraph,* 15 October 1854.
72. Frederick Maurice, *Life of Frederick Denison Maurice* (New York: Scribners, 1884).
73. Bessie Raynes Parkes to Barbara Smith (Bodichon), 27 March 1852. Barbara Bodichon Papers, Girton College Archives.
74. Excerpt from Wood, *Bees,* reported in *Haverfordwest Telegraph,* 22 October 1854.
75. Report on George Wilson. *Haverfordwest Telegraph,* 23 August 1854.
76. Many years later, Royer mentioned that her initial discussion of atomic theory in 1858 was intended for exactly this kind of scientific prize.
77. Smith, *Selections,* including a discussion on "Female Education and Conduct of the Understanding," as reported in the *Haverfordwest Telegraph.*
78. Royer, "Rectifications," 5.

Chapter 2 *The Question of Abuse*

1. Royer, *Autobiography,* 49.
2. *Haverfordwest Telegraph* carried almost daily reports from 24 September through October 1854, as did the *Pembrokeshire Herald* during the same period.
3. Royer, "*Rectifications,*" 6.
4. Royer, *Les Jumeaux d'Hellas* (1864); the first version was written in 1858.
5. James Hannay, "Lectures on Byron," quoted in *Haverfordwest Telegraph* and probably drawn from his *Satires and Satirists* (London, 1854).
6. See Patrick Kay Bidelman, *Pariahs Stand Up! The Founding of the Liberal Feminist Movement in France, 1858–1889* (Westport, CT: Greenport Press, 1982). There is a lengthy discussion here of Léon Richer.
7. For details about Maria Deraismes's life and writings and those of Léon Richer, see Patrick Kay Bidelman, "Maria Deraismes, Léon Richer, and the Founding of the French Feminist Movement, 1866–1878," in *Third Republic/Troisième République,* nos. 3–4 (1977): 20–73, Bidelman, *Pariahs Stand Up!* and Moses, *French Feminism,* 179–184.
8. In Royer's novel, *Les Jumeaux d'Hellas.*
9. Royer, *Autobiography,* 49.
10. Royer, *Les Jumeaux d'Hellas.*
11. Royer discussed her writing the novel in a letter about her relationship with Duprat, written at the end of her life to Ghénia Avril de Sainte-Croix, n.d. [1899?], Correspondence Clémence Royer, BMD. Both her initial decision to write the novel and the contents of this letter are examined in greater detail in chapter 3.
12. Preface to Royer, *Les Jumeaux d'Hellas.*
13. The novel of Elizabeth Gaskell, *Ruth* (London: Chapman and Hall, 1853), may provide a model here.
14. This may have been an indirect reference to Alexander Dumas's *Count of Monte Cristo* (1846), in which the hero is held in the Château d'If for many years. It is not clear why Royer adopted the name *Oeuf,* or egg, for this prison.
15. "La République de Parthénope," in Royer, *Les Jumeaux d'Hellas,* vol. 2.
16. "La Victoire des dieux," in Royer, *Les Jumeaux d'Hellas,* 2:523 ff.
17. Ibid.
18. Royer, preface to *Les Jumeaux d'Hellas.*
19. Ibid.
20. Ibid.
21. Ibid.
22. Ibid.
23. "Album d'un voyageur," in Royer, *Les Jumeaux d'Hellas,* 1:199–325. On the whole, this section is an account of an intellectual rather than a physical progress.
24. The early discussions of science are discussed at greater length in chapter 3.
25. "Révélations," in Royer, *Les Jumeaux d'Hellas,* 2:171.
26. Ibid.
27. Ibid., 2:175.
28. Ibid.
29. Ibid.
30. Ibid., 2:125. Another long description of Mathilde, Lady Howard, in the grip of

depression following her divorce trial shows a very similar pattern of behavior to that of Lucie listening to music with her elbows on the clavier so she can feel the vibrations or sitting with her head in her lap. "Mathilde à la reine," in Royer, *Les Jumeaux d'Hellas,* 2:351. The vivid manner of this description of depression, coupled with her reports of her own exaltations in "mystical crisis," leads us naturally to wonder whether Royer was prey to cyclical mood swings.

31. "Révélations," in Royer, *Les Jumeaux d'Hellas,* 2:125.
32. Ibid.
33. Ibid., 2:172.
34. Ibid., 2:179.
35. Ibid.
36. See appendix and a discussion of related issues in chapter 7, "Woman Is Not Made Like This."
37. "Révélations," in Royer, *Les Jumeaux d'Hellas,* 2:179—180.
38. Ibid., 2:180.
39. "Stefano à Matteo," in Royer, *Les Jumeaux d'Hellas,* 2:369–170.
40. Jules Michelet, *La Femme* (Paris: Lévy, 1860), 37–38.
41. See her comments in "Sur la natalité," translated in the appendix to this volume.
42. "Mathilde à la reine," in Royer, *Les Jumeaux d'Hellas,* 2:352.
43. Ibid., 2:356. It is possible that this cold-shouldering is something that also happened to Royer at some point in her brief teaching career, or at least to a close colleague.
44. Cited in Acland, *Caroline Norton.* On reactions to Norton's epigram see Longford, "The Sex," and Herstein, *A Mid-Victorian Feminist.*
45. Barbara Smith, *A Brief Summary in Plain Language of the Most Important Laws of England Concerning Women* (London: Holyoake, 1854). For the context of this book see Herstein, *A Mid-Victorian Feminist.*
46. Longford, "The Sex."
47. Mdlle [*sic*] Clémence Royer, "Women in French Switzerland, 49–57.
48. These laws are included in "La République de Parthénope," in Royer, *Les Jumeaux d'Hellas,* 2:499–507. While insisting that these are "liberties" rather than rights and that they carry "duties" with them, her republic assigns women the right to bring up their own children and tutor them. Children also bear the mother and not the father's name. The father can assign his property to his recognized child or children. The right of divorce is maintained, prostitution forbidden, and adultery considered to be like rape, requiring punishment and remarriage. The man is presumed to be the initiator of force or seduction. Unmarried men are disenfranchised. Although the husband and wife together are considered to form a single citizen and have a single vote, *the husband is allowed to cast that vote.* All religions, arts, theater, and sciences depend on the subsidies of their members, not of the state. Not surprisingly, the citizens of her little republic of Naples are somewhat dubious of the constitution.
49. Letter of Clémence Royer to Ghénia Avril de Sainte-Croix, n.d. [1899?]. Correspondence Clémence Royer, BMD.
50. Royer, "Rectifications," 6. William Ellery Channing's nephew, W. H. Channing, was touring Bristol and other British cities in the mid-1850s, lecturing on Channing's style of Unitarianism, on whom he had published six years before.

See Channing, *Memoir of William Ellery Channing.* Channing is said to have had a profound sympathy for France and its revolutionary movements.

51. Michelet, *Jeanne d'Arc.*
52. Royer, "Rectifications," 6.
53. Royer, *Autobiography,* 51.
54. Royer, "Rectifications," 6.
55. Royer, *Autobiography,* 51–53.
56. Royer, "Rectifications," 6.
57. Ibid.
58. Royer, *Autobiography,* 53.
59. Ibid., 54.
60. Daubié, "L'enseignement secondaire," 382–402. This was the first of two articles.
61. Royer, *Autobiography,* 54. These sentences, unlike the main text, are written in her own handwriting.
62. Ibid., 55.
63. Milice, *Clémence Royer.* 42.
64. Royer, "Rectifications," 6–7.

CHAPTER 3 ***Mind and Love Awaken***

1. *Lausanne Guide Officiel,* 1990–1991.
2. Victor Hugo, as quoted in *Lausanne Guide Officiel,* 1990–1991 (my translation).
3. Royer, *Autobiography,* 59–60.
4. Royer, *Les Jumeaux d'Hellas.*
5. See her later extension of these ideas in her paper "De la nature du beau," 71–87. She summarized these arguments in a note to the fourth edition of her translation of Charles Darwin, *De l'origine des espèces,* (Paris: Flammarion, 1882), 537–538 n. Q.
6. Royer, *Autobiography,* 59–60.
7. Ibid., 60–61.
8. Clémence Royer to Victor Considérant, Considérant Archives, Archives Nationales, 10 AS 41; letter no. 1, n.d. [March 1882]. According to Milice, in 1857 she read Lyell, Blumenbach, Hollard, Geoffroy Saint-Hilaire, Humboldt, De la Bêche, Agassiz, Beudant, Tacitus, the Bhagavad-Gita, Laws of Manu, Ossian, Zend-Avesta, and Plato. Milice, *Clémence Royer,* 44.
9. Royer, *Autobiography,* 60–61. This text on Maine de Biran no longer exists.
10. See chapters 4, 8, and 9 for a discussion of her concepts of matter.
11. Album d'un voyageur, in *Les Jumeaux d'Hellas,* 1:199–325.
12. Ibid., 1:231–234.
13. Ibid., 1:232.
14. Ibid., 1:233.
15. Ibid.
16. "Ibid., 1:234.
17. Ibid., 1:267–272. This section of the "Album" is subtitled "Une Expérience" (an experiment).
18. Ibid., 1:200.
19. Ibid., 1:201.

20. Ibid.
21. Royer, *Autobiography,* 57.
22. In the Dossier Clémence Royer, Archives Historiques, Préfecture de Police, Paris, a report records many years after the fact (in the 1880s) that Royer was thought to dress in an eccentric manner in both Switzerland and Italy. Also cited in Clark, *Social Darwinism in France.*
23. René Bray, *Sainte-Beuve à l'Académie de Lausanne: Chronique discours sur Port-Royal* (Paris: E. Droz; Lausanne: F. Rouge, 1937).
24. For a discussion of Marie Forel and the other women auditors of Sainte-Beuve, see Bray, *Sainte-Beuve.*
25. In the Charles Secrétan Correspondence, the letters to Marie Forel begin in 1851 and extend into the 1870s. They cover the books exchanged, the manuscript she was preparing of Alexandre Vinet's lectures, upon which he commented, and, increasingly frankly, his personal life. Fonds Charles Secrétan, Bibliothèque Cantonale et Universitaire de Lausanne, IS 3760.
26. The wide interest of the Forel family in both science and literature is shown by the experiments of her sister-in-law, Adèle Forel, who raised ten generations of silkworms as a method of studying the effects of "open-air education." Her experiments, conducted at Chigny near Morges from 1862 to 1871, "obtained a complete success" in curing silkworm diseases, "applying artificial selection to this problem," as her son later claimed. F. A. Forel, "La Sélection naturelle et les maladies parasitaires des animaux et des plantes domestiques" (1877), sent to Darwin" with "*hommage* and respectful admiration and devotion." Darwin Pamphlet Collection, Darwin Archive. One cannot help wondering about the influence, if any, of Royer's discussion of evolution on Adèle Forel's research.
27. Royer, *Autobiography,* 65. By 1861 she was living at 2, place de la Madeleine, as noted by Charles Darwin in his address book in 1861 and in a letter requesting the publisher John Murray to send her a copy of the third edition of the *Origin of Species.* Burkhardt et al., Darwin Archive; and Charles Darwin to John Murray, 10 September [1861], *Correspondence of Charles Darwin,* vol. 9.
28. Royer, *Autobiography,* 65.
29. Ibid.
30. Brigitta Holm, "Life in the Drawing Room: A Chapter of a Study on Frederika Bremer as a Novelist," in *Suppression, Struggle, and Success: Studies in Three Representations of Cultural Life in Sweden: Frederika Bremer, Andreas Kempe, and Linnaeus,* ed. Claes-Christian Elert and Gunaar Eriksson, *Acta Universitas Umensis Umea (Studies in the Humanities)* 47 (1982): 101.
31. Royer, *Autobiography,* 65–67.
32. See, among other sources, Moufflet, "L'Oeuvre," 658–693.
33. Royer, "Rectifications," 7.
34. The only account by Royer of her relationship with Duprat is in a typewritten letter to Ghénia Avril de Sainte-Croix [1899?] beginning "Chère Amie, Dans la biographie que je vous ai fait remettre, il n'est jamais question de mes liens avec Pascal Duprat." Correspondence Clémence Royer, BMD.
35. Moufflet, "L'Oeuvre."
36. Letter to Ghénia Avril de Sainte-Croix [1899?], Correspondence Clémence Royer, BMD.

37. Pascal Duprat, *Essai historique sur les races anciennes et modernes de l'Afrique septentrionale: Leur origine . . . depuis l'antiquité la plus reculée jusqu'à nos jours* (Paris: Labitte, 1845). For biographies of Duprat see *La Grande Encyclopédie Universelle* (Paris: Larousse, [1890?]), 15:92 s.v. "Duprat, Pascal." Nigoul, *Pascal Duprat.*
38. Clémence Royer, "La vie politique de François Arago," *Revue Internationale* 15, 3e année. Dossier Cléemence Royer, BMD.
39. Ibid., 13.
40. For an interesting view of the circle of French republicans just before and during the 1848 revolution, see Lovett, *Giuseppe Ferrari.* Duprat's association with Ferrari is discussed on pages 51–52, 61.
41. Pascal Duprat, *De l'état: Sa place et son rôle dans la vie des sociétés* (Brussels, 1852).
42. Royer, letter to Ghénia Avril de Sainte-Croix, n.d. [1899?]. Correspondence Clémence Royer, BMD.
43. "Duprat, Pascal," *La Grande Encyclopédie.*
44. Royer, letter to Ghénia Avril de Sainte-Croix, n.d. [1899?]. Correspondence Clémence Royer, BMD.
45. Royer, preface to Charles Darwin, *De l'origine des espèces,* 1st ed., 1862.
46. Marie d'Agoult, letter to Dolfuss of 5 August 1857, cited in *La Comtesse d'Agoult,* Vier, 3:120.
47. Royer, *Les Jumeaux d'Hellas,* 1:201.
48. Ibid., 201–202.
49. Royer, letter to Ghénia Avril de Sainte-Croix, n.d.[1899?]. Correspondence Clémence Royer, BMD.
50. Ibid.
51. Ibid.
52. Royer, "Héloise et Abélard," in *Les Jumeaux d'Hellas,* 2:139–141.
53. For an interesting discussion of the party given in honor of Hugo's book *Les Misérables* by his publishers on 16 September 1862, see Alfred Barrou, *Victor Hugo et son temps* (Paris: G. Charpentier, 1881). Among the writers who attended were Texier, Pelletan, Nefftzer, Nadar, Ferrari, the Italian francophile, friend of Duprat, and "Royer," who may well have been Clémence (308–309). Although Duprat is mentioned as an editor with Hugo and others for the journal *L'Homme,* the journal of expatriate Frenchmen in Jersey (271), his name does not appear in this list of those attending the celebration, although he was probably there.
54. Mlle A.C.R. [Clémence Royer], "Introduction à la philosophie des Femmes (opening lecture of the course given in Lausanne by Royer), 1–34. This text has been reprinted as an appendix to Fraisse, *Clémence Royer,* 105–125. (I have paged to the original source.)
55. Royer, "Introduction à la philosophie," 13.
56. Ibid., 18.
57. Ibid., 16.
58. Ibid., 4.
59. Ibid., 11–12.
60. Ibid.

61. Ibid.
62. Ibid.
63. Marcet, like Harriet Martineau, included social science in her lessons for children, which she published under the pseudonym "John Hopkins." For a contemporary account, see Auguste de la Rive, "Madame Marcet."
64. Royer, "Introduction à la philosophie," 17.
65. Ibid., 18.
66. She told Ghénia Avril de Sainte-Croix many years later that once the journal moved to Geneva, "my assistance ceased." Letter to Ghénia Avril de Sainte-Croix [1899?], Correspondence Clémence Royer, BMD. However, when Joseph Garnier was introduced to her by Duprat at the international conference on taxation in Lausanne in 1860, it was as Duprat's collaborator on the journal.
67. Letter of Clémence Royer to the director of the Bibliothèque Publique et Universitaire de Genève, 9 January 1861. Bibliothèque Publique et Universitaire Archives. She gives an address in Geneva.
68. Royer gives the debts of his wife as a reason for Duprat's flight in her letter to Ghénia Avril de Sainte-Croix [1899?], but claims were made by Duprat's political opponents in the 1870s that he had incurred large debts from speculations in Swiss railroad stock during this period. Dossier Pascal Duprat, Préfecture de Police, Paris.
69. Royer, *Autobiography,* 73.
70. Marie d'Agoult, unpublished journal, quoted in Vier, *La Comtesse d'Agoult,* 3:358 n.818. We know no more about this intriguing "discovery."
71. The most detailed life of the Comtesse d'Agoult is that of Vier, *La Comtesse d'Agoult.*
72. Duprat had published a piece by Marie d'Agoult entitled "Gervinus et son histoire dans le XIXe siècle" in the first issue of his Brussels journal, *Libre Recherche.* In the third number in 1857, an article praised her work as a novelist.
73. See Marie d'Agoult, unpublished journal, 31 May 1862, cited in Vier, *La Comtesse d'Agoult.* This and Royer's letters to the Countess d'Agoult are in the Charnacé manuscripts in the Bibliothèque de Versailles. Juliette Lamber Adam discusses Marie d'Agoult's enthusiastic response to them in her memoirs, *Mes premières armes.*
74. Clémence Royer, "Origine et développements des facultés mentales," in *Origine de l'homme,* 54.
75. For a tribute to Guillaumin, see Garnier, "Nécrologie," 108–121. His friendship with the economist Adolphe Blanqui resulted in his establishing a bookstore and publishing house specialising in economics and political economy. The *Journal des Économistes* first appeared in December 1841. Royer maintained a friendship with Guillaumin's daughters, Félicité (who died in 1885) and her much younger sister, Pauline, who continued to direct the publishing house of Guillaumin and Company. (This is mentioned in a report in the Dossier Clémence Royer, Préfecture de Police.)
76. Joseph Garnier, in this report to the Société d'Économie Politique, also praised "Madame Marcet, Miss Harriet Martineau, and Madame Maynieu," *Journal des Économistes,* 2d ser., 28 (1860): 142.
77. Adam's anti-Proudhon book was published as Juliette Lamber, *Idées anti-Proudhoniennes.*

78. Royer, *Théorie de l'impôt ou la dîme sociale.* Although I have focussed on Royer's discussion of women in society, for a much broader analysis of her economic theories see Fraisse, *Clémence Royer.*
79. Royer, *Théorie de l'impôt,* 1:25–27.
80. Ibid., 2:285.
81. Ibid.
82. Ibid., 1:147. In spite of the military metaphor, she objected to permanent professional armies and preferred the Swiss system of required participation by all citizens.
83. Ibid., 2:287.
84. Ibid., 2:286.
85. Ibid., 2:287. The image of the woman as a doll in her husband's house prefigures Nora in Ibsen's play *A Doll's House.*
86. Ibid., 2:289.
87. Royer, *Autobiography,* 73. Marie d'Agoult, for example, seemed to assume she was Swiss before she met her for the first time.
88. "Société d'Économie Politique," *Journal des Économistes* 5 (1862): 305–307. This same volume contains an article by another brilliant woman, Julie-Victoire Daubié, discussing means of subsistence for women (361–378). Daubié, like Royer, regularly wrote for the journal in the 1860s.
89. Clark, *Social Darwinism,* 13–14.
90. Royer (Discussion of the Société d'Économie Politique), *Journal des Économistes* 5 (1862): 305–307. There is a resonance here with the belief of Lucie's mother, Joanna, in *Les Jumeaux d'Hellas,* who imparted sexual information to her daughter to allow her to protect herself. See chapter 2.
91. For a further discussion of this society and the failure to admit Royer, see Fraisse, *Clémence Royer.*
92. Royer, *Autobiography,* 67.
93. Ibid. For the *Origin of Species* Royer uses the date of the copy she translated (the third edition of 1860), which was sent to her in 1861, rather than that of the first edition of 1859. Her lectures in Geneva took place in 1861.
94. Royer, "Rectifications," 7. She added that this was not the reason why she left Switzerland, because although she had adversaries among the orthodox there, she also had suppporters.
95. Ibid., 8.
96. For a discussion of the Darwin translations and the later encounter between Naville and Royer, see chapters 4 and 5.

Chapter 4 ***"True Science"***

1. François Jules Pictet, "Sur l'origine de l'espèce."
2. Claparède, "M. Darwin," 523—559.
3. Royer, "Rectifications," 8.
4. A series of letters from Carl Vogt to Charles Darwin from 1867 to 1868 are in the Charles Darwin Archives. Vogt proposed first a German and then a French translation of Variation and put Darwin in contact with his former student, Colonel J. J. Moulinié, and the French publisher Charles Reinwald. See F. Burkhardt and S.

Smith, eds., *Calendar of Darwin Correspondence,* rev. ed. (Cambridge: Cambridge University Press, 1994).

5. Carl Vogt, *Lectures on Man, 1863* (London: Anthropological Society of London, 1864).
6. Clémence Royer, preface to Charles Darwin, *De l'origine des espèces,* translated by Mlle A. C. Royer from the third English edition (Paris: Guillaumin and Masson, 1862), lxv (page citation as reprinted in the 3d French edition).
7. Royer, *Autobiography,* 67.
8. Louise Swanton Belloc, wife of the painter Hilaire Belloc, had first written to Darwin in November 1859, offering to translate Origin of Species. Louise S. Belloc to Charles Darwin, in Burkhardt and Smith, *Correspondence of Charles Darwin,* vol. 7. By January she had decided the science was too difficult. See letter from Charles Darwin to Charles Lyell of 14 January [1860] in Burkhardt and Porter, *Correspondence of Charles Darwin,* vol. 8.
9. See letter of Charles Darwin to Edward Cresy of 15 January [1860] concerning Pierre Talandier in Burkhardt et al., *Correspondence of Charles Darwin,* vol. 8. The answer was apparently satisfactory, since Darwin replied with some pleasure to the report on 20 January 1860. He also wrote to Quatrefages about these negotiations. Letters to Armand de Quatrefages of 21 January and 31 March [1860]. The quotation is from the letter of 31 March. Burkhardt and Porter, *Correspondence of Charles Darwin,* vol. 8.
10. See chapter 3.
11. Burkhardt et al., *Correspondence of Charles Darwin* (1861), vol. 9. The original can be found in the John Murray Archive, John Murray Publishers, London.
12. See the advertisements and listings for the Darwin translation in *Journal Général de l'Imprimerie et de la Librarie*, 2d ser., 6 (Paris: Guillaumin and Masson, 1862). The first section, "Bibliographie," lists the translation among publications for 21 June 1862 (275). Earlier dates are given in the advertisements. The printer was Moulin of Saint-Denis. The third section, "Feuilleton commercial," contains the advertisements from publishers and booksellers on a weekly basis. The issue for 3 mai 1862 (p. 294) includes a large advertisement for "*Théorie de l'impôt ou la dîme sociale* par Mlle Cl. Aug. Royer, ouvrage couronné par le Congrès de Lausanne, 2 volumes . . . prix 12 francs, Librarie de Guillaumin et Cie, rue de Richelieu, 14." In the issue of 24 Mai 1862, under the heading of "Nouvelles publications," Royer's *Théorie de l'impôt* is listed at Fr 10 (p. 341). At the bottom of the same page is a large advertisement: "En vente le 31 mai chez Guillaumin et Cie et Victor Masson et Fils: *De l'origine des espèces ou des lois du progrès chez les êtres organisés* par Ch Darwin, traduit en français sur la 3e édition avec l'autorisation de l'auteur par Mlle Cl-Aug Royer avec une préface et notes du traducteur." In the 7 June 1862 issue is a half-page advertisement for the Darwin edition, listed only under Guillaumin but with both Guillaumin and Masson listed at the head of the page. Advertised as containing "plus de 720 pages," it adds that it is "avec l'autorisation de l'auteur" and includes "une table analytique." The translator is listed as "Mlle Clem. Aug. Royer." Note that Masson did not independently advertise the book.
13. The best summary of the life and work of René-Édouard Claparède (1832–1871) is provided by the publication of his letters by Morsier, *Lettres.*

14. Royer "Rectifications," 8.
15. Royer, preface *Origine des espèces,* 1st ed.
16. Ibid.
17. Ibid.
18. In Darwin's copy of the preface he has marked this passage with a number of lines. The copy is in the Darwin Pamphlet Collection, Darwin Archive. Her raillery however is—in her case—in reference to a satirical view of God fashioning the human being "like a poor worker who, having ruined his work, is reduced to repenting that he has ever made it." Ibid., lvi.
19. Royer, preface to *Origine des espèces,* 1st ed.
20. See "Table analytique" following the table of contents at the end of the first edition of Darwin, *Origine des espèces.*
21. Pictet, review.
22. Royer, preface to *Origine des espèces,* 1st ed., lvii, liii. She is quoting Claparède, "M. Darwin."
23. Ibid., liii–lv. She continues to quote him at great length.
24. Ibid., lvi.
25. Ibid., lvii. See chapter 5 for her insistence in 1867 to Naville that her comments on the weak had been misunderstood.
26. Was this a tacit comment about the strength that she believed her mother inherited from her sea captain father, rather than from her beautiful and "lazy" mother? In Royer's own case, she seemed to believe that she had derived most of her "racial characteristics" from her Breton mother.
27. Marie d'Agoult, unpublished journal, 11 June 1862. Cited in Vier, La Comtesse d'Agoult.
28. Darwin to Asa Gray, 10 June 1862 (Gray Herbarium 66), in Burkhardt et al., *Correspondence of Charles Darwin,* vol. 10 (forthcoming).
29. Royer to Ghénia Avril de Sainte-Croix [1897]. Dossier Clémence Royer, BMD.
30. Charles Darwin to Armand de Quatrefages, 11 July 1862. Wellcome Institute for the History of Medicine. Burkhardt et al., *Correspondence of Charles Darwin,* vol. 10 (forthcoming).
31. Edouard Claparède to Charles Darwin, Cologny près Genève, 6 September 1862. Burkhardt et al., *Correspondence of Charles Darwin,* vol. 10 (forthcoming). The original is in the Darwin Archive, DAR 161.1.149.
32. Ibid.
33. Ibid. Yvette Conry was the first modern historian to question the Royer translation and see it as the source of French scientific hostility and Lamarckian readings. Conry, *Introduction du Darwinisme.* Recently, Sara Joan Miles has looked extensively at Royer's first French edition, reanalyzing her translation, her notes, and her preface with somewhat less censorious conclusions. Miles, "Evolution and Natural Law," and Miles, "Clemence Royer," 61–83. Claude Blanckaert has examined these and other arguments and comes down on the side of Conry; Blanckaert, "Les Bas-Fonds," 115–130. These arguments and others are examined in the afterword.
34. Burkhardt et al., *Correspondence of Charles Darwin,* vol. 10 (forthcoming).
35. "Instinct," in chapter 7, Darwin, *Origin of Species,* 3d ed. (London: Murray, 1860). This passage by Darwin contains a rather involved geometrical argument

posed in a complex manner so that Royer's problem may have been one of language rather than of science.

36. Edouard Claparède to Charles Darwin, 6 September 1862. Darwin Archive. Burkhardt et al., *Correspondence of Charles Darwin,* vol. 10 (forthcoming).
37. Ibid. In a replacement note for the one Claparède cites, Royer carefully remarked that the electric organs developed in a parallel manner, and then cited the experiments by the Italian physiologist Carlo Mattuecci that indicated that vertebrate muscle fibers were capable of producing electrical discharges.
38. Morsier, *Lettres de René-Édouard Claparède.* The letter to Darwin is not included among these.
39. Charles Darwin to J. D. Hooker, 11 September 1862. Darwin Archive, DAR 115:162. Burkhardt et al., *Correspondence of Charles Darwin,* vol. 10 (forthcoming). Darwin continues by laughing at his own conceit in telling a botanist, Hooker, about flower homologies.
40. See the presentation list for Orchids prepared by Charles Darwin, included as an appendix in Burkhardt et al., *Correspondence,* vol 10 (forthcoming).
41. "Mademoiselle C. A. Royer, who accepts and comments on the theory of the author, sees in this law of selection [*élection*] the generalization from that of Malthus and at the same time the condemnation of the consequences that Malthus drew from it for the human species. This merits examination." Garnier, "Société d'Économie Politique," 153. Garnier was the editor in chief of the *Journal des Économistes,* although for a time he had turned over the regular editorship to others. See Clark, *Social Darwinism,* 189 n. 32.
42. See chapter 3, where her connection to Marie d'Agoult is discussed in greater detail.
43. Royer, "Association internationale," 63–100.
44. Ibid., 89–90. The congress included discussions on state education and on the possibility of the state underwriting public lecturers and writers. Pascal Duprat rose to plead eloquently that in a society that was not free this support could result in intellectual control by the state (p. 83). Issues of welfare and public hygiene were also raised, including the issue of "women's work," for which few commentators offered a solution
45. Vier, *La Comtesse d'Agoult.*
46. Ronchaud, "Chronique Littéraire: *Les Jumeaux d'Hellas,*" 557–560.
47. Clémence Royer to Ghénia Avril de Sainte-Croix [1899?], Correspondence Clémence Royer, BMD.
48. Royer, "Congrès International des Sciences Sociales," 224–241. See pp. 227–230 for Royer quotations.
49. Ibid. See p. 232 for Duprat quotation.
50. Royer, *Le Bien.*
51. Clémence Royer to Marie d'Agoult, 28 August 1863, cited in Vier, *La Comtesse d'Agoult,* 4:282. The original is in the Fonds Charnacé, Bibliothèque de Versailles, F 768.
52. Clémence Royer to Marie d'Agoult, 10 October 1863. Fonds Charnacé, Bibliothéque de Versailles, F 768. Quoted in Vier, *La Comtesse d'Agoult.*
53. Mdlle [*sic*] Clémence Royer "Women in French Switzerland," 49–57.
54. Jane Rendall, "A 'Moral Engine'? Feminism, Liberalism, and the *English*

Woman's Journal," Equal or Different? Women's Politics, 1800–1914, ed. Jane Rendell (Oxford: Blackwell, 1987).

55. Royer, "Women in French Switzerland," 55–56.
56. Editorial comment, *The English Woman's Journal* 11 (1863): 57.
57. Clémence Royer to Ghénia Avril de Sainte-Croix, n.d. [1899?], BMD.
58. Gabriel de Mortillet noted Royer's lectures on Darwinism in his journal *Materiaux pour l'Histoire de l'Homme,* which he founded and edited from 1866 to 1868.
59. See Vier, *La Comtesse d'Agoult.*
60. Clémence Royer to Victor Considérant [1882]. Correspondence Victor Considérant, Archives Nationales 10 AS 41.
61. Lovett, *Giuseppe Ferrari.* Ferrari was a Francophile and had spent time in Paris during the Second Republic.
62. Clémence Royer to Ghénia Avril de Sainte-Croix [1899?], BMD. This is partly supported by three letters from Mme Pascal Duprat to Jules Simon—mistakenly listed as letters from Pascal Duprat—of 28 June 1866, July 1866, and 6 August 1866. Archives Nationales, Correspondence Jules Simon, AP 87/3 and AP 87/6. She asks for an interview and then money to enable her and her daughter to return to Geneva to teach, although they remained in Paris and seem to have never had any intention of teaching.
63. Clémence Royer to Ghénia Avril de Sainte-Croix [1899?], BMD. Later notes in Dossier Pascal Duprat in the files of the Préfecture de Police indicate that he and his wife had separated and that she was running a *bureau de tabac* at various locations in Paris.
64. Adam, *Mes premières armes.*
65. Ibid.
66. Ibid. Perhaps Royer was the more annoyed since she knew Texier professionally both from the celebration of Victor Hugo's novel given by his publisher and as a fellow member of the Société d'Ethnologie.
67. Royer praised Jenny d'Héricourt at length to Léopold Lacour in a letter written in 1897. This is discussed at length in chapter 9. Juliette Adam's depiction of Royer and d'Héricourt as her enemies can be found throughout her books. For further information on Jenny d'Héricourt, see Offen, "French Feminist Rediscovered," 144–157.
68. Block, "Revue," 413–414. Duprat always dated his contributions to journals. His articles on economic ideas in Italy place him in Turin from 1 September 1864 through December 1864. Duprat, "Idées économiques en Italie," 431–448, and Duprat, "Mainmorte," 172–190, which refers to his Italian statistical journal.
69. By September 1865 Gicca took over the journal, which became *L'Economista Nazionale, Revista di Economia Politica et di Statistica,* and was the organ of the Italian Society of Political Economy. This is reviewed as "founded recently at Florence" with Duprat one of the founding editors. "Revue des principales publications économiques de l'étranger," *Journal des Économistes,* 3d ser., 1 (1866): 103.
70. Duval, "Review," 421.
71. Royer, "Avvenire di Torino." This was published as a brochure, probably by Duprat's printer. Some years before, Marie d'Agoult had published on the role of Florence and Turin in the new Italy.

72. A copy of this photo is in the Nadar collection, n.a.fr., Bibliothèque Nationale, dated 1865. (fig. 3). Many years later, Nadar made a photographic portrait of Royer's son just before his departure for the colonies, for which she was very grateful. It is not known who took the less well known portrait of her with elaborately coiffed hair and presented it to the Société d'Anthropologie probably the year of her admission, 1870. Unusually, she smiles and looks sideways at the camera, which gives her a more coquettish look. This has been published recently in Blanckaert, "Les Bas-Fonds de la Science Française," 115–130.
73. Letter of Royer to Ghénia Avril de Sainte-Croix, n.d.[1899?].
74. This journal, founded by Mortillet, was first published in 1866.
75. Agoult, *Dante et Goethe* (taken from articles written between 1864 and 1865 for the *Revue Germanique* and *Revue Moderne* (the continuation of the *Revue Germanique*).
76. Clémence Royer to Ghénia Avril de Sainte-Croix [1899?], BMD.
77. Ibid.
78. For a more objective view of this congress, see review of "Congès International des Sciences Sociales, Bern," *Journal des Économistes* 46 (1865).
79. Clémence Royer to Ghénia Avril de Sainte-Croix [1899?], BMD.
80. Ibid.
81. Duprat, *Encyclopédistes.*
82. Charles Darwin, *De l'origine des espèces par sélection naturelle, ou des lois de transformation des êtres organisés,* 2d French ed. (Paris: Guillaumin and Masson, 1866).
83. The subtitle changes in the French editions from "or the laws of progress of organized beings" to "by natural selection, or laws of transformation of organized beings."
84. Royer, "Avant-propos" to Darwin, *Origine des espèces,* 2d French ed., ix.
85. Pierre Flourens, *Examen du livre de M. Darwin,* (Paris, 1864). Darwin wrote a letter to Alfred R. Wallace about this book: "Le big gun Flourens has written a little dull book against me." Charles Darwin to A. R. Wallace, 16 September [1864]. Burkhardt et al., *Correspondence, of Charles Darwin* vol. 12 (forthcoming).
86. Royer, "Avant-propos" to Darwin, *Origine des espéces,* 2d French ed. Sara Joan Miles has spotted this comparison as one made by Darwin himself in defending natural selection in the third English edition. Miles, "Clémence Royer," 61–81.
87. Prosper Lucas, *Traité . . . de l'hérédité naturelle.*
88. This note has been identified by the author as being from Clémence Royer on the basis of handwriting and content. It will be published as a letter/memorandum from Clèmence Royer to Charles Darwin, written between March and late June 1865, in Burkhardt et al., *Correspondence,* vol. 13 (forthcoming). The memorandum extends a note to the first French edition (p. 57), referring to the Hindu caste rules, the Laws (or Institutes) of Manu. The French publication of this Hindu text was in 1833, the English in 1828. Loiseleur-Deslongchamps, *Manava-Dharma-Sastra.* Darwin seems to have preserved it, intending to use it in *Descent of Man*, but his notes about it (based on the translation by Emma Darwin) attribute the source to Prosper Lucas, *Traite . . . de l'hérédité,* who also refers to the Hindu text. The original is in the Darwin Archive, DAR 80.44. The transla-

tion (incomplete) by Emma Darwin is included, DAR 80.42–43. Darwin annotated only the translation, indicating that he did not find relevant information in the first two references.

89. Darwin's first mention of the second French edition is in a letter to John Murray of 31 March [1865], in which he comments that he has just heard that a new French edition was required. On 10 April 1865 he wrote to J. D. Hooker that he was working on the edition, but his illness postponed his work until June. Burkhardt et al., *Correspondence of Charles Darwin,* vol. 14 (forthcoming).
90. Emma Darwin to Henrietta Darwin [June 1865]. Charles Darwin Archives, DAR 219.
91. Royer, "Avant-propos" to Darwin, *Origine des espèces,* 2d French ed. Darwin thought the second edition would appear by the end of September, as he wrote to Alfred Russel Wallace on 22 September [1865], but the edition bears the date 1866. Burkhardt et al., *Correspondence of Charles Darwin,* vol. 13 (forthcoming).
92. Ibid.
93. Ibid.
94. Royer, (reprinted with modifications). "Préface à la première édition," in Darwin, *Origine des espèces,* 2d French ed.
95. Royer, "Avant-propos" to Darwin, *Origine des espèces,* 2d French ed.
96. Ibid.
97. Letter of Clémence Royer to [Paul Broca], n.d. (written before 22 December 1865); received 22 December 1865. Société d'Anthropologie de Paris Archives, F1–796.
98. Ibid.
99. Clémence Royer, "Avant-propos" to Darwin, *Origine des espéces,* 2d French ed., ii.
100. Paul Broca to Carl Vogt, 24 May 1867. Correspondence Carl Vogt, Bibliothèque Publique et Universitaire, MS 2188, no. 154.
101. Broca had his reasons for wanting open support of Darwinism to be muted in the society. See Harvey, "Races Specified, Evolution Transformed." See also Harvey, "Evolutionism Transformed: Positivists and Materialists before the Société d'Anthropologie de Paris."

Chapter 5 ***Motherhood, Social Theory, Social Realities***

1. See Lovett, *Giuseppe Ferrari,* 157–159.
2. Ibid.
3. Alexandre Dumas, *Voyage à Florence.*
4. Cobbe, *My Life,* vol. 2. She describes the other English intellectuals in some detail.
5. The Herzen family in Florence is beautifully described by Carr, *Romantic Exiles.*
6. See chapter 6.
7. Pancaldi, *Darwin in Italy.* Pancaldi, unfortunately, is weak on a discussion of the many non-Italian Darwinists located in Italy at that time, discussed in Landucci, *Darwinismo a Firenze,* who looks at Schiff, Herzen, and the Italian anthropologist Mantegazza among others. For a discussion of the scientific materialists in-

cluding Jacob Moleschott, see Frederick Gregory, *Scientific Materialism in Nineteenth-Century Germany* (Dordrecht/Boston: Reidel, 1979).

8. Pancaldi, *Darwin in Italy.*
9. Landucci, *Darwinismo,* discusses this group and Mantegazza in his study of Darwinists in Florence. Schiff wrote to Darwin about some of his experiments from Florence, 8 May 1876. Darwin Archive, DAR 86 (ser. 2): 8–9.
10. Paolo Mantagazza to Charles Darwin, 19 March 1868; 10 June 1871. Darwin Archive, DAR 171.
11. See Harvey, "*Races Specified.*" The families of Broca, Mantegazza, and Letourneau sometimes met in the summer by the sea in Spezia. Letourneau, who was a colleague of Royer on the scientific materialist journal *La Pensée Nouvelle* and later a strong supporter of her in the Société d'Anthropologie, worked with Mantegazza during his period of exile in Florence following the Paris Commune. Here Letourneau also developed a close tie to the Herzen family, as Edward Carr has detailed in *Romantic Exiles.*
12. Carlo Darwin, *Sull'origine delle specie per elezione naturale, ovvero conservazione delle razze perfezionate nella lotta per l'esistenza,* trans. Giovanni Canestrini and Leonardo Salimbeni (Modena: Zanichelli, 1864). See preface.
13. Pancaldi, *Darwin in Italy,* 79–80.
14. Cobbe, *Life,* vol. 2. For a more sympathetic look at the work of Schiff and Herzen and the controversy over vivisection, see Landucci, *Darwinismo a Firenze.*
15. Cobbe, *Life,* vol. 2.
16. Royer, *Origine de l'homme.*
17. See a long discussion of these groups in Judith Jeffrey Howard, "Patriot Mothers in the Post-Risorgimento: Women after the Italian Revolution," in *Women, War, and Revolution,* ed. Carol R. Berkin and Clara M. Lovett (New York: Holmes, 1980), 237–258.
18. Royer, "Sur la natalité" (see appendix for my translation).
19. Royer, *Origine de l'homme.* 236–237. She cites her earlier article, "La Tristesse dans l'art."
20. Royer, *Origine de l'homme.* She remarked that the nineteenth century had become "more delicate" in its expression of ideas about human origins.
21. This date, not listed in any biography, is based on the reported age of René in later letters and reports and a notation in a letter to Ghénia Avril de Sainte-Croix on 12 March [1900], to whom she regularly wrote about her later worries about her son, "Today is the birthday of my big son" (C'est l'anniversaire de le [*sic*] grand fils). Correspondence Clémence Royer, BMD.
22. Moufflet, "L'Oeuvre de Clémence Royer," 658–693.
23. Royer, "Sur la natalité." For the full text see Ducros and Blanckaert, "L'animal de la création." See appendix for my translation of this memoir.
24. Ibid.
25. Royer, *Théorie de l'impôt* (discussed in chapter 3).
26. Howard, "Patriot Mothers."
27. Royer, *Origine de l'homme,* 382.
28. Ibid. See the beginning of this discussion for her attack on Rousseau's idea of primitive promiscuity (369–385).

29. Ibid.
30. Ibid. Spencer discussed exclamation as the origin of language in his essay "Progress: Its Law and Cause," in *Essays,* vol. 1, but without reference to observations of young children.
31. Clémence Royer, "La Race blonde primitive," *Bulletin de la Société d'Anthropologie de Paris* (1874): 622–636.
32. Royer, *Origine de l'homme,* 64.
33. Royer, preface to *Origine de l'homme,* viii.
34. Naville, "Des variations," 1–22.
35. Ibid., 7–8.
36. Ibid.
37. Clémence Royer, "Á Monsieur le Rédacteur en chef de la Revue Chrétienne" (Florence, 17 February 1867), *Revue Chrétienne* 14 (1867): 246–247.
38. Ibid.
39. Ibid.
40. Ibid.
41. Naville, "Lettre à l'éditeur," 247. In Naville's published reply, he quite accurately noted that the greatest changes had been to pages xiii and xiv of Royer's preface, which discussed exactly these issues.
42. Ibid.
43. Clémence Royer to Ernest Naville, Florence, 17 March 1867. Naville Correspondence, Bibliothèque Publique et Universitaire, Geneva, MS fr 5425, no. 341–342.
44. Ibid.
45. Ibid. An unfair assessment by Royer.
46. Ibid.
47. Royer, "La Tristesse."
48. Royer, *Origine de l'homme,* 236.
49. Ibid., 547.
50. In her article "Amazones," written for *Encylopédie générale,* 2:39–41.
51. Darwin, *Descent of Man.* The second half of this book expands Darwin's ideas of sexual selection. For Royer's discussion of sexual selection in *Origine de l'homme,* see 386–388.
52. Royer, *Origine de l'homme,* 381.
53. Gilman, *Herland.*
54. Royer, *Origine de l'homme,* 379.
55. See, for example, Royer, "La Tristesse," which appeared in that journal.
56. Her name appears as a collaborator on the first page of this journal in 1868. It was first published as *Libre Pensée* in 1866.
57. For a discussion of this alliance, see Harvey, "Evolutionism Transformed."
58. Royer, "Lamarck," 3:173–205, 333–372; 4:5–30. Émile Littré was a famous linguist, dictionary writer, and commentator on Hippocrates and would soon become a member of the Institut de France and a republican senator. He was a renowned freethinker. The Russian-born crystallographer Wyrouboff would hold the first chair of history of science in France by the end of the century.
59. Royer, *Origine de l'homme,* 25.
60. Ibid., 25–26. The reference is to the physiologist Maurice Schiff, who published a series of physiological experiments on the energy of work based on animal experiments.

61. Royer, *Origine de l'homme,* 27.
62. Ibid., 28–29.
63. Ibid.
64. To what degree does this derive from the primitive forms of life described in Haeckel's *Generelle Morphologie* She cites, however, in these passages F. Pouchet, *Nouvelles expériences,* rather than Haeckel, although Haeckel appears in her bibliography. She doubted whether such monads could result in organized forms like infusoria, which then reproduce sexually.
65. Royer, *Origine de l'homme,* 30.
66. Ibid., 34–38.
67. Georges Pouchet, the son of Felix Pouchet, who upheld spontaneous generation, insisted on the link between polygenism and spontaneous generation in his important book *Pluralité des races humaines* (1858). The second edition (1864) attempted to bring Darwinian concepts into accord with his theories. He was an active member of the Société d'Anthropologie, of the first to be elected after its founding in 1859. For a further discussion of this, see Harvey, "Evolutionism transformed."
68. Royer, *Origine de l'homme,* 58. See for example, the opening statements of the scientific materialist Ludwig Büchner, *Kraft und Stoff (Force and Matter),* and a discussion of varieties of materialism in Lange, *History of Materialism.*
69. Royer, *Origine de l'homme,* 60–61. Some of this analysis of passion and thought may have been in direct response to Charles Letourneau's evolutionary psychology, *La Physiologie des Passions.* This section includes Royer's earlier quoted comment, "No passion, no action; no action, no thought" (54).
70. See chapter 9.
71. Royer, *Origine de l'homme,* 364–365.
72. Royer, preface to *Origine de l'homme,* v–xiii.
73. Royer, *Origine de l'homme,* 582–583.
74. Royer cites only Spencer's *Essays* (almost certainly *Essays: Scientific, Political, Speculative*), first published in two volumes in 1858 and 1863. She makes very little use of his other concepts here, except for a reference to the nebular hypothesis (the title of one of Spencer's essays) and an occasional reference to the move from homogeneity to heterogeneity, to which she does not give the same weight as Spencer does.
75. Royer, preface to *Origine de l'homme,* xii.
76. Ibid.
77. Royer, *Origine de l'homme,* 385.
78. Ibid., 580.
79. Ibid., 587.
80. Ibid.
81. It is curious that Royer did not introduce the references to the Hindu Laws of Manu that she had cited in her first Darwin edition, (57) which explain the laws structuring castes. She used these in her preface to demonstrate the selection of women with particular characteristics. Possibly, since Darwin had retained them for future use, she had lost the references.
82. Royer, *Origine de l'homme,* 574. See also 576–577.
83. Ibid., 576.

84. Ibid., 531.
85. Ibid., 532.
86. Georges Clemenceau to Jules Ferry, as quoted in Duroselle, *Clemenceau,* 223.
87. Royer, *Origine de l'homme,* 540.
88. Ibid., 99–101. In 1868, Haeckel had published an evolutionary tree in which human national groups and races were shown branching like subspecies, with the Papuan and Bushman at the bottom and the German at the top. Ernst Haeckel, *Natürliche Schöpfungsgeschichte,* 1868. (Human evolutionary trees are included at the back of this book.)
89. Ibid., 142.
90. Royer, *Origine de l'homme.*
91. Ibid., 587. These are the last words of her book.
92. Pascal Duprat, dedication, "Á la Jeunesse française," in *L'Esprit des révolutions.*
93. Ibid.
94. Duprat, "La Révolution," 41–56. Written as letter to Joseph Garnier, "Mon cher Garnier," Madrid, 30 December 1868.
95. Ibid. Duprat starts his letter, "I am watching this revolution that has astonished all of Europe from close up." He signs "with friendship and devotion."
96. Nigoul, *Pascal Duprat.*
97. Royer, *Origine de l'homme,* 547.
98. Ibid., 515–516.
99. Royer, "Lamarck, sa vie, ses travaux et son système." *La Philosophie Positive* 3:173–205, 333–372; 4:5–30.
100. Royer, preface to the third edition of the French translation of Darwin, *Origine des espèces.*
101. J. D. Hooker to Charles Darwin, 3 March 1868. Darwin Archive, DAR 102:204–207.
102. A lengthy discussion of Federico Delpino can be found in Pancaldi, *Darwin in Italy,* 79–80.
103. Royer, preface to the third edition of Darwin, *Origine des espèces,* xviii.
104. Ibid. Royer refers to the English physicist Michael Faraday, the French chemist Adolphe Wurtz, and the German physicist Julius Robert Mayer, whose investigations on conservation of force (or energy) had been discussed by Hermann von Helmholtz.
105. Ibid.
106. Pancaldi, *Darwin in Italy,* 115–116.
107. Royer, preface to to third edition of *Origine des espèces.* She published this some eight years later as "Deux hypothèses," 443–484, 660–685.
108. See letter from V. O. Kovalevsky to Charles Darwin, 13 September 1869. Emma's diary and a letter from Darwin to T. H. Huxley of 1 October [1869] establish Kovalevsky's presence at Down in late September. Although there is no proof that this was Darwin's source for the new Royer edition, Darwin's hostile reaction followed immediately after this visit.
109. See Armand de Quatrefages, *Les Précurseurs de Darwin,* published as a series of articles in the *Revue des Deux Mondes* throughout 1868 and 1869. See chapter 6,

footnote 23, for a citation to the specific article in this series that discussed Royer on spontaneous generation (abiogenesis).

110. Victor Masson *fils* to Charles Darwin, 29 September 1869 under the letterhead "V. Masson et fils, Paris, Place de l'École de Médecine." Darwin Archive, DAR 96.
111. Charles Darwin to J. J. Moulinié, 23 October [1869]. Bibliothèque Publique et Universitaire, Geneva. See also a letter to Charles Darwin from J. J. Moulinié of 5 November 1869 from Geneva, in which Moulinié says Reinwald will be pleased to publish *Descent of Man,* as well as a Moulinié translation of the latest English edition of the *Origin.* Darwin Archive, DAR 171.
112. John Murray to Charles Darwin, 17 November 1869. Darwin Archive, DAR 171:6.
113. Charles Darwin to J. D. Hooker, 19 November 1869, Darwin Archive, DAR 94:159–161. By November 20, Darwin had already sent the corrections of Moulinié's translation of the first part of *Origin.*
114. J. D. Hooker to Charles Darwin, 21 November 1869, Darwin Archive, DAR 103:39–41.
115. See Paul Broca's praise of Royer's use of the French language (including her earlier term "élection naturelle") and criticism of Moulinié's awkward translations of *Descent of Man* in his article "Les sélections," 691.
116. Charles Darwin to J. J. Moulinié, 15 November [1869]. Bibliothèque Publique et Universitaire, Geneva.
117. Charles Reinwald to Charles Darwin, 4 March 1873. Darwin Archive, DAR 176.
118. Darwin cited Royer in *Descent of Man.* In his copy of her book, he made a number of comments on her text. For example, next to her discussion of language as an outgrowth of social behavior, Darwin wrote, "No. Rabbit silent but social." He seems to have misunderstood her discussion of men and women, commenting on her remark upon the greater physical strength of men over women, "No, men stronger." Darwin Archive, Charles Darwin Library. For a transcription of this and other Darwin notes, see di Gregorio and Gill, *Charles Darwin's Marginalia,* vol. 1.
119. See list in Darwin's handwriting headed "Moral and Social Evolution." Darwin Archive, DAR 80.
120. This date of 1870 appears on a number of copies of the book, including my own and that in the Bibliothèque Nationale, although the copy in the Société d'Anthropologie de Paris library bears the earlier date that Royer claimed in her autobiography. The volume was reviewed at the end of 1869 by at least one reviewer.
121. Royer, *Autobiography.* Certainly it was Juliette Adam's impression that Royer was primarily a translator. See Adam, *Mes premières armes,* 257. "Mademoiselle [*sic*] Clémence Royer was an admirable translator. She had besides this talent more capacity for demolition than creation, just like her rival Proudhon."
122. See Royer's mention of this arrangement about the rental of apartments in her letter to Ghénia Avril de Sainte-Croix [1899?], BMD.
123. Royer, *Origine de l'homme,* 547.

Chapter 6 *"A Little Scientific Church"*

1. Royer, *Origine de l'homme,* 73. My own copy and the copy in the Bibliothèque Nationale bear the 1870 date, but a copy in the Société d'Anthropologie holdings is dated 1869.
2. Clémence Royer, "Moyens d'améliorer le sort des classes ouvrières," *Journal des Economistes,* 3d ser., 13 (1869): 404–429. In this same article she ends with a rejection of state aid for workers, but voices her strong belief in free education for all children: "Nothing from the state for the adult but everything for the child" (429).
3. Clémence Royer to Ernest Havet, 19 July 1881. Correspondence Ernst Havet, Bibliothèque Nationale.
4. Nigoul, *Pascal Duprat,* 122–126.
5. A. Milice in his biography *Clémence Royer,* 74, gives the title of the newspaper as *Le Citoyen,* but as Geneviève Fraisse points out in her bibliography, that was its subtitle.
6. Royer's unfinished novel appeared from 4 March to 24 April 1870. She apparently then offered it to the popular liberal newspaper *Le Temps,* which refused it. Fraisse, *Clémence Royer,* 53.
7. Royer, *Origine de l'homme,* 192. For a delightful recent account of the early days of the Paris crèches, see Ann La Berge's recent article "Medicalization," 65–87.
8. Mme le Docteur (Madeleine) Brès, speech given at the Clémence Royer banquet, 10 March 1897 (MSS). Dossier Clémence Royer, BMD.
9. Harvey, "Evolutionism Transformed."
10. Charles Letourneau, "Banquet Tribute," unpublished speech given at the Clémence Royer banquet of 1897. Dossier Clémence Royer, BMD.
11. Marks, "Attitudes of French Physicians."
12. "I love little churches, which are small and free, I hate large churches. . . . Royer's speech given at the Clémence Royer banquet, 10 March 1897. Dossier Clémence Royer, BMD.
13. See Harvey, "Races Specified," chapter 3, in which I detail the early discussion of Darwinism by Broca, Bertillon, Dareste, and Dally before 1868. Dareste had been in communication with Darwin, and Quatrefages even quoted a letter from Darwin to him in a debate about environmental influence on the formation of domestic varieties in 1863. *Bulletin de la Société d'Anthropologie de Paris* 4 (1863): 378–379.
14. Huxley, *La Place de l'homme*, criticized by Letourneau, "Variabilité," 99–121.
15. Gaudry, *Animaux fossiles.* In spite of his disclaimers, Gaudry had written to Darwin that his writings had been a source of inspiration to him. Albert Gaudry to Charles Darwin, 11 January 1868, Darwin Archive, DAR 165.
16. Letourneau, "Variabilité," 99–121.
17. Dally, "Primates," 673–712.
18. Dally, "Introduction" to Huxley, *La Place de l'homme,* 1–95. This introduction is almost as long as the book he translated.
19. Ibid., 80.
20. Conry, *Introduction du Darwinisme.* Conry discusses Dally's interpretations in this manner, and later those of Albert Giard among others.

21. Armand de Quatrefages in a discussion of Carl Vogt, *Les Émules de Darwin* (Paris, 1894).
22. For an analysis of these debates see Harvey, "Evolutionism Transformed," 289–310. For a more extensive discussion of this, see chapter 3 of Harvey, "Races Specified."
23. Quatrefages, *Darwin et ses précurseurs français.* This had appeared in 1868 and 1869 as a series of articles in the popular literary and philosophical journal *Revue des Deux Mondes* under the general title "L'Origine des espèces, animales et végétales." Part 1, "Les Précurseurs de Darwin," 78 (1868): 832–860; part 2, "Théorie de Darwin," 79 (1869): 208–240; part 3, "Discussion des théories transformistes," 80 (1869): 64–95. This includes a discussion of Dally's introduction to Huxley and Royer's divergence from Darwin on abiogenesis (spontaneous generation); part 4, "Darwin et les théories transformistes: L'Espèce et la race," 80 (1869): 495–532 (Broca's theory of hybridity was discussed here); part 5, "Théories de la transformation progressive et de la transformation brusque: L'Origine simienne de l'homme," 80 (1869): 638–672.
24. Royer, "Transformisme," 275.
25. Ibid., 273.
26. Ibid., 285–286.
27. Ibid., 273–279; quotation on p. 279.
28. Quatrefages, "Transformisme," 312–317.
29. Royer, "Transformisme," 284–285.
30. Ibid., 293–294. Here Royer argues against the scientific tendency to divide the world into male and female polar opposites. See chapter 7.
31. Ibid., 294.
32. Ibid., 297.
33. Ibid., 301.
34. Mortillet, "Transformisme," 360.
35. Bertillon, "Transformisme," BSAP, 488–528.
36. Royer, "Transformisme," 309.
37. See Royer,"Lois mathématiques," 725–737. This article includes a number of diagrams.
38. Royer, "Transformisme," 311–312.
39. Quatrefages "Transformisme," 314.
40. Broca, "Sur le transformisme," 168–239. It is worth noting that Bertillon, Dally, and Broca all used the term "séléction naturelle" in 1863 before Clémence Royer produced her second edition in which she, too, conformed to the use of "séléction" rather than "éléction."
41. Bertillon, "Transformisme," 488–528.
42. Darwin's discussion of Broca's emphasis on the power of the environment on organisms and his own doubts about the exclusivity of natural selection as an agent can be found in Darwin, *Descent of Man,* 68–69, as well as in later editions of *Origin of Species.*
43. Hector George, "Un dernier mot sur Darwinisme," Bulletin de la Société d'Anthropologie de Paris, 2d ser., 5 (1870): 622–627 (see 626). Yvette Conry has echoed this comment in her book *L'Introduction du Darwinisme.*
44. Ibid., 626.

45. Ibid., 627.
46. For a life of Letourneau see the biographical memoir that prefaces his last book, Papillault, "Notice biographique." For a discussion of his link to Alexander Herzen, see Carr, *Romantic Exiles.*
47. Letters of Paul Broca to Ernest Hamy (1870–1871), Correspondence to Ernest Hamy, Musée d'Histoire Naturelle Archives.
48. Letter from Clémence Royer to members of the Défense Nationale (after 4 September 1870). Dossier Clémence Royer, Préfecture de Police. This letter was found among the papers of Charles Delescluze, who was first a member of the National Defense and then killed on the last barricades as a leader of the Paris Commune in 1871. It appears to have been placed in Royer's dossier on 12 September 1872, since a note accompanying it gives that date.
49. This comment may have been meant as an attack against Henri de Rochefort, whose role as an agitator has never been satisfactorily explained. It may also reflect Duprat's suspicion of demagogues.
50. Edmond Lepelletier in *L'Echo de Paris* (1885), quoted by Nigoul, *Pascal Duprat,* 248.
51. Fraisse mentions the visits of Lafargue to Royer. Marx was apparently rather relieved that she did not wish to translate his book, since he thought her "bourgeoise," as demonstrated in her Darwin preface.
52. For an interesting discussion of the view of Gambetta as a potential dictator during this period, see J.P.T. Bury, *Gambetta and the National Defense: A Republican Dictatorship in France* (London: Longmans Green, 1936).
53. Clémence Royer to Ernest Havet, 19 July 1881. Correspondence Ernest Havet, Bibliothèque Nationale, n.a.fr. 24478, fols. 183–187.
54. Duprat, *L'Esprit des révolutions,* 1st ed., 20.
55. Ibid., 69.
56. See chapter 8 for a further discussion of this antagonism and its effects.
57. Edmond Lepelletier in *L'Echo de Paris* (1885), quoted by Nigoul, *Pascal Duprat,* 57–59.
58. After Thiers resigned from the government, he still contacted Duprat to conduct this kind of survey according to police reports in the Dossier Pascal Duprat Préfecture de Police.
59. See the series of reports signed "Jack" from 4 June 1872 to 8 July 1874 on Royer's contributions to the Russian newspaper *Goloss,* signed K. R. in the cyrillic alphabet. Dossier Clémence Royer, Préfecture de Police.
60. Émile Calmette, Duhosset, Marquis d'Hervey-Saint-Denys, Charles de Labrathe, Léon de Rosny, and Clémence Royer, "Instructions ethnographiques. Projet de questionnaire concernant les caractères ethniques particuliers du système reproducteur chez les diverses races humaines et leur différence ou variations particulières." *Actes de la Société d'Ethnographie Américaine et Orientale* 2d ser., 3 (1873): 13–26. Royer was apparently the reporter on this project.
61. Maurel, "Gustave Flourens," *Bulletin de la Société d'Ethnographie* 3 (1873): 26–31. This includes a description of his publications in ethnography.
62. A drawing depicting the square des Batignolles from 1867 is in Hillairet, *Dictionnaire: Histoire des rues de Paris.* 1:319. This shows the railroad running along the far end of the square. In this drawing the outline and the layout of the square are the same as they are today without the gates that currently surround it.

63. François Lenoir to Clémence Royer, [September] 1872. Correspondence of François Lenoir, Bibliothèque Nationale, n.a.fr. 21481, no. 152–153.
64. Clémence Royer to François Lenoir, 21 September 1872, Correspondence of François Lenoir, Bibliothèque Nationale, nos. 158–160.
65. François Lenoir to Clémence Royer, 7 January 1874. Correspondence of François Lenoir, Bibliothèque Nationale, 191. He ends with thanks to M. Duprat for his kind remembrances and reminds her that they are coming to visit her next Saturday.
66. Royer reprinted both her letters to the Académie des Sciences Morales et Politiques and the reply to her as a pamphlet. See Royer, "Lettre."
67. Royer, "Lettre à M. le Président, 1. Although no letter from Darwin to Royer has survived, this is a totally believable statement. Darwin was in the habit of assuring his supporters that they alone had plumbed the depths of his thought. He was capable of telling both Asa Gray (a very religious teleologist) and Ernst Haeckel (a materialist) that they understood him best. Royer had no direct knowledge of Darwin's great discomfort with her long notes and his rage at her preface to the third edition of *Origine des espèces.*
68. Ibid., 3.
69. Moufflet, "L'oeuvre," 658–693.
70. Louis Lartet to Ernest Hamy, February 1874, correspondence Ernest Hamy. Muséum d'Histoire Nationale, Bibliothèque. MS 2254, nos. 230–231.
71. Ibid., February 1875, Correspondence Ernest Hamy, 246–248.
72. One should recall that the first woman member of any branch of the Institut de France was the writer Marguerite Yourcenar in 1981.
73. Report of a lecture by Royer at the boulevard des Capuchines in December[?] 1874. Dossier Clémence Royer, Préfecture de Police Archives. Harry Paul has given the most detailed account of this reaction by French scientists in *The Sorcerer's Apprentice: The French Scientists' Image of German Science, 1840–1919.* (Gainsville: University of Florida Press, 1972).
74. Ibid., "un panier vide." For further discussion of the importance of science to the Third Republic, see Georges Weill, *L'Histoire de l'idée laïque au XIX*e siècle (Paris: Alcan, 1925), and J.P.T. Bury, *Gambetta and the Making of the Third Republic* (London: Longman, 1973).

CHAPTER 7 ***"Woman Is Not Made Like This"***

1. Clémence Royer, "Sur la condition des femmes dans l'antiquité," *Bulletin de la Société d'Anthropologie de Paris* 7th ser., 2 (1872): 638–641.
2. Royer, *Origine de l'homme,* 23.
3. Royer, "Transformisme," 291.
4. Ibid., 292.
5. Charles Letourneau was also a notable exception, but he was in exile in Italy and became a faculty member of the school only upon his return at the end of the 1870s.
6. Clémence Royer to Armand de Quatrefages, April 1891. Correspondence of Armand de Quatrefages, Muséum d'Histoire Naturelle, MS 2258. Yvette Conry quotes only part of this letter in the appendix to her book *l'Introduction du Darwinisme en France,* 437.

7. L.-A. Bertillon, "La Population française," in *Association Française pour l'Avancement de la Science,* 2d Conference (Lyon, 1873), 45–66.
8. Broca, "Sur le transformisme," 187. These are Broca's italics. Broca went on to discuss in detail the various translations of "struggle for existence" (*combat pour la vie; lutte pour la vie*) and Clémence Royer's more satisfactory term *concurrence vitale,* partly derived from the use of the term *concurrence* (competition) in economics.
9. Broca, "Sélections," 691.
10. Bertillon, "La Population française," 45–66.
11. Royer, "Sur la natalité," 135. This is a suppressed communication in the archives of the society intended for the *Bulletin de la Société d'Anthropologie de Paris,* 2d ser., 9 (1874). Archives of the Société d'Anthropologie, B1, 1891. This paper exists in corrected galleys and in page proofs, indicating that it would have run on pages 598 to 613 if it had been published. First located in the archives by Claude Blanckaert and Joy Harvey in 1979, the text has been recently published in French in the new series of the *Bulletin et Mémoires de la Société d'Anthropologie de Paris* by Albert Ducros and Claude Blanckaert, who also put it into context within the Société d'Anthropologie. Ducros and Blanckaert, "L'Animal de la création," 131–144. They have included Royer's letter to Paul Broca objecting to the suppression (143–144). (Page numbers refer to the text published by Ducros and Blanckaert.) The full text is given in my translation in the appendix.
12. Royer, "Sur la natalité," 135.
13. Ibid.
14. Ibid.
15. Ibid.
16. Ibid., 136.
17. Ibid.
18. Ibid.
19. Ibid.
20. Ibid.
21. This appears to be a reference to William Hepworth Dixon, *New America.* (1867). But although there is a discussion of the new immigrants, he does not discuss abortion or even the lowered birth rate. Royer may have confused this with a book by the New York surgeon Edward Henry Dixon, who discussed various common methods of causing miscarriages (which he condemmed) in his book on women's diseases. Dixon, *Woman and her Diseases,* with an appendix on the propriety of limiting the increase in family.
22. Royer, "Sur la natalité," 137. The woman may have been her old friend Jenny d'Héricourt, who studied medicine in Chicago during the late 1860s. See Karen Offen, "French Feminist Rediscovered."
23. Ibid. Royer says "from the moment the flower is set," by which she seems to mean from the first stopping of menstruation.
24. Ibid., 137.
25. Ibid.
26. Ibid., 138.

27. Ibid.
28. Ibid.
29. Ibid.
30. Ibid.
31. Ibid.
32. Ibid., 139.
33. Ibid.
34. Ibid.
35. Ibid.
36. Ibid., 140.
37. Ibid.
38. Ibid.
39. Ibid.
40. Ibid.
41. Ibid.
42. Ibid.
43. Ibid.
44. Ibid., 140–141.
45. Ibid., 141.
46. Ibid.
47. Ibid.
48. Ibid.
49. Ibid.
50. Ibid.
51. Ibid.
52. Ibid.
53. Ibid., 142.
54. Ibid.
55. Ibid.
56. Ibid.
57. Ibid.
58. Ibid.
59. Naville's comments are discussed in chapter 5. Broca wrote his comments in a review of various forms of selection, "Les sélections," 691.
60. Royer, "Sur la natalité," 142.
61. Ibid.
62. Ibid.
63. Clémence Royer to Paul Broca, 3 May 1875. Correspondence files, Société d'Anthropologie de Paris Archives. Also see Ducros and Blanckaert, "L'Animal de la création," 143–144.
64. Quoted in Bidelman, *Pariahs Stand Up!* He describes the suppression of feminist journals.
65. Royer, *Origine de l'homme.* See chapter 4.
66. Royer, "Introduction à la philosophie."
67. Broca, "Sélections."
68. For this crucial moment in the society, see Harvey, "Evolutionism Transformed."

69. Clémence Royer to Paul Broca, 3 May 1875. Correspondence files, Société d'Anthropologie de Paris Archives. Also see Ducros and Blanckaert, "L'Animal de la création," 143–144.
70. Ibid., 143.
71. Ibid., 144.
72. The note on the society's letterhead is dated first May and then July 1875. See Ducros and Blanckaert, "L'animal de la création," and Harvey, "Strangers,"
73. See, for example, her discussion "Sur la fécondité relative des différentes classes de société," Bulletin de la Société d'Anthropologie de Paris, 2d ser., 9 (1874): 585–591.
74. Royer, "Deux hypothèses," 443–484, 660–685.
75. Ibid., 467.
76. Ibid., 476.
77. Ibid.
78. Ibid.
79. Ibid., 482. Royer might have appreciated the stimulation of frog eggs with sea water to produce haploid individuals, as done in the 1930s.
80. She devotes the last section of the article, "Contingence de la sexualité," to the contingent evolution of sexuality. Royer, "Deux hypothèses," 660–685.
81. Ibid., 662.
82. Ibid., 665.
83. Ibid., 668.
84. Ibid., 670.
85. Ibid.
86. Ibid.
87. Royer, *Origine de l'homme,* 582. For a discussion of this, see chapter 5.
88. This, like many reports in the police files, reads like nasty local gossip motivated by personal and political dislike. For example, the same report details as recent news that Duprat left his legitimate wife and "children" to live with a concubine [*sic*] and gives an incorrect previous address (5, not 3, rue de Brochant). It may be worth noting that a future political enemy, Lockroy, lived around the corner from their address at the rue de Brochant, on rue Truffaut.
89. Clémence Royer to Céline (Renooz) Muro, 28 March 1877. Correspondence Céline Renooz, Fonds Bouglé, Bibliothèque Historique de la Ville de Paris (listed as no. 74, 1877). This will be discussed at greater length in chapter 8.
90. Clémence Royer, "Les Rites funéraires aux époques préhistoriques et leur origine, *Revue d'Anthropologie* 5 (1876): 437–478.
91. Royer's mother, however, also had retained her own apartment close to the rue de Brochant, according to the information provided to the Préfecture de Police on the occasion of Royer's application for a *bureau de tabac* license.
92. Royer, "Rites funéraires," 452.
93. Ibid., 442.
94. bid., 442–443.
95. Clémence Royer to Céline (Renooz) Muro, 28 March 1877, Bibliothèque Historique de la Ville de Paris (listed as no. 74, 1877). This is one of three letters to Céline Renooz around this time. The first is dated 19 February 1877, the last has no date.

96. Report of the Préfecture de Police, Dossier Clémence Royer, April 1877. She was forbidden to speak at Céline (Renooz) Muro's conference. See also report dated 8 March 1877 (stamped 12 March) on the letterhead of the Ministère de l'Intérieur, Direction Générale de la Surété Générale, signed by the director. Her address is given as 105, rue de Rome, and her talk as "Les Moeurs et la loi morale." Dossier Clémence Royer, Préfecture de Police.
97. Clémence Royer to Céline (Renooz) Muro, 28 March 1877. Bibliothèque Historique de la Ville de Paris.
98. *Congrès International des Droits des Femmes: Compte rendu des séances plenières,* (Paris: Auguste Chio, 1878). This was organized by Maria Deraismes and Léon Richer. See Bidelman, *Pariahs Stand Up!*
99. Dumas *fils, L'homme-femme.* Maria Deraismes had written a scathing reply to this in *Ève contre M. Dumas.*
100. Le Bon, "Recherches anatomiques," 27–104. Stephen Jay Gould has discussed the arguments about brain volume in *Mismeasure of Man.* See my own discussion in Harvey, "Races Specified," 288–292.
101. Central Committee, Procès verbaux, Archives of the Société d'Anthropologie, vol. 2, meeting record for 27 March 1879. Paul Broca had long believed that education had a direct effect on the brain, increasing its size as well as its knowledge, as he stated first in "Les Sélections."
102. Manouvrier, "Anthropologie des sexes, 41–61. If this claim was true, she hesitated to put it to the test and have her brain preserved for posterity. She studied briefly in Broca's Laboratoire d'Anthropologie under Manouvrier's instruction, something that may have given her a distaste for the process of brain dissection and cranial measurement, although she did propose some improvements in cranial measurement to the society.

Chapter 8 ***Years of Trial***

1. The address is given in the dossier of both Royer and Duprat at the Préfecture de Police, as well as in letters written by Royer in 1881 and 1882.
2. Duprat, *Esprit,* 2d ed. It is possible to detect in his chapter "Types et portraits" satirical portraits of Gambetta, Littré, Hugo, de Rochefort, Lamennais, Lamartine, Thiers, and possibly even Marx's son-in-law, Paul Lafargue. Some of these are flattering (in the case of Lamartine, Hugo, and Thiers). The others hit a little too close to the skin. A possible description of Marx's son-in-law, Paul Lafargue (or of Marx himself) describes a vehement socialist addicted to the German philosophy of "thesis, antithesis, and synthesis," who speaks on behalf of violent social revolution but who then goes home and dines with his delightful family and plays with his children.
3. Bury, *Gambetta's Final Years,* 234. Bury is one of the few historians of this period who regularly cites the important role of Duprat in the systematic opposition to Gambetta.
4. All this is detailed in his dossier at the Préfecture de Police.
5. The Dossier Pascal Duprat at the Préfecture de Police includes further details of this attack.

6. As reported in the newspaper *L'Intransigeant* (1881) and extracted in Dossier Pascal Duprat, Préfecture de Police.
7. The report of the police informant "Grégoire," 8 February 1880, included his own statements at a meeting in support of Henri Maret in which he suggested that it was time to give Duprat "his walking papers."
8. One complication was Duprat's severe illness, which necessitated that he leave Paris and live with his brother's family in Landes during part of this period according to Nigoul. Nigoul also claimed that the change of the election date from October to July meant that Duprat had no chance to prepare his campaign properly. Nigoul, *Pascal Duprat.* The reports at the Préfecture de Police, however, show him meeting most of his speaking engagements, although he cancelled some in March and April, 1880.
9. The description of Duprat during this period by Toussaint Nigoul makes no direct mention of Royer or René.
10. *Petit Caporal,* 14 November 1882, copied into Dossier Pascal Duprat, Préfecture de Police.
11. Clémence Royer to Ernest Havet, 19 July 1881, Bibliothèque Nationale, no. 183.
12. "Prima vivere par philosophia," Clémence Royer to Ernest Havet, 27 July 1881, Bibliothèque Nationale, no. 185.
13. Ibid.
14. This letter could not be found in the Darwin Archive.
15. Charles Darwin, *De l'origine des espèces par sélection naturelle, ou des lois de transformations des êtres organisés,* traduction de Mme Clémence Royer avec préface et notes du traducteur 4th ed., revue d'après l'édition stéréotypée anglaise, avec les additions de l'auteur (Paris: C. Marpon and E. Flammarion, 1882). Royer mentions a fifth edition possibly in 1892, published, according to Clémence Royer, with the agreement of Darwin's astronomer son, George Darwin. This continued to be printed, with no additional changes, well into the twentieth century by Ernest Flammarion, except for the removal of the "Avertissement aux lecteurs de la 4e édition." Royer's original preface to the first edition was retained, with the language modifications and corrections made in her second edition.
16. See appendix 1 and 2 of Darwin, *Origine des espèces,* 4th ed.
17. Ibid. "Notice to Readers of the Fourth Edition" (Avertissement aux lecteurs de la 4e édition). As an example, she adds that in response to one anti-Darwinian piece "in a widely read journal" she was able to point out to the author "seven errors of fact" made in an article only two columns long.
18. Royer, "De la nature du beau."
19. Clémence Royer to Ernest Havet, 19 July 1881, no. 183.
20. Ibid.
21. Royer, preface to *Le Bien et la loi morale.*
22. Ibid.
23. Royer, preface to Darwin, *Origine des espèces,* 1st ed., lxii.
24. Royer, preface to *Le Bien et la loi morale.*
25. Royer, "Congrès International," 227–228.
26. Ibid., 230.
27. Ibid., 231. As a reporter, she apologized for the lengthy discussion of her own

ideas but added that "the gravity of the subject" required it and that she was only repeating what she had said in the meeting.

28. Ibid. For the context of this discussion of a morality based on science, see Clark, *Social Darwinism in France,* who relates these attempts as a response to murder cases in which young perpetrators quoted Darwin's "law of struggle" as justification.
29. Royer, preface to *Le Bien et la loi morale.*
30. Ibid., viii.
31. Ibid.
32. Ibid., xxxiii.
33. Ibid., xiii.
34. She cites her first preface to Darwin, *Origine des espèces* (1862), lxii.
35. Royer, preface to *Le Bien et la loi morale,* xxi.
36. Ibid., xxiv.
37. Royer, *Le Bien et la loi morale,* 58–59.
38. Ibid.
39. Royer, preface to *Le Bien et la loi morale,* xxviii.
40. Royer, *Le Bien et la loi morale,* 106–107.
41. Ibid.
42. Her discussion within the body of the text lists sensory responses: to light, sound, and so forth, by nerves in which "nervous activity places a central and positive role." *Le Bien et la loi morale,* 130–135.
43. Ibid., 275.
44. Ibid., 302.
45. "Clemence Royer," *Les Hommes d'aujourd'hui* 4, no. 170 (1881). This included a short biographical piece and a list of her publications to date. Among those caricatured over the next ten years were Gambetta, Paul Bert, Jules Ferry, Maria Deraismes, Sarah Bernhardt, Juliette Adam, and Jean Charcot, as well as some of her colleagues from the Société d'Anthropologie: Henri Thulié, Abel Hovelacque, and Mathias Duval.
46. Clémence Royer to Ernest Havet, Bibliothèque Nationalle,n.a.fr. 224478, n.a.fr. 224478, See fig. 7. 27 July 1881. Havet Correspondence, no. 27 July 1881. 185.
47. Ibid., 19 July 1881, no. 183.
48. Ibid.
49. Ibid.
50. bid.
51. Janet, "Rapport sur le concours relatif à la doctrine de l'évolution" (Report on the competition relating to the doctrine of evolution), read at the meeting of September 1, 1883. 489–497. Note the long time lag between the award and the published report (1888).
52. Paul Janet, called a "spiritualist" by Conry, was a professor of the history of philosophy at the Sorbonne. He had such strong anti-Darwinist and religious convictions that he had objected to the teleological and materialist implications of natural selection in 1863. In 1869 he had also criticized Quatrefages's antievolutionist, but even handed, discussion of Darwinism in the *Revue des Deux Mondes,* 1868–1869.
53. Janet, "Doctrine de l'évolution," 489.

54. Ibid., 491.
55. Ibid., 493.
56. Ibid., 495.
57. Ibid.
58. Ibid., 497.
59. Ibid.
60. According to the report of 21 April 1882 on the meeting of 20 April 1882. Dossier Clémence Royer, Préfecture de Police.
61. An announcement of the Société d'Études Philosophiques et Morales exists for 1882, in which Royer is listed as offering a series of lectures on (1) "Unity of Substance of World Force, Matter, Mind," 17 May; (2) Theory of Cohesion and Affinity through Repulsion, 28 May; (3) Theory of Gravitation through Repulsion, 4 June; (4) Theory of Calorific Vibration, 18 May; (5) Theory of Luminous Vibration, 2 July; (6) Theory of Electricity and Magnetism, 16 July. A copy of this is in Correspondence François Lenoir, Bibliothèque Nationale, no. 215, but by mistake someone has incorrectly inserted it in the Boban Correspondence. See also Lenoir, no. 226, "Statutes Société d'Études Philosophiques et Morales," which list Royer as secretary-general and M. Mesnil as treasurer.
62. Royer, *Constitution du monde.*
63. Report on the meeting of 20 April 1882. At almost the same time as this meeting, Duprat had been too ill to give a lecture on the origins of revolution (a topic on which he was regularly speaking throughout the arrondissement and the provinces). Dossier Pascal Duprat, Préfecture de Police.
64. Report of 6 May 1882 on Clémence Royer as secretary-general of the Société d'Études Philosophiques et Morales. Dossier Clémence Royer, Préfecture de Police.
65. "Direction de la Presse," 21 April 1882, sent information that Royer "declared to the préfet de la Seine on 22 September [1881] that she intended to publish a weekly journal entitled *Le Progrès Moral,* a journal for reforms of legislative laws, social economics, politics, literature, and arts." The notice adds that the journal will be printed by M. Hennuyer, rue Farcet, Paris. Dossier Clémence Royer, Préfecture de Police.
66. Clémence Royer to Victor Considérant, 8 May [1882], Archives Nationales, Archives Sociétaires, Correspondence Victor Considérant, 10 AS 41.
67. Clémence Royer to Victor Considérant, 12 May [1882], and after, Archives Nationales 10 AS 41. (1) after 12 May 1882 (8 pp.), (2) 12 May [1882] (8 pp.), (3) 8 May [1882] (6 pp.). These letters carry the address of 82, avenue des Ternes. An undated card from "Madame Clemence Royer" is included, asking that her work (not specified) be sent to Considérant.
68. Clémence Royer to Victor Considérant, 12 May [1882], Archives Nationales.
69. Ibid.
70. Ibid. She refers to Haeckel, *Essais.*
71. Clémence Royer to Victor Considérant, 12 May [1882], Archives Nationales.
72. Ibid.
73. Ibid.
74. Clémence Royer to Victor Considérant (after 12 May 1882). This letter, undated, appears from the content to have followed the letter dated 12 May [1882]. Fraisse

reads Royer's difficult handwriting somewhat differently here, interpreting the phrase as "as 'massif' as Chevreul," but given that Chevreul lived well past the age of one hundred, "ancien" seems the appropriate term.

75. Ibid.
76. Clémence Royer, "Attraction et gravitation," 206–226. The editors at the time were Charles Robin, the histologist, and G. Wyrouboff, the Russian-born crystallographer and historian of science. Littré had died in 1875. There appears to be a copy of this article with manuscript notes among the Ernest Renan collection of books in the Bibliothèque Nationale, but I have not had the opportunity to consult these notes. See Bibliothèque Nationale, Ernest Renan, 8641.
77. See a list of these talks in Correspondence François Lenoir.
78. Milice quotes in his biography from a 1885 article by Royer published in this *Bulletin,* but no copies appear to have survived in the Marguerite Durand library.
79. Royer, *Autobiography.*
80. This suprisingly favorable report was dated 17 September 1883 and printed in *Mot d'Ordre,* Rochefort's journal, which commonly attacked him. It is included as an excerpt in the Dossier Pascal Duprat, Préfecture de Police.
81. Nigoul, *Pascal Duprat,* 245.
82. Ibid. Nigoul uses the phrase "sa gouvernante," which can be read as "housekeeper" or "mistress."
83. Clémence Royer, "L'abolition de l'esclavage au Brésil," *Journal des Économistes,* 4th ser., 43 (1888): 17–33; and "La République argentine et ses progrès récents," *Journal des Économistes,* 4th ser., 46 (1889): 59–75.
84. Some controversy followed in the press over the failure to embalm him, but the ship was not a military vessel and had no facilities for embalming. See Nigoul, *Pascal Duprat,* 247.
85. Ibid., 249.
86. See lengthy reports on the death and funeral of Admiral Courbet in *L'Illustration,* 22 August, 29 August, and 5 September 1885.
87. See Clémence Royer to Ghénia Avril de Sainte-Croix [1899], BMD, and a mention of Duprat's death by the president of the Anthropological Society in his annual report. *Bulletin Société d'Anthropologie* 3d ser., 5 (1885): 595. See also Nigoul, *Pascal Duprat,* 241.
88. Royer's unsigned articles for the science columns of Gambetta's daily newspaper, *La République Française*, appeared under the editorship of Paul Bert: "L'Homo primigenius et son industrie," 9 December 1873; "La Transition de l'âge de la pierre taillée à l'âge de la pierre polie," 22 September 1874; "La Civilisation mégalithique," 24 June 1875; "La Céramique primitive," 27 July 1875; "La Civilisation de la pierre polie," 30 November 1875. These are identified as her work at the end of her *Autobiography,* 83. Fraisse adds "L'Archéologie préhistorique," 18 February 1873, and gives the date of "La Civilisation mégalithique" as 24 June 1873. Fraisse, *Clémence Royer,* 181.
89. Royer explains this in one of her (undated) letters to the ministry. Archives Nationales (now designated CARAN), Ministère d'Instruction Publique; Indemnités littéraires, dossiers individuels, 1829–1931; Dossier Clémence Royer, F17 3216.
90. This is detailed in a large number of letters to the ministry, some sent by friends,

colleagues, political men, and scientists who wrote on her behalf, sending her letters along. The one with this quotation is undated and was sent by Jules Dévolle; it specifically mentions that (after Bert had gone to Tonkin, and she had received an initial grant) "in the year that Pascal died, I found myself in a very difficult situation. I wrote to Paul Bert, and he sent his card to the ministry."

91. Ministère d'Instruction Publique, Dossier Clémence Royer, F17 3216.
92. In 1886, René was still "in her charge," soon to start at "a state school." A later appeal to the Ministry of Public Education in 1888 gives René's age as 22 and mentions that as a sublieutenant he could not contribute anything to cover her expenses.
93. Milice, *Clémence Royer.*
94. The address, 2, quat. boulevard Jourdan, and the yearly rental come from the files of the Préfecture de Police, Dossier Clémence Royer.
95. Parc Montsouris, opened in 1878, has a number of trees now living that date back more than a century. The man responsible for the construction of the artificial lake committed suicide when the lake drained dry on the day of formal opening due to a fault in construction, according to a notice posted in the park.
96. Royer, "Dépopulation de France" 681–99. The parc Montsouris is mentioned on p. 689.
97. Clémence Royer "Laboratoire d'experiences transformistes à Montsouris," *Bulletin de la Société d'Anthropologie de Paris* (1887): 461–462.
98. Royer, "L'Instinct social," 710.
99. Ibid., 719. Her reference is probably to Jean-Charles Houzeau, *Études sur les facultés mentales des animaux comparées à celle de l'homme.* Mons: Manceaux, 1872.
100. Ibid., 726.
101. "Discussion sur l'instinct social," *Bulletin de la Société d'Anthropologie de Paris,* 3d ser., 5 (1882). Dally's comments are on p. 729. Royer replies with some heat on pp. 730–732.
102. Ibid., 734–736.
103. See a delightful series of pictures, "Les Orangs-Outangs du Jardin d'Acclimatation" in *L'Illustration* 90 (45e année) (July 1887): 212. This shows the young apes playing with eggs, cups, etc., around their mother.
104. Royer, "Facultés mentales," 257–270. This article was published in English as "Faculties of Monkies: Mental Evolution," *Popular Science Monthly* 30 (1887): 17–24.
105. Clémence Royer, "Notions du nombre," 649–658. Published in English as "Animal Arithmetic," *Popular Science Monthly* 30 (1887): 252–262.
106. Harvey, "Races Specified." See also the discussion of this debate in Clark, *Social Darwinism.*
107. Royer, "Évolution mentale," 39:749–758, 40:70–79.
108. Ibid., 39:750. Royer praised her colleagues' earlier presentations.
109. In a letter written in 1890, Royer mentions her difficulty in climbing the stairs. Her observations on population repeat some of her remarks suppressed in 1875. Royer, "Dépopulation," 681–699.
110. Procès Verbaux, Bureau Central, vol. 2 (1900).
111. Royer, "Évolution mentale," Archives Société d'Anthropologie de Paris (MSS). 39:756.

112. Ibid., 757.
113. Ibid.
114. Ibid., 758. See the discussion by Edwin Clarke and L. S. Jacyna of William B. Carpenter's ideas of adaptation to the environment by plants in his attempt to show a correlation between plant response and nervous system response in animals in the 1840s. *Nineteenth-Century Origins of Neuroscientific Concepts* (Berkeley: University of California, 1987, 139. Carpenter also made a distinction between ideomotor actions (stimulated by an idea) and "emotional" actions (stimulated by a feeling) (141). Royer had been interested in the connection between nervous action and muscular activity as early as her first translation of *Origin of Species,* as shown in her extensive notes on electric fish that cite Carlo Matteucci.
115. She did not use, as one might have expected, the studies of comparative brain anatomy of primates done by her colleague in the Société d'Anthropologie Paul Broca shortly before his death in 1880. These studies focussed on the limbic lobe and had been recently edited and published by Paul Broca's student Samuel Pozzi in Paul Broca, *Mémoires d'Anthropologie,* vol. 5 (Paris: Reinwald, 1888).
116. Royer, "Facultés mentales." See also Milice, *Clémence Royer,* 177.
117. Royer, "Domestication des singes," 170–181.
118. Royer, "Discours," *Congrès des Droits des Femmes.*
119. For a discussion of this point of view, which follows the liberal feminist line, see the section on Maria Deraismes and liberal feminism in Moses, *French Feminism.*
120. Léonce Manouvrier recalls his involvement with the congress and his explicit reasons to support the moderate feminist movement in "Anthropologie des sexes," 41–61. For a discussion of this in relation to Gustave Le Bon's claims about women's limited brain size, see Harvey, "Races Specified," and "Strangers to Each Other," and Gould, *Mismeasure of Man.*
121. Royer, "Toast," *Congrès des Droits des Femmes* 268.
122. For Céline Renooz's life history, see her memoirs and collection of letters in the Bibliothèque Historique de Paris, Fonds Louise Bouglé. I thank Professor James Allen for calling her and her connection to Royer to my attention.
123. Renooz describes Charcot as a physician "devoted to a kind of human vivisection on women under the pretext of studying an illness for which he knew neither the cause nor the treatment" (a reference to Charcot's rather theatrical demonstrations of women's hysteria). Céline Renooz, "Charcot dévoilé" (Charcot unmasked), *Revue Scientifique des Femmes* 1 (1888): 245. This objection prefigures later feminist criticisms of Charcot.
124. Céline Renooz, *La Nouvelle Science* (Paris: [self-published], 1890) discusses at length this new "feminist" science. Her earlier book, *L'Évolution de l'homme et des animaux,* depicts itself as an evolutionary book based on embryology, but is actually neither evolutionary in any acceptable sense nor does it show an understanding of either human or plant development. Baillière published this book but later apologized, saying no one had actually read it before publication.
125. Céline Renooz, "Mémoires," (unpublished manuscript); her quotation. Bibliothèque Historique de Paris, box 17, fol. 181, October 1896. The American physician Mary Putnam Jacobi, trained in French medicine and a strong sup-

porter of women in science and medicine, thought that the reason that her review had not lasted for more than a year was because it had rushed in "waving a red flag" in every sentence and making extreme claims that it couldn't sustain instead of slowly building up its readership. Mary Putnam Jacobi, "Woman in Medicine," 163 n.

126. Renooz, *La Nouvelle Science.*
127. Archives Nationales (now designated CARAN), Ministère d'Instruction Publique; Indemnités Littéraires, Dossier Clémence Royer, F17 3216.
128. The award of Fr 500 was made 31 December, 1890. The letter from Hovelacque et al. (he was a deputy at the time as well as an important member of the Société d'Anthropologie) is dated 16 January 1891. The note granting the award is dated 17 January 1891, and Hovelacque's thanks are dated the same day. The amount was paid almost two weeks later. See Archives Nationales, Dossier Clémence Royer, F17 3216.
129. Archives Nationales, Dossier Clémence Royer, F17 3216. List of indemnities for Clémence Royer: Fr 1,200, 13 April 1885, P. Bert; Fr 1,200, 31 November 1887, M. Carnot *père* (he was a senator); Fr 1,000, 7 June 1887, M. Hovelacque; Fr 800, 2 May 1888; Fr 500, 13 May 1889; Fr 800, 22 February 1890; Fr 500, 31 December 1890; Fr 500, 31 January 1891; Fr 500, 15 March 1892 (at this point the list of indemnities notes that "Mme Clémence Royer is, it appears, a pensioner at the Galignani asylum"); Fr 600, 3 April 1893; Fr 500, 16 April 1894; Fr 500, 6 April 1895, M. Léon Say, deputy; Fr 600, 8 February 1896; Fr 500, 31 December 1896; Fr 500, 26 July 1897; Fr 500+, 28 August 1899. The final entry reads: "Annual indemnity of Fr 2,000 from 1 June ordered 22 May 1900. G. Leygues." Although letters are included in 1889 from Yves Guyot, who was minister of Public Works, from Marey at the Institute, and from others, they are not noted on this list, which heads the dossier.
130. Royer, "L'Assistance publique d'après 1888," *Académie des Sciences Morales et Politiques* 131 (1889): 187, 812–814, submitted for the competition, the article won a prize of Fr 1,000, not awarded until some time later. Linda Clark has interpreted this essay as reflecting a greater sympathy for the underclass during Royer's period of privation. See Clark, *Social Darwinism,* 57.
131. Clémence Royer to Armand de Quatrefages, April 1891. Correspondence to Quatrefages, Muséum d'Histoire Naturelle, Bibliothèque, MS 2258. Yvette Conry prints only the first part of this letter in the appendix to her book *Introduction du Darwinisme,* 437.

CHAPTER 9 ***"I See Young and Old"***

1. This was repeated in the listings of titles of work presented to the Académie des Sciences by the *Revue Scientifique,* although the papers themselves were not included.
2. See Royer, *Autobiography.* She published many of her articles on physics in this journal in the 1890s, for example, "La Matière," *Société Nouvelle (Revue Internationale),* (Brussels) (1895): 334–350, 507–523. By the mid-1890s, as she became better known again, she also regularly published short articles on science in *La Science Française.*
3. Clémence Royer, "An American Philosopher" (translated from the *Revue de*

Belgique), *The Open Court* 4 (1890–1891): 2413–2414; Paul Carus, "The Ethics of the New Positivism": A Letter to the *Revue de Belgique* in Reply to the Article 'Un Philosophe américain' by Clémence Royer," *Open Court* 4 (1890–1891): 2414–2415; "Is the Idea of God Tenable? A Letter from Madame Clémence Royer to the *Revue de Belgique,*" *Open Court* 4 (1890–1891): 2526–2427.

4. See, for example, a review by Carus of "Les Notions de force de la matière et de l'esprit selon la science moderne," by Clémence Royer, *Bulletin Mensuel d'Études Philosophiques et Sociales,* n.d., printed in *Open Court* 4 (1890–1891): 2387–2389, with note stating that "The *Open Court* has received several valuable scientific articles from this well-known French lady, among which we notice an exhaustive essay 'On the molecular constitution of water in its three physical states and concerning the properties of gases according to a new hypothesis' and further the above mentioned essay on the notions of force, of matter, and of mind according to modern science."
5. See, for example, a brief discussion of Royer's physical theories in the companion journal to *Open Court,* Lucien Arréat, "Literary Correspondence, France," *The Monist* 1 (1890–1891): 126–127.
6. Was Mary Lacour the woman distracted by her naughty children whom Royer had so vividly described that year in the bulletins of the Anthropological Society? See chapter 8. Royer, "Dépopulation," 681–699.
7. Royer mentions that Nadar's brother is "like a child" but well looked after by the women at the Galignani home. Clémence Royer to Félix Nadar [1899?].
8. If any of the proposed retired persons had a pension, they had to contribute Fr 750 a year for their keep. Half the places were free to men and women "of letters." A copy of the rules of the "maison de retraite" is in the Bibliothèque Marguerite Durand.
9. This date is given by Milice, Clémence Royer, 185.
10. Ibid., 186.
11. Léopold Lacour, "Les Femmes à l'Institut," *L'Événement,* 18 December 1892. Léopold Lacour recalled that the articles appeared not only in *L'Événement* but in *Gil Blas* and other newspapers in his laudatory speech at Royer's banquet of 1897. Dossier Clémence Royer, BMD.
12. A handwritten copy of the article by Lacour is in Dossier Clémence Royer, BMD. Also see her letter to Léopold Lacour, 18 August [1900], at the time of her Legion of Honor award. Letters to Mary and Léopold Lacour, Correspondence Clémence Royer BMD.
13. Clémence Royer to Léopold Lacour, 18 August [1900], Correspondence Clémence Royer, BMD.
14. According to the report for May 1892 in the Préfecture de Police dossier.
15. Fraisse, *Clémence Royer,* 97.
16. This is according to a report of "Officer of the Peace Girard," 15 May 1881, in Dossier Clémence Royer, Préfecture de Police.
17. For a discussion of Deraismes's ties to the Masonic movement see Bidelman, *Pariahs Stand Up!*
18. Her will was written at the Maison Galignani, 5 May 1895, a copy of which is in the Bibliothèque Marguerite Durand.
19. Clémence Royer, "Testament," Dossier Clémence Royer, BMD. It may be worth

noting that in this will she excluded any collateral relative from inheriting from her, something that reminds us of the suspicion of seduction or rape by a near relative.

20. Clémence Royer to Ghénia Avril de Sainte-Croix [1897?]. "Je sais depuis longtemps que Marie Durand . . ." Copies of the letters to Ghénia Avril de Sainte-Croix are in the Correspondence of Clémence Royer, BMD.
21. Ibid.
22. "The Dreyfus Case," *La Fronde,* 9 December 1897. This was the first number of that daily paper. Royer would remark some years later: "After the closure of the Zola affair [Dreyfus case], the journal [*La Fronde*] is empty of interest." Clémence Royer to Ghénia Avril de Sainte-Croix, 21 March [1900?], BMD.
23. Clémence Royer to Ghénia Avril de Sainte-Croix, 13 January [1898?], BMD. Ghénia Avril de Sainte-Croix became the secretary-general of the Conseil National des Femmes Françaises (CNFF), an amalgamated group of moderate feminist societies, founded in 1901, that had a membership in the thousands. This group later supported suffrage for women. For more on Sainte-Croix, see Steven C. Hause and Anne R. Keeney, *Women's Suffrage and Social Politics in the French Third Republic* (Princeton, NJ: Princeton University Press, 1984).
24. Ghénia Avril de Sainte-Croix, like Josephine Butler in England, was involved in philanthropic schemes to improve the lot of prostitutes. Royer took an interest, although she had no direct involvement in this work, and informed her friend that Mrs. Chapman, widow of the editor of the *Westminster Review,* was interested in discussing this work. Clémence Royer to Ghénia Avril de Sainte-Croix, Monday, March 21 [1899?]. The letter starts out, "Bien chérie, Mme Chapman . . ." BMD.
25. These have not been found in the Darwin Archive, but as George Darwin's letters are more thoroughly catalogued, they may yet turn up.
26. Clémence Royer to Ghénia Avril de Sainte-Croix, n.d., February [1897]. BMD.
27. Clémence Royer to Ghénia Avril de Sainte-Croix, n.d., February [1897]. BMD.
28. Charles Letourneau to Ghénia Avril de Sainte-Croix, 26 February 1897. "Banquet 1897," Dossier Clémence Royer, BMD.
29. Alfred Giard to the organizers of the banquet, 22 February 1897, BMD. "Socialist ideal," speaking of someone known to be in opposition to socialism?
30. The theme of admiration for Royer as Darwin's first translator ran as a thread through the banquet tributes on the evening of the celebration, 10 March 1897, as one speaker after another rose to sing her praises. See the report on the front page of *L'Événement,* 11 March 1897, headed "Le Banquet Clémence Royer: Imposante manifestation," which begins with a quotation from Ernest Renan, "She was almost a man of genius," but drops the word "almost." This piece refers to her as having "one of the most powerful and fertile brains of our time" and mentions the request to the French Third Republic for a Legion of Honor award three years earlier. Two hundred people attended the banquet. Levasseur of the Collège de France, member of the Institute, presided, "having on his right Mme Clémence Royer, on his left Mlle [Mme] de Sainte-Croix, the true instigator of this family fête." Others included senators; the president of the Grand Orient de France, the central Masonic lodge; the publisher of the journal *L'Événement;* Georges Clemenceau, "the brilliant writer" Clovis Hughes, "deputy and exquisite poet"; and many others including her friends, Léopold Lacour and Albert Colas;

colleagues like Charles Letourneau; the secretary-general of the Société d'Anthropologie Léonce Manouvrier; Dr. Capitan; her son, now Captain René Duprat, "a brilliant engineering officer"; and a variety of women doctors and women lawyers, artists, and writers. The list included Maude Gonne, a friend of Ghénia Avril de Sainte-Croix (later Yeats's great friend); Mme Feresses-Deraismes, the sister of Maria Deraismes and a delegate from the Masonic lodge Le Droit Humain; and a large number of journalists. Telegrams came from Mantegazza on behalf of the Italian Anthropological Society of Florence and from Deputy Charles Beauquier, and there were letters from Enrico Ferri, Alfred Naquet, Gabriel de Mortillet, Th. Ribot, Anatole France, John Lubbock (now Lord Aveling), Émile Zola, and representatives from various feminist groups. Among the speakers were Dr. Madeleine Brès, Ghénia Avril de Sainte-Croix, and Maria Chéliga representing "the foreign press and several groups of the Union Internationale des Femmes." Amélie Kammer, president of the Ligue des Droits des Femmes (League of the Rights of Women) presented Royer with "a superb bouquet." "At the moment at which Clémence Royer ended her improvisation there was a terrific salvo of applause. Every hand reached towards her," according to Hugues Bargeret, *L'Evenement,* 11 March 1897.

31. Charles Letourneau, Banquet tribute to Clémence Royer, 10 March 1897. "Banquet 1897" MSS, Dossier Clémence Royer BMD.
32. This is quoted at length in chapter 6.
33. Dr. Madeleine Brès, Banquet tribute to Clémence Royer, Banquet 10 March 1897. "Banquet 1897" MSS, Dossier Clémence Royer, BMD.
34. Léopold Lacour, Notes on "Banquet 1897" speech.
35. Clémence Royer, Speech for "Banquet 1897" 10 March 1897.
36. Ibid.
37. Ibid.
38. Ibid.
39. Ibid.
40. Eugène Tavernier, "Madame Clémence Royer," *L'Univers,* 9 March 1897. It is interesting that this article, written before the banquet, was included in the Ministry of Education files, but not the favorable article by Clemenceau, "Madame Clémence Royer."
41. Desiré Louis, "Clémence Royer," *La Justice,* 17 March 1897.
42. Clemenceau, "Madame Clémence Royer," 194–195. The lithograph that accompanies this article shows a rather thoughtful Royer, grown heavy, possibly as a consequence of the asthma and her general ill health, which rendered her inactive.
43. Ibid.
44. Ibid., 195.
45. Clémence Royer to Mary Lacour; undated, typewritten letter [1897?] beginning, "Carina, René m'a donné une machine à écrire." BMD. The reference is to Lacour, *Humanisme intégral.*
46. Clémence Royer to Léopold Lacour [1897]. BMD. She added some detailed information about the men and women as well as booksellers that might have a copy of d'Héricourt's book. Héricourt, *La Femme affranchie.*
47. During the 1890s she is listed as one of the founders of the journal *Bulletin de l'Union Universelle des Femmes.* An interview with her appears in *Bulletin,* no.

15 (January-February 1891). See the bibliography in Fraisse, *Clémence Royer,* 178.

48. Clémence Royer to Ghénia Avril de Sainte-Croix, n.d. [1899?], beginning, "Que devenez-vous, chère amie?" BMD.
49. Le Bon, *Évolution de la matière* and *Évolution des forces.* These were included in his series Bibliothèque de Philosophie Scientifique, which included French physicists. I thank Bob Nye for his discussion with me of Le Bon's later work.
50. Royer, preface to *Constitution du monde.* The full title of the book is *La Constitution du monde: Natura rerum. Dynamique des atomes. Nouveaux Principes de philosophie naturelle* (Paris: Schleicher Frères, 1900). [The publisher was Reinwald's publishing house continued under this new name by his two adopted sons.]
51. Ibid., xx.
52. Ibid.
53. Ibid.
54. Quoted by John Theodore Merz, *A History of European Thought in the Nineteenth Century,* vol. 2, *Scientific Thought* (Edinburgh and London: Blackwood and Sons, 1905), 740.
55. Clémence Royer to Ghénia Avril de Sainte-Croix, 6 July 1898. BMD.
56. A current soap bubble model of the universe has been suggested by members of the Smithsonian Astrophysical Labs at Harvard, especially by Margaret J. Geller and her colleagues.
57. He was, interestingly enough, the great-uncle of Henri Becquerel whose interest in radioactivity sparked the Curies' study of uranium and led to their discovery of other radioactive elements.
58. Royer, *Constitution du monde,* 74. Soury's translation of Haeckel had employed the word *âme* (soul, or mind) for Haeckel's concept of cell consciousness.
59. Ibid.
60. Ibid.
61. Ibid. The French language seems to have encouraged her to conflate "radiation" with "radius" so that her idea of "radiating out" is more like that of spokes on a wheel.
62. Royer, *Constitution du monde.* For a recent discussion of ether in connection with older ideas of force and mind, see G. N. Cantor and M.J.S. Hodge, "Major Themes in the Development of Ether Theories from the Ancients to 1900," in *Conceptions of Ether: Studies in the History of Ether Theories, 1740–1900,* ed. G. N. Cantor and M. J. S. Hodge (Cambridge: Cambridge University Press, 1981), 1–60.
63. Royer, *Constitution du monde.*
64. Clémence Royer to Ghénia Avril de Sainte-Croix, n.d. [1899?], beginning "Je trouve toujours . . . " BMD.
65. She thanks this woman in her dedication to *Constitution du monde.* Milice identifies Barrier as "a friend of Hippolyte Laroche."
66. Clémence Royer to Ghénia Avril de Sainte-Croix, n.d. [1900], BMD.
67. Clémence Royer to Ghénia Avril de Sainte-Croix, 10 April [1900], BMD. Unfortunately many of these letters no longer exist, having been destroyed by her ex-

ecutors, Albert Colas and his wife, along with all letters from her son, Duprat, friends, and colleagues.

68. See Howard Stein, "'Subtler Forms of Matter' in the Period Following Maxwell," in Cantor and Hodge, *Conceptions of Ether.*
69. Review of *La Constitution du monde,* by Clémence Royer, *Science* 2 (1900): 785.
70. G.B.H., review of *La Constitution du monde* by Clémence Royer, *Nature* 63 (1901): 534. A review signed T. J. McC. with two portraits of Royer appeared in *The Open Court* 14 (1900): 562–564. He called her a *Naturphilosophe* but adds that the book "is aglow with faith in science."
71. Banquet for Clémence Royer by Bleus de Bretagne, as reported by Jeanne Brémond, *La Fronde,* 17 November 1900.
72. Clémence Royer speech before the banquet of Bleus de Bretagne, as reported in *La Fronde,* 17 November 1900. Copy in Archives Nationales, Dossier Clémence Royer, F17 3216.
73. See note 129, chapter 8, detailing the indemnities from the ministry from 1885 up to her award following the presentation of the Legion of Honor.
74. Banquet for Clémence Royer by Bleus de Bretagne.
75. Clémence Royer speech before the banquet of Bleus de Bretagne, Archives Nationales.
76. Ibid.
77. Royer, "La Vérité sur Madagascar," signed with the pseudonym "Lux" and printed as a separate pamphlet. Léopold Lacour identified the article as Royer's in the Bibliothèque Marguerite Durand. See, Fraisse, *Clémence Royer,* 65.
78. Clémence Royer to Ghénia Avril de Sainte-Croix, n.d., beginning, "C'est gentil à voir . . ." BMD.
79. Clémence Royer to Félix Nadar, March 1899 and 19 November 1899. These letters describe René's journey to Indochina. Nadar had taken a number of photographs of her son in uniform that he presented to her at no cost, for which she thanked him. One of these was later printed in the memorial issue of *La Fronde.* Nadar Archive, Bibliothèque Nationale, n.a.fr. 24285, nos. 691, 694.
80. Milice, *Clémence Royer,* 107.
81. Clémence Royer to Ghénia Avril de Sainte-Croix, 2 July 1901, BMD.
82. Ibid.
83. Clémence Royer to Ghénia Avril de Sainte-Croix, n.d. [1898?], beginning, "Je vous ai expectée [*sic*] sur samedi, bonne amie . . ." BMD.
84. Clémence Royer to Ghénia Avril de Sainte-Croix, 18 June 1901, BMD.
85. Albert Wiert to "Madame" [Ghénia Avril de Sainte-Croix or Marguerite Durand?], Paris, 13 Jan 1903, BMD. Wiert says about René Duprat's death in Hanoi on 13 November 1902 that he had been diagnosed as having a bilious fever and that a liver abscess was later discovered and operated on without success. His friends had stayed with him at the hospital until the end. Although the funeral itself was "rather good" and the various branches of engineering and of the colonial army were represented, no farewell speeches were made over his tomb to the dismay of his friends, who felt that some recognition of his work should have been given by his commanding officers. He was awarded a posthumous Legion of Honor. René Duprat's life and death are described in Moufflet, "L'oeuvre de

Clémence Royer"; Milice, *Clémence Royer;* and Fraisse, *Clémence Royer.* Fraisse considers the liver disorder to have been a cancer.

86. Blanche Edwards-Pilliet, discussion as president of sec. 5, Arts, Letters, Sciences, 22 June 1900, *Congrès International des Oeuvres et Institutions Féminins: Compte rendu par Madame Pégard.* (Paris: Charles Blot, 1902), 4:304. Royer was listed as honorary president of the sister conference, Congrès des Droits des Femmes, the same year.
87. Clémence Royer to Ghénia Avril de Sainte-Croix, 2 February 1901, BMD.
88. Clémence Royer to Mary Lacour [1897?], BMD.
89. Royer to Ghénia Avril de Sainte-Croix, [1901?], BMD.
90. Milice, *Clémence Royer,* 210–212.
91. Ibid.
92. Sara Joan Miles has visited her grave there. (Personal communication).
93. Milice, *Clémence Royer,* 214.

Afterword

1. Moufflet, L'Oeuvre de Clémence Royer, 658–693.
2. Saulze, "L'atomisme dynamigne de Mlle Cl. Royer," 35–58, 121–151.
3. Pratelle, "Clémence Royer," 263–276.
4. Harlor, "Clémence Royer, une savante," 525–535.
5. Stebbins, "France."
6. Conry, *Introduction du Darwinisme,* 40. Does the French acceptance of Conry's interpretation explain why in the new evolution galleries at the Muséum d'Histoire Naturelle it is not Royer's translation of the first or even the second French edition in the 1860s but the Barbier translation of 1873 that is on display?
7. Clark, *Schooling the Daughters of Marianne.*
8. Fraisse, Clémence Royer.
9. For this she credits the influence of the study of her dissertation advisor, Richards, *Darwin.*
10. Miles, "Clémence Royer," 61–81. This is drawn from Miles's dissertation, but since it is put more concisely in this article, I have discussed it here.
11. Richards, *Meaning of evolution.*
12. Without a discussion of the many readings of *Origin of Species* arguing this point, I might add that Huxley also pointed out the various teleological and nonteleological interpretations by his contemporaries in 1864. Thomas Henry Huxley, "Criticisms on the *Origin of Species, Natural History Review* (1864), reprinted in *Collected Essays* (London: Macmillan, 1893), 2:80–106.
13. Blanckaert, "L'anthropologie au féminin," 23–38.
14. Blanckaert, "Les Bas-Fonds de la science française." 115–130.
15. Ibid.
16. Ducros and Blanckaert, "L'Animal de la création que l'homme connaît le moins," 131–144.
17. Shapin, *A Social History of Truth.*

Appendix

1. Société d'Anthropologie de Paris Archives, Folder B1, 1891. The suppressed memoir and the letter from Royer have been recently published in the journal of the society by Ducros and Blanckaert, "L'animal de la creation que l'homme connaît le moins," 131–144.
2. The most likely reference is to the feminist Jenny d'Héricourt, who moved to Chicago in the 1860s and qualified herself as a doctor. See Karen Offen on her life, *French Feminist Rediscovered.* Juliette Adam describes the friendship between d'Héricourt and Royer, both of whom she considered her enemies, in her autobiographical books, especially in *Mes premières armes.* For a discussion of Hepworth Dixon, see chapter 7.

Bibliography

Archives

French Archives

Archives Nationales de France (CARAN), Paris

Ministère d'Instruction Publique; Indemnités littéraires
Dossier Clemence Royer, F^{17} 3216
Archives Sociétaires
Correspondence to Victor Considérant, 10 AS 4
Correspondence Jules Simon AP 87/3

Bibliothèque Marguerite Durand, Paris

Dossier Clémence Royer
Correspondence Clémence Royer

Bibliothèque Historique de la Ville de Paris, Paris

Fonds Louise Bouglé
Céline Renooz Papers

Bibliothèque Nationale, Paris

Département de Manuscrits; Nouvelles acquisitions françaises
Collection Félix Nadar, n.a.fr. 24285.
Correspondence Ernest Havet, n.a.fr. 24478
Correspondence François Lenoir, n.a.fr. 21481

Muséum d'Histoire Naturelle, Bibliothèque, Paris

Correspondence to Ernst Hamy, MS 2254
Correspondence to Armand de Quatrefages, MS 2258

Préfecture de Police, Paris

Dossier Pascal Duprat
Dossier Clémence Royer

Société d'Anthropologie de Paris Archives, Paris
(held at Musée de l'Homme, Paris)

BRITISH ARCHIVES

University of Cambridge, Cambridge, UK

Girton College Archives
Bessie R. Parkes Papers
Barbara Bodichon Papers
Cambridge University Library
Darwin Archive (DAR); Charles Darwin Papers

Pembrokeshire County Archives, Haverfordwest, UK

SWISS ARCHIVES

Bibliothèque Publique et Universitaire, Geneva

Correspondence René-Édouard Claparède
Correspondence Carl Vogt
Correspondence Ernest Naville
Correspondence de Bureau, Bibliothèque Publique et Universitaire

Published Sources

Acland, Alice. *Caroline Norton.* London: Constable, 1948.

Adam, Juliette Lamber. *Idées anti-Proudhoniennes sur l'amour, la femme, et le mariage.* 1st ed. Paris: Lévy, 1858; 2d ed., enl., 1862.

———. *Mes premières armes littéraires et politiques.* Paris: Alphonse Lemerre, 1904.

Agoult, Marie de Flavigny, comtesse d' [Daniel Stern, pseud.]. *Histoire de la Révolution de 1848.* 3 vols. Paris: G. Sandré, 1850–1853.

———. *Jeanne d'Arc: Drame historique en cinq actes et en prose.* Paris: M. Lévy, 1857.

———. *Dante et Goethe.* Paris: Didier, 1866.

———. *Mes souvenirs, 1806–1833.* Paris: Calmann Lévy, 1877.

Beale, Dorothea. *Reports Issued by the School's Inquiry Commission on the Education of Girls.* London: David Nutt, [1870].

Bertillon, L.-A. "Valeur de l'hypothèse du transformisme." *Bulletin de la Société d'Anthropologie de Paris,* 2d ser., 5 (1870): 488–528.

Bidelman, Patrick. *Pariahs Stand Up! The Founding of the Liberal Feminist Movement in France, 1858–1889.* Westport, CT: Greenwood Press, 1982.

Blanckaert, Claude. "L'Anthropologie au féminin: Clémence Royer (1830–1902)." *Revue de Synthèse,* 3d ser., 105 (1982): 23–38.

———. "'Les Bas-Fonds de la science française': Clémence Royer, *L'Origine de l'homme,* et le Darwinisme social." *Bulletin et Mémoires de la Société d'Anthropologie de Paris,* n.s., 3 (1991): 115–130.

Block, Maurice. "Revue des publications de l'étranger." *Journal des Économistes* 41 (1864): 413–414.

Bodichon, Barbara Smith. *A Brief Summary in Plain Language of the Most Important Laws of England Concerning Women.* London: Holyoake, 1854.

Boyer, Jacques. "Clémence Royer." *Popular Science Monthly* 54 (1899): 690–698.

Brisson, Adolphe. "Clémence Royer." In *Portraits Intimes.* Series no. 3. Paris: Colin, 1897.

Broca, Paul. "Sur le transformisme. *Bulletin de la Société d'Anthropologie de Paris,* 2d ser., 5 (1870): 168–239.

———. "Les Sélections." *Revue d'Anthropologie* 1 (1872): 683–710.

———. *Mémoires d'anthropologie.* Vols. 1–5. Paris: Reinwald, 1878–1888.

Büchner, Ludwig. *Kraft und Stoff: Empirisch-naturphilosophische Studien.* Frankfurt: Meisinger Sohn, 1855.

Burkhardt, Frederick, and Sydney Smith, eds. *Correspondence of Charles Darwin (1821–1859).* Vols. 1–7. Cambridge: Cambridge University Press, 1984–1991.

Burkhardt, Frederick, and Duncan Porter, eds. *Correspondence of Charles Darwin (1860).* Vol. 8. Cambridge: Cambridge University Press, 1993.

Burkhardt, Frederick, Duncan Porter, Joy Harvey, and Marsha Richmond, eds. *Correspondence of Charles Darwin (1861).* Vol. 9. Cambridge: Cambridge University Press, 1994.

Burkhardt, Frederick, et al. eds. *Correspondence of Charles Darwin* 1862–1870. Vols. 10–19. Cambridge: Cambridge University Press, 1997–.

Bury, J.P.T. *Gambetta's Final Years: "The Era of Difficulties," 1877–1882.* Longman: London and New York, 1982.

Carr, Edward Hallett. *Romantic Exiles: A Nineteenth-Century Portrait Gallery.* 1933. Reprint, New York: Beacon Press, 1961.

Channing, W. H. *Memoir of William Ellery Channing with Extracts from His Correspondence and Manuscripts.* 3 vols. London: Williams and Norgate 1848.

Claparède, René-Édouard. "M. Darwin et sa théorie de la formation des espèces." *Revue Germanique* 16 (1861): 523—559.

Clark, Linda L. *Social Darwinism in France.* Tuscaloosa, AL: University of Alabama Press, 1984.

———. *Schooling the Daughters of Marianne: Textbooks and Socialization of Girls in Modern French Primary Schools.* Albany, NY: State University of New York Press, 1984.

Clemenceau, Georges. "Madame Clémence Royer." *L'Illustration,* 13 March 1897, 194–195.

Cobbe, Frances Power. *Life of Frances Power Cobbe by Herself.* 2 vols. London: R. Bentley & Son, 1894.

Colenso, John William. *Village Sermons.* Cambridge: Macmillan, 1853.

Congrès International des Droits des Femmes: Compte rendu des séances plénières. Paris: Auguste Chio, 1878.

Conry, Yvette. *L'Introduction du Darwinisme en France au XIXe siècle.* Paris: Vrin, 1974.

Dally, Eugène. "L'Ordre des primates et le transformisme." *Bulletin de la Société d'Anthropologie de Paris,* 3d ser., 2 (1868): 673–712.

———. "Introduction" to *De la place de l'homme dans la nature,* by T. H. Huxley, 1–95. Paris: Baillière, 1868.

Darwin, Charles. *De l'origine des espèces, ou des lois du progrès chez les êtres organisés.* Trans. Clémence Royer. 1st French ed. Paris: Guillaumin and Masson, 1862.

———. *De l'origine des espèces par sélection naturelle, ou des lois de transformation des êtres organisés.* Trans. Clémence Royer. 2d French ed. Paris: Guillaumin and Masson, 1866.

———. *Variation under Domestication in Animals and Plants.* London: Murray, 1868.

———. *Descent of Man and Selection in Relation to Sex.* 2d ed. London: Murray, 1874.

Daubié, Julie-Victoire. "L'enseignement secondaire pour les femmes." *Journal des Économistes,* 2d ser., 46 (1865): 382–402.

Deraismes, Maria. *Ève contre M. Dumas.* Paris, 1872.

Di Gregorio, Mario A., ed., with N. W. Gill. *Charles Darwin's Marginalia.* Vol. 1. New York: Garland, 1990.

Dixon, Edward H. *Woman and Her Diseases from the Cradle to the Grave Adapted Exclusively to Her Instruction in the Physiology of Her System.* 10th ed. New York: Ranney, 1857.

Dixon, William Hepworth. *New America.* Philadelphia: Lippincott, 1867.

Ducros, Albert, and Claude Blanckaert "'L'Animal de la création que l'homme connaît le moins': Le Mémoire refusé de Clémence Royer sur la femme et la natalité." *Bulletins et Mémoires de la Société d'Anthropologie,* n.s. 3 (1991): 131–144.

Dumas, Alexandre. *Une année à Florence: Impressions de voyage.* 2 vols. Paris: Dumont, 1841–1844.

Dumas *fils,* Alexandre. *L'homme-femme.* Paris: Michel Lévy Frères, 1872.

Duprat, Pascal. "Les Principaux Représentants des idées économiques en Italie." *Journal des Économistes* 43 (1864): 431–448.

———. "De la mainmorte en Italie et de sa suppression." *Journal des Économistes* 45 (1864): 172–190.

———. *Les Encyclopédistes.* Paris: Librairie Internationale, 1866.

———. "La Révolution et les problèmes économiques en Espagne." *Journal des Économistes,* 3d ser., 13 (1869): 41–56.

———. *L'Esprit des révolutions.* Paris: A. LeChevalier, 1869.

———. *L'Esprit des révolutions.* 2d ed. Paris: A. LeChevalier, 1879.

Duroselle, Jean-Baptiste. *Clemenceau.* Paris: Fayard, [1988].

Duval, Jules. "Société d'Économie Politique." *Journal des Économistes* 44 (December 1864): 421.

Duval, Mathias. *Le Darwinisme.* Paris: Lehaye and Ducrosnier, 1886.

Fraisse, Geneviève. *Clémence Royer: Philosophe et femme de sciences.* Paris: Éditions de la Découverte, 1985.

Garnier, Joseph."Société d'Économie Politique." *Journal des Économistes,* 2d ser., 25 (1862): 153.

———. "Nécrologie: Guillaumin, ses funerailles, sa vie, et son oeuvre." *Journal des Économistes,* 2d ser., 45 (January 1865): 108–121.

[Garnier, Joseph]. "Revue des principales publications économiques de l'étranger." *Journal des Économistes,* 1st ser., 3 (1866).

Gaudry, Albert. *Animaux fossiles et géologie de l'Attique.* 2 vols. Paris: F. Savy, 1862–1867.

Gilman, Charlotte Perkins. *Herland.* New York: Pantheon Books, 1979.

Gould, Stephen Jay. *Mismeasure of Man.* New York: Norton, 1981.

Haeckel, Ernst. *Generelle Morphologie des Organismus.* Berlin: Reimer, 1866.

———. *Natürliche Schöpfungsgeschichte: Gemeinverständliche wissenschaftliche Vorträge über die Entwicklungslehre* . . . . Berlin: Reimer, 1868.

———. *Essais de psychologie cellulaire.* Trans. and with a preface by Jules Soury. Paris: Baillière, 1880.

Harlor, [Thérese Hammer]. "Clémence Royer, une savante." *Revue des Deux Mondes* 5 (1954): 525–535.

Harvey, Joy. "Evolutionism Transformed: Positivists and Materialists in the Société d'Anthropologie de Paris." In *Wider Domain of Evolutionary Thought,* ed. David Oldroyd and Ian Langham, 289–310. Dordrecht, Holland, and Boston: Reidel, 1983.

———. "'Doubly Revolutionary': Clémence Royer before the Société d'Anthropologie de Paris." In *Proceedings, Sixteenth International Congress History of Science* (Bucharest: Academy of Socialist Republic of Romania, 1981) Symposia B: 250–256.

———. "Races Specified, Evolution Transformed: The Social Context of Scientific Debates Originating in the Société d'Anthropologie de Paris, 1859–1902." Ph.D. diss. Harvard University, 1983.

———. "'Strangers to Each Other': Male and Female Relationships in the Life and Work of Clémence Royer, 1830–1902." In *Uneasy Careers and Intimate Lives: Women in Science, 1789–1979,* ed. Pnina G. Abir-Am and Dorinda Outram, 147–171, 322–330. New Brunswick, NJ, and London: Rutgers University Press, 1987.

Heilbrun, Carolyn. *Writing a Woman's Life.* New York: Norton, 1988.

Herstein, Sheila R. *A Mid-Victorian Feminist: Barbara Leigh Smith Bodichon.* New Haven, CT: Yale University Press, 1985.

Héricourt, Jenny P. d'. *La Femme affranchie: Réponse à MM Michelet, Proudhon, E. de Girardin, A. Comte, et aux autres novateurs modernes.* Brussels: F. van Meenan, 1860.

Hillairet, Jacques. *Dictionnaire Histoire des rues de Paris.* Vol. 1. Paris: Éditions de Minuit, 1963.

Holmes, Richard. *Coleridge: Early Visions.* New York: Viking, 1982.

Hugo, Victor. *Les Misérables.* Brussels: A. Lecroix, Verboeckhoven, 1862.

Huxley, T. H. *De la place de l'homme dans la nature.* Trans. Eugène Dally. Paris: Baillière, 1868.

Jacobi, Mary Putnam. "Woman in Medicine." In *Woman's Work in America,* ed. Annie N. Meyer, 139–205. New York: G. P. Putnam's Sons, 1891.

Janet, Paul. "Le Matérialisme contemporain: Une théorie anglaise sur les causes finales." *Revue des Deux Mondes* 48 (1863): 556–586.

———. "Rapport sur le concours relatif à la doctrine de l'évolution." Presented at the meeting of 1 September 1883. *Mémoires de l'Académie des Sciences Morales et Politiques* 15 (1888): 489–497.

La Berge, Ann. "Medicalization and Moralization: The Crèches of Nineteenth-Century Paris." *Journal Social History* 25 (1991): 65–87.

Lacour, Léopold. *Humanisme intégral: Le duel des sexes.* Paris: Stock, 1897.

Lamartine, Alphonse de. *Histoire des Girondins.* Paris: Furne, 1847.

Landucci, Giovanni. *Darwinismo a Firenze: Tra scienza e ideologia (1860–1900).* Florence: Olschki, 1977.

Lange, Friedrich Albert. *The History of Materialism.* 3 vols. London: Trubner, 1877–1881.

Le Bon, Gustave. *L'Homme et les sociétés.* Paris: Flammarion, Bibliothèque de Philosophie Scientifique, 1877.

———. "Recherches anatomiques et mathématiques sur les lois des variations du volume des cerveaux." *Revue d'Anthropologie,* 2d ser., 2 (1879): 27–104.

———. *L'Évolution de la matière.* Paris: Flammarion, 1905.

———. *L'Évolution des forces.* Paris: Flammarion, 1908.

Letourneau, Charles. "Variabilité des êtres organisés." *La Philosophie Positive* 3 (1868): 99–121.

———. *La Physiologie des passions.* Paris: Baillière, 1868.

Loiseleur-Deslongchamps, Auguste Louis Armand, ed. and trans. *Manava-Dharma-Sastra: Lois de Manou,* comprenant les institutions religieuses et civiles des Indiens . . . . Paris, 1833.

Longford, Elizabeth. "The Sex." In *Eminent Victorian Women.* New York: Knopf, 1981.

Lovett, Clara M. *Giuseppe Ferrari and the Italian Revolution.* Chapel Hill: University of North Carolina, 1979.

Lucas, Prosper. *Traité philosophique et physiologique de l'hérédité naturelle dans les états de santé et de maladie du système nerveux* . . . . Paris: Baillière, 1847–1850.

Manouvrier, Léonce. "Sur l'Anthropologie des sexes et applications sociales III," *Revue de l'École d'Anthropologie* 9 (1909): 41–61.

Marks, Harry P. "Attitudes of French Physicians toward Women, 1840–1900." Master's thesis, University of Wisconsin, 1972.

Maurel, F. "Gustave Flourens." *Bulletin Société d'Ethnographie* 3 (1873): 26–31.

Maurice, Frederick D. *Lectures on the Ecclesiastical History of the First and Second Centuries.* Cambridge: Macmillan, 1854.

Michelet, Jules. *Histoire romaine: République.* Paris: Hachette, 1831.

———. *Jeanne d'Arc.* Paris: Hachette, 1853.

———. "Les Femmes de la Révolution." In *Histoire de la Révolution.* Paris: A. Delahays, 1855.

———. *La Femme.* Paris: Hachette, 1860.

Michelet, Jules, and E. Quinet. *De les Jésuites.* Paris: Hachette, 1843.

Miles, Sara Joan. "Evolution and Natural Law in the Synthetic Science of Clémence Royer." Ph.D. diss., University of Chicago, 1988.

———. "Clémence Royer et *De l'origine des éspèces: Traductrice ou traîtresse?*" *Revue de Synthèse,* 4th ser., (1989): 61–83.

Milice, Albert. *Clémence Royer et sa doctrine de la vie.* Paris: J. Peyronnet, 1926.

Moers, Ellen. "Performing Heroinism: The Myth of Corinne." In *Literary Women,* 173–210. New York: Doubleday, 1976.

Morsier, Georges de, ed. *Lettres de René-Édouard Claparède.* Basel/Stuttgart: Schwabe, 1971.

Mortillet, Gabriel de. "Transformisme et paléontologie." *Bulletin de la Société d'Anthropologie de Paris,* 2d ser., 5 (1870): 360–368.

Moses, Claire Goldberg. *French Feminism in the Nineteenth Century.* Albany: State University of New York Press, 1984.

Moufflet, André. "L'Oeuvre de Clémence Royer." *Revue Internationale de Sociologie* 13 (1910): 658–693.

Naville, Ernest. "Des variations de la conscience morale." *Revue Chrétienne* 14 (1867): 1–22.

———. "Lettre à l'éditeur." *Revue Chrétienne* 14 (1867): 247.

Naylor, B. S. *Time and Truth Reconciling the Moral and Religious World to Shakespeare.* London: Kent, 1854.

Néron, Marie-Louise. "Clémence Royer." *La Fronde,* 18 August 1900.

Nigoul, Toussaint. *Pascal Duprat: Sa vie, son oeuvre.* Paris: Dentu, 1887.

Nye, Mary Jo. "The Nineteenth-Century Atomic Debates and the Dilemma of an 'Indifferent Hypothesis' " *Studies History and Philosophy of Science* 7 (1976): 245–268.

Nye, Robert. *Origins of Crowd Psychology; Gustave Le Bon and the Crisis of Mass Psychology in the Third Republic.* London: Sage, 1975.

———. *Crime, Madness, and Politics in Modern France: The Medical Concept of National Decline.* Princeton, NJ: Princeton University Press, 1984.

Offen, Karen. "A Nineteenth-Century French Feminist Rediscovered: Jenny P. d'Héricourt, 1809–1875." *Signs: Journal of Women in Culture and Society* 13 (1987): 144–157.

Pancaldi, Giuliano. *Darwin in Italy: Science across Cultural Frontiers.* Trans. Ruey Brodine Morelli. Bloomington: Indiana University Press, 1991.

Papillault, Georges. "Notice biographique." In *La Condition de la femme,* by Charles Letourneau. Paris: Giard et Brière, 1903.

Paul, Harry W. *The Edge of Contingency: French Catholic Reaction to Scientific Change from Darwin to Duhem.* Gainesville: The University Presses of Florida, 1979.

Pictet, François Jules. "Sur l'origine de l'espèce." *Bibliothèque Universelle,* n.s., 7 (1860): 233–255.

Pouchet, Felix A. *Nouvelles Expériences sur la génération spontanée.* Paris: Masson, 1861.

Pouchet, Georges. *De la pluralité des races humaines.* 1st ed. Paris: Baillière, 1859; 2d ed. Paris: Masson, 1864.

Pratelle, Aristide [Albert Milice]. "Clémence Royer: Notice biographique." *Revue Anthropologique* (1918): 263–276.

Quatrefages, Armand de. "L'Origine des espèces, animales et végétales." 1. "Les Précurseurs de Darwin." *Revue des Deux Mondes* 78 (1868): 832–860; 2. "Théorie de Darwin," 79 (1869): 208–240; 3. "Discussion des théories transformistes," 80 (1869): 64–95; 4. "Darwin et les théories transformistes: L'Espèce et la race," 80 (1869): 495–532; 5. "Théories de la transformation progressive et de la transformation brusque. L'Origine simienne de l'homme," 80 (1869): 638–672.

———. *Darwin et ses précurseurs français.* Paris: Baillière, 1870.

———. "Remarques sur le transformisme." *Bulletin de la Société d'Anthropologie de Paris,* 2d ser., 5 (1870): 312–317.

———. *Les Émules de Darwin.* Paris: Alcan, 1894.

Renan, Ernest. *Vie de Jésus.* Paris: Michel Lévy Frères, 1863.

Report of Commissioners of Inquiry into the State of Education in Wales, South Wales. London: Her Majesty's Stationery Office, 1847.

Richards, Robert J. *Darwin and the Emergence of Evolutionary Theories of Mind and Behavior.* Chicago: University of Chicago Press, 1987.

———. *The Meaning of Evolution. The Morphological Construction and Ideological Reconstruction of Darwin's Theory.* Chicago: University of Chicago Press, 1992.

Richardson, Joanna. *Rachel.* New York: G. P. Putnam's Sons, 1957.
Rive, Auguste de la. "Madame Marcet." *Bibliothèque Universelle* 4 (1859): 445–468.
Roger, Jacques. "Les Néo-Lamarckiens français". *Revue de Synthèse* 95–96 (1979): 279–468.
Ronchaud, L. de. "Chronique littéraire: *Les Jumeaux d'Hellas.*" *Revue Germanique* 30 (1864): 557–560.
Saulze, J.-B. "L'atomisme dynamique de Mlle Cl. Royer." In *Le Monisme matérialiste en France . . . MM le Dantec, Mlle C. Royer, Jules Saury, . . .* Foreword by Ernst Haeckel. Paris: Beauchesne, 1912.
Shapin, Steven. *A Social History of Truth: Civility and Science in Seventeenth-Century England.* Chicago: University of Chicago Press, 1994.
Smith, Sydney. *Selections from the Writings of Sydney Smith.* London: Longman, 1854.
Spencer, Herbert. *The Principles of Psychology.* London: Longman, Brown, 1855.
———. *Essays: Scientific, Political, Speculative.* 3 vols. London: Longman, Brown, 1858–1874.
———. *First Principles.* 2 vols. London: Williams and Norgate, 1860–1862.
———. *The Principles of Biology.* 2 vols. London: Longman, Brown, 1864–1867.
———. *The Principles of Psychology.* 2d ed. 2 vols. London: Williams and Norgate, 1870–1872.
Staël, Anne-Louise-Germaine de. *Corinne, or Italy.* Trans. Auriel Goldberger. New Brunswick, NJ: Rutgers University Press, 1987.
Stebbins, Robert E. "France." In *Comparative Reception of Darwinism,* ed. Thomas F. Glick. Austin, TX: University of Texas Press, 1972.
Strauss, David Friedrich. *The Life of Jesus Criticially Examined.* Trans. Marian Evans. London: Chapman, 1846.
Stuart, James. "The Teaching of Science." In *Women's Work and Women's Culture,* ed. Josephine Butler, 121–151. London: Macmillan, 1870.
Verneau, René. "Discours prononcé aux obsèques de C. Royer." *Bulletins et Mémoires de la Société d'Anthropologie de Paris,* 5th ser., 3 (1902): 75–78.
Vier, Jacques. *La Comtesse d'Agoult et son temps.* 6 vols. Paris: Armand Colin, 1960–1962.
Wood, John George. *Bees: Their Habits, Management, and Treatment.* London: G. Routledge, 1853.

Major Articles and Books by Clémence Royer

"Introduction à la philosophie des femmes: Leçon d'ouverture par Mlle A.C.R." Lausanne: A. Larpin, 1859.
"Préfaces" and "Avant-propos" to Royer's translation, *De l'origine des espèces,* by Charles Darwin. 1st ed., 1862; 2d ed., 1866; 3d ed., 1869; 4th ed., [1882]; 5th ed., [1892?].
"Association Internationale pour le Progrès des Sciences Sociales." *Journal des Économistes,* 2d ser., 36 (1862): 63–100.
Théorie de l'impôt ou la dîme sociale. 2 vols. Paris: Guillaumin, 1862.
"Congrès International des Sciences Sociales." *Journal des Économistes,* 2d ser., 40 (1863): 224–241.

"Women in French Switzerland: The Laws Relating to Them." *The English Woman's Journal* 11 (1863): 49–57.

Les Jumeaux d'Hellas. 2 vols. Brussels: Lacroix, Verbroecken, 1864.

"Avvenire di Torino, sua transformazione in citta industriale." Brochure. Turin: Typografia Nazionale, 1864.

"La Tristesse dans l'art." *Revue Moderne,* 1 May 1867.

"Lamarck: Sa vie, ses travaux et son système." *La Philosophie Positive* 3 (1868): 173–205, 333–372; 4 (1869): 5–30.

"Amazones." In *Encylopédie générale,* Paris: Lacroix, Verbroecken, 1869–[1871], 2:39–41.

"Remarques sur le transformisme." *Bulletin de la Société d'Anthropologie de Paris,* 2d ser., 5 (1870): 265–312.

L'Origine de l'homme et des sociétés. Paris: Guillaumin and Masson, [1869] 1870.

"Lettre à M. le Président de l'Académie des Sciences Morales et Politiques." Magny-en-Vexin: O. Petit, August 1873. Pamphlet.

"De l'origine des diverses races humaines et de la race aryénne en particulier." *Bulletin de la Société d'Anthropologie de Paris,* 2d ser., 8 (1873): 905–936.

"Lois mathématiques de réversion par l'atavisme convergent." *Bulletin de la Société d'Anthropologie de Paris,* 2d ser., 8 (1873): 725–737.

(with Émile Calmette, marquis d'Hervey-Saint Denys, Charles de Labrathe, Léon de Rosny). "Instructions ethnographiques: Projet de questionnaire concernant les caractères ethniques particuliers du système reproducteur . . . ." *Actes de la Société d'Ethnographie Amèricaine et Orientale,* 2d ser., 3 (1873): 13–26.

"Origine et migrations des diverses races humaines." *Bulletin de la Société d'Anthropologie de Paris,* 2d ser., 9 (1874): 54–63.

"Sur la natalité." Suppressed article intended for publication in *Bulletin Société d'Anthropologie de Paris,* 2d ser., 9 (July 1874): 597–614.

"La Nation dans l'humanité et dans la série organique." *Journal des Économistes,* 3d ser., 39 (1875): 234–249.

"Deux Hypothèses sur l'hérédité." *Revue d'Anthropologie* 6 (1877): 443–484, 660–685.

"De la nature du beau." *La Philosophie Positive* 22 (1879): 71–89, 201–229.

Le Bien et la loi morale: Éthique et téléologie. Paris: Guillaumin et Cie, 1881.

"L'Instinct social." *Bulletin de la Société d'Anthropologie de Paris,* 3d ser., 5 (1882): 707–727.

"Attraction et gravitation d'après Newton." *La Philosophie Positive* 31 (1883): 206–226.

"Darwinisme." In *Dictionnaire encyclopédique des sciences médicales,* ed. A. Dechambre, 698–767. Paris: G. Masson and P. Asselin, 1883.

"Facultés mentales et instincts sociaux des singes." *Revue Scientifique,* 3d ser., 38 (1886): 257–270.

"La Domestication des singes." *Revue d'Anthropologie,* 2d ser., 3 (1887): 170–181.

"Les Notions du nombre chez les animaux." *Revue Scientifique,* 3d ser., 40 (1887): 649–658.

"L'Évolution mentale dans la série organique." Conférences transformistes de la Société d'Anthropologie. *Revue Scientifique,* 3d ser., 39 (1887): 749–758; 40 (1887): 70–79.

"Discours" and "Toast." In *Congrès Français et International des Droits des Femmes,* 21–23, 267–269. Paris: Dentu, 1889.
"Discussion sur la dépopulation de la France." *Bulletin de la Société d'Anthropologie de Paris,* 4th ser., 1 (1890): 680–701.
La Constitution du monde: Natura rerum. Paris: Schleicher Frères, 1900.

Index

About the Author

Joy Harvey is a historian of science. She received her Ph.D. in History of Science from Harvard University and was a recipient of a Rockefeller Fellowship from the Department of History of Science at the University of Oklahoma, to complete this biography of Clémence Royer. Most recently she has been working as associate editor with the Darwin Correspondence Project at the Cambridge University Library. She has taught history of science at Harvard, Skidmore, Sarah Lawrence, and Virginia Polytechnic Institute and State University. Currently she is working on a number of projects that include a biographical dictonary of women scientists (with Marilyn Ogilvie), a biography of Dr. Mary Putnam Jacobi, and a book on Darwin and his French correspondents.